Healing Elements

T0256804

Healing Elements

Efficacy and the Social Ecologies of Tibetan Medicine

Sienna R. Craig

UNIVERSITY OF CALIFORNIA PRESS

Berkeley · Los Angeles · London

University of California Press, one of the most distinguished university presses in the United States, enriches lives around the world by advancing scholarship in the humanities, social sciences, and natural sciences. Its activities are supported by the UC Press Foundation and by philanthropic contributions from individuals and institutions. For more information, visit www.ucpress.edu.

University of California Press
Berkeley and Los Angeles, California

University of California Press, Ltd.
London, England

© 2012 by The Regents of the University of California

Library of Congress Cataloging-in-Publication Data

Craig, Sienna R.
    Healing elements : efficacy and the social ecologies of Tibetan medicine / Sienna R. Craig.
        p. ; cm.
    Includes bibliographical references and index.
    ISBN 978-0-520-27323-8 (cloth : alk. paper) —
    ISBN 978-0-520-27324-5 (pbk. : alk. paper)
    I. Title.
        1. Medicine, Tibetan Traditional—Tibet. 2. Asian Continental Ancestry Group—ethnology—Tibet. 3. Holistic Health—Tibet. WB 55.T5
    610.51'5—dc23   2012007775

Manufactured in the United States of America

21   20   19   18   17   16   15   14   13   12
10   9   8   7   6   5   4   3   2   1

In keeping with a commitment to support environmentally responsible and sustainable printing practices, UC Press has printed this book on Rolland Enviro100, a 100% post-consumer fiber paper that is FSC certified, deinked, processed chlorine-free, and manufactured with renewable biogas energy. It is acid-free and EcoLogo certified.

In memory of Yeshi Chödron Lama (1969–2006)

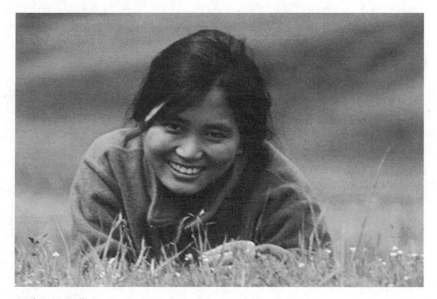

© Thomas Kelly

Contents

Illustrations

Preface

This book is dedicated to Yeshi Chödron Lama (1969–2006), a friend and colleague who died tragically, along with twenty-three others, in a helicopter crash in eastern Nepal on September 26, 2006. The daughter of a Tibetan lama, Yeshi joined the World Wildlife Fund–Nepal program in 1997 and began working on a project that aimed to document the ethnobotanical knowledge of *amchi*, Tibetan medical practitioners, in Dolpa District. What began for Yeshi as a project management assignment turned into a deep personal and professional commitment to *amchi*, to the environments they steward and on which they rely, to the cultural and scientific knowledge they hold, and to the communities they serve. She earned a bachelors degree from Middlebury College in Middlebury, Vermont, and an advanced degree in anthropology from the School of Oriental and African Studies in London, where her work focused on *amchi* experiences of and involvement with conservation and development in Nepal.

Wry, ironic, and smart, Yeshi was intimately aware of the profound differences between life in Kathmandu and life in the mountains. She saw clearly the challenges faced by the *amchi* with whom she worked. They were her friends and collaborators, not simply "local informants." Her fluency in Tibetan and her comfort in the villages along Nepal's northern edge served her well. Yeshi bridged many worlds with grace. She was marked by her years in Nepal and her educational experiences in the United States and the United Kingdom. She held fast to her family's history in Tibet even as she made her peace, as so many Tibetans do, with the lived experience of exile. She was a scholar, inquisitive and skeptical, with a deeply collaborative spirit and a commitment to the exchange of knowledge across divides of language and culture. She was also a practitioner, dedicated and filled with a sense of duty to the people with whom she worked. Friend, you are remembered, and missed.

Acknowledgments

Books often feel like singular endeavors, but they require a network of encouragement and critical feedback to produce. David Holmberg guided me with skill and kindness through the Ph.D. process and through many other scholarly and personal transitions. Davydd Greenwood and Vincanne Adams have been true exemplars. Mona Schrempf has been as gracious to me as she has been wise. Mark Unno and Harold Roth provided clarity and compassion at critical junctures, both in writing and in life. I owe a great deal to Tshampa Ngawang, not the least of which for his willingness to let me in, to be my teacher. I owe a similar debt of gratitude to Gyatso and Tenzin Bista and Mingkyi Tsomo (Mingji Cuomu).

I am fortunate to be part of a smart, collaboratively minded, and sincerely fun group of people engaging with Tibetan medicine across continents, languages, and disciplines. I've benefited from dialogues, on and off the page, with Florian Besch, Calum Blaikie, Alessandro Boesi, Alejandro Chaoul, Carroll Dunham, Frances Garrett, Barbara Gerke, Suresh Ghimire, Denise Glover, Kim Gutschow, Susan Heydon, Theresia Hofer, Stephan Kloos, Alex McKay, Colin Millard, Laurent Pordié, Audrey Prost, Jan Salick, Geoffrey Samuel, Martin Saxer, Herbert Schwabl, Brion Sweeney, Yildiz Thomas, and Claudia Witt.

I have also benefited from the collegiality, friendship, and insightful scholarship of others in Tibetan and Himalayan studies: Ann Armbrecht, Cynthia Beall, Mary Cameron, Geoff Childs, Andrew Fischer, David Germano, Melvyn Goldstein, Janet Gyatso, Ian Harper, Amy Heller, Toni

Huber, Leonard van der Kuijp, Todd Lewis, Kabir Mansingh-Heimsath, Charlene Makley, Kathryn March, Carole McGranahan, Stacy Leigh Pigg, Anne Rademacher, Charles Ramble, Tashi Rapgay, Françoise Robin, Volker Scheid, Sara Shneiderman, Nicolas Sihlé, Mark Turin, and Emily Yeh. I owe particular thanks to those who participated in a May 2011 manuscript review hosted by the John Sloane Dickey Center for International Understanding at Dartmouth College, during which the scope, meaning, and form of this project came into clearer view: Rebecca Biron, Douglas Haynes, James Igoe, Craig Janes, Kirin Narayan, Theodore Levin, John Watanabe, and Christiane Wohlforth.

Other colleagues, friends, and practitioners of Tibetan medicine who live and work in Nepal and Tibetan areas of China have contributed in innumerable ways to this book. In Nepal, I am particularly grateful to Amchi Nyima and his teacher, the late Amchi Gege, as well as Menla Phuntsok, Amchi Wangchuk, Lama Namgyal, Tenzin Darkye, and the late Lama Drukgye. I also thank Jigme S. P. Bista, Tsewang Bista, Raju Bista, Nirmal and Laxmi Gauchan, Kunzom Thakuri, Chimi Dolkar Bista and Tshampa Angyal, Dawa and Mahendra Bista, and Angya and Palsang Gurung.

In Qinghai Province, China, I thank colleagues at Arura, specifically Dhondrup Drotsang, Renchen Dhondup, Kunchok Gyaltsen, O Tsok-chen, Lusham Gyal, and Dorje. In Yunnan, I thank Samdrup Tsering and Ma Jiangzhong (Tibi Tsering). In the TAR, I thank members of the NIH and OneHeart teams as well as other Tibetan colleagues who remain un-named but who have worked tirelessly to practice, document, and teach Tibetan medicine and provide compassionate, high-quality health care in Tibetan areas of China during uncertain times. Although India has not been a central focus of my fieldwork, Dr. Dawa, former director of the Dharamsala Men-tsee-Khang, and expert in *materia medica*, has always been generous with his time and as humble as he is learned.

Others have taught me much about medicine, global health work, and Tibet. I acknowledge Sibylle Christensen, Tim Dye, Bernhard Fassl, Suellen Miller, Michael Varner, and especially Arlene Samen. Enrico Dell'Angelo, Elena McKinley, Ursula Rechbach, Gerald Roche, Kevin Stewart, Paula Vanzo, Phuntsok Wangmo, and Yangga have offered sound advice and invaluable perspectives over the years.

Andrea Clearfield and Maureen Drdak inspire me and were great travel companions to Mustang in 2008. Cherry Bird has been a reliable colleague in efforts to support Tibetan medicine in Nepal. Tenzin Norbu remains a wonderful friend and collaborator over many years and several joint projects. I thank him for his lovely line drawings of Dolpo *amchi* presented in this book. Likewise I am grateful to Thomas Kelly for his beautiful photographs. I could not have completed this book without the adept and good-natured research assistance of Liana Chase, Phagmo Droma, Rinchen Dorje, Ngawang Tsering Gurung, Tara Kedia, and Tshewang Norbu Lama.

I have benefited from the following grants and fellowships in researching and writing this book: a NSF Graduate Student Fellowship, a Social Science Research Council Dissertation Fellowship, a Wenner-Gren Foundation for Anthropological Research Dissertation Fellowship and an International Collaborative Research Grant, travel and research support from the Cornell and Dartmouth departments of anthropology, Cornell's Mario Einaudi Center for International Studies and the South Asia Program, and Dartmouth's Nelson A. Rockefeller Center, John Sloane Dickey Center for International Understanding, and Dean of Faculty. Support for related projects from the Trace Foundation and the International Association for the Study of Traditional Asian Medicines has also been indispensible.

It has been a pleasure to work with the University of California Press. I am particularly indebted to Stan Holwitz, who first suggested I send him something, and to Reed Malcolm, who has shepherded this book through the publication process since Stan's retirement. I thank Judith Hoover for her meticulous and thoughtful copyediting. Debbie Masi and Stacy Eisenstark have also been delights to work with through the production process.

As with any substantial piece of lifework, writing a book demands support and sacrifice. I am deeply indebted to my family: Steve Craig, Mary Heebner, Charles Rowley, Macduff Everton, Robert Everton, Larry and Sylvie Bauer, and Regina and Brian Mair. This book could not have come to be without the support of my husband, Ken Bauer, or our daughter, Aida, with whom life is always more fun. Any inaccuracies or inconsistencies in what follows are my own.

Notes on the Use
of Non-English Terms

This book uses the system of phonetic pronunciation (transcription) for Tibetan language of the Tibet Himalayan Library's Simplified Phonetic Transcription of Standard Tibetan (www.thl.org). This is for the benefit of those who do not read Tibetan, because transliterations using the standard scholarly method (Wylie 1959) can be cumbersome. As one notable exception, I use "Sowa Rigpa" rather than "Sowa Rikpa" for the Tibetan "science of healing," as this reflects common usage. The Glossary lists Tibetan words in simplified phonetics, followed by Wylie transliteration.

The Tibetan language does not differentiate between plural and singular nouns. I do not use an *s* at the end of plural Tibetan terms, for example *amchi* (medical practitioner[s]/doctor[s]); exceptions include Tibetan terms that have entered English lexicon, such as lama(s). Tibetan terms are not italicized if they are part of a person's name, such as Amchi Namgyal. I use capital letters for Sowa Rigpa, as one would use capitals for Ayurveda or Chinese medicine. Sanskrit terms that have entered English lexicon—mandala, mantra, and karma, for example—are rendered without diacritics or italics. Chinese terms are provided in Pinyin. Titles of Tibetan literary works are given in English translation, with Tibetan transliterations of titles in the glossary. The one exception to this rule is the *Fourfold Treatise* or *Gyüshi*, the texts comprising the core Tibetan medical canon. I alternate between the English and Tibetan titles throughout the text. *Materia medica* are rendered in simplified Tibetan. Botanical and common English names are sometimes given in the text as well; all are listed in the glossary, along with transliterated Tibetan spellings.

Since Tibetan is the language to which I most commonly refer, the reader can assume that if a non-English word is given in the text it is Tibetan unless it has been labeled otherwise. Chinese terms are designated by Ch. prior to the word or phrase, while N. stands for Nepali and Skt. references Sanskrit.

Acronyms

CAM	Complementary and Alternative Medicine
CMS	Cooperative Medical System (China)
CTEVT	Council on Technical Education and Vocational Training (Nepal)
FBO	Faith-based Organization
FDA	Food and Drug Administration (U.S.)
GCP	Good Clinical Practices
GMP	Good Manufacturing Practices
HAA	Himalayan Amchi Association (Nepal)
IASTAM	International Association for the Study of Traditional Asian Medicines
ICDP	Integrated Conservation and Development Project
IRB	Institutional Review Board
MCH	Maternal and Child Health
NAHC	Nepal Alternative Health Council
NGO	Nongovernmental Organization
NIH	National Institutes of Health (U.S.)
NITM	National Institute of Traditional Medicine (Bhutan)
PPH	Postpartum Hemorrhage
PI	Principal Investigator

RCT	Randomized Controlled Trial
SBA	Skilled Birth Attendant
SLC	School Leaving Certificate (Nepal and India)
SFDA	State Food and Drug Administration (China)
TAR	Tibet Autonomous Region (China)
TCM	Traditional Chinese Medicine
TM	Traditional Medicine
TMP	Traditional Medicine Practitioner
UNDP	United Nations Development Program
WHO	World Health Organization
WSR	Whole Systems Research
WTO	World Trade Organization
WWF	World Wildlife Fund

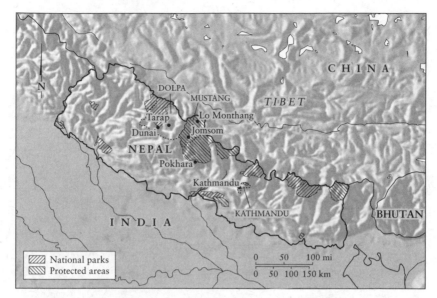

Map of Nepal, with primary sites where the author conducted fieldwork named.

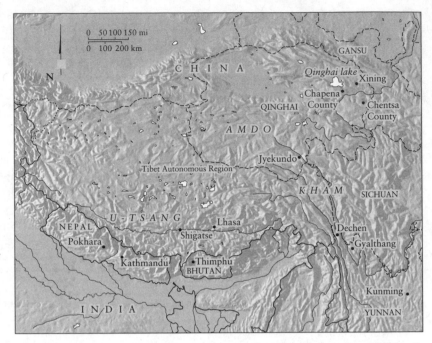

Map of Tibetan areas of China, with primary sites where the author conducted fieldwork named.

Introduction

Translations are a partial and precious documentation of the
changes the text suffers.
—Jose Luis Borges, *Some Versions of Homer*
  [*Las Versiones Homéricas*]

BUT DOES IT WORK?

On a warm summer day in 2004, a friend comes into the Lhasa café
where I'm having breakfast. This American nurse practitioner has spent
many years in Tibet, working with local colleagues to improve the health
of women and children. She has just returned from a trip to a region Tibetans call Kham, in the Chinese province of Sichuan. She made this trip
with several other Western clinicians and Tibetan staff to conduct a field
assessment of an American-funded Nongovernmental Organization's
(NGO) public health program. This team returned to Lhasa, the capital
of China's Tibet Autonomous Region (TAR), the previous evening. My
middle-aged friend has seen a lot of suffering during her years here, from
untimely deaths to politically motivated arrests. Though compassionate,
she is not easily flustered. So I am surprised that, despite a hot shower,
a night of sleep in a bed instead of a tent, and a cappuccino, she still
looks travel-worn and agitated.

"The situation in some of those villages is just abysmal," she begins
her debriefing. "Kids with rickets and pneumonia, women dying in childbirth. And I can only imagine the TB rates! You should have seen the
township clinics this NGO has supposedly helped to improve. Used needles and broken glass bottles from IV antibiotics lying around. Health
workers with, like, eighth-grade educations and hardly any medical training. Some places were better than others, but overall it was awful."

I begin to formulate questions—about the politics of the place, about the relationship between the NGO's local staff, government health workers, and foreign project managers, about how far away the nearest referral hospital might be and the road conditions to get there—but before I voice such queries, my friend continues.

"And I just do not understand why the NGO insists on supporting Tibetan doctors." She is turning to me as a confidant, but also as an anthropologist who has conducted research on Sowa Rigpa, the Tibetan "science of healing," and has worked with *amchi,* Tibetan medical practitioners, in Nepal and the TAR.

Before allowing me to respond, she adds, "Those medicines look like rabbit droppings to me, or balls of dirt. I can't tell them apart. The village and township doctors who say they know Tibetan medicine don't seem to have much training. Or they read someone's pulse and then just hand over whatever antibiotics might be on the shelf. I mean, it is great that Tibetan medicine is a part of Tibetan culture—and *of course* I want to support Tibetan culture—but what are those little brown pills supposed to do? Do they work? Can Tibetan medicine cure pneumonia or TB? Most of the doctors don't even give blessings with their medicine. At least lamas do that."

I know my friend has good intentions and that she is speaking from a raw, impassioned place. As a nurse-practitioner, her mind and hands *know* the extent to which relatively simple interventions could improve basic health and limit the devastation of disease. As a Buddhist practitioner and someone who has dedicated much of her life to working in underserved communities in the United States and abroad, she brings awareness and compassion to her work. I know all these things.

Even so, first instinct is to respond defensively, to volley back the language of science and clinical evidence. I could mention Randomized Controlled Trials (RCTs) that have been performed on Tibetan formulas—research on diabetes, irritable bowel syndrome, hepatitis, palliative care for cancer patients—and say that, yes, according to these parameters, Tibetan medicines do indeed "work."

My next thought is less of a gut reaction, but more personal. I put a hand on my belly and feel the child growing inside, recalling how I found out about this pregnancy from doctors at Mentsikhang, the TAR's Tibetan medical hospital. In my mind's eye, I see images of conception and gestation as depicted in Tibetan medical *thanka* paintings, recalling how these seventeenth-century illustrations portray the marvelous process of becoming human with a great deal of physiological accuracy and philosophical insight. I consider the ways I've been cared for through my pregnancy by both Tibetan physicians and biomedical practitioners.

Then my mind turns to the Tibetan doctors I know well: their commitment to the patients they serve, the rugged environment in which they live, the plants they harvest and trade for, the medicines they prepare, the young people they train, and the ways they make sense of the causes and conditions of illness. I think about their struggles to support their families and pass on what they know in the face of rapid socioeconomic change and political instability and repression. Here in China, the government's support for Sowa Rigpa is coupled with the cultural, economic, and ecological impacts of a commercial industry for Tibetan medicines that is swiftly scaling up. Meanwhile *amchi* in Nepal make the effort to engage their government, seeking recognition for their work in regions that are chronically underserved by the state's health care system and also intertwined with the country's dependence on foreign aid.

Why, in her moment of exasperation, does my friend allow herself the quick self-assuredness that Tibetan medicine is not worth investing in and that its therapies are dubious, instead of examining the structures that give rise to the health care inequities she describes and considering the place of rural Tibetan medical practitioners therein? I weigh the implications of granting value to Tibetan medicine *only* by virtue of what it accomplishes culturally. Can the work of culture and the work of healing be so easily parsed?

In our ensuing conversation, we touch on these themes. I ask my friend to consider the significance of passing judgment on the effectiveness of a diverse body of knowledge and practice by virtue of what it looks like in one place on the map—and an impoverished place, at that. Would one ever think to ask, by contrast, if biomedicine "really works"? While we might chalk up a medical or public health failure to problems within the system—maybe even to problems with the doctor, the patient, the treatment prescribed, or some combination thereof—we would probably not question the inherent value of the system itself.

As my friend and I talk, the challenge from Paul Farmer, a physician-anthropologist and global health activist, rings in my ears: Do not conflate cultural difference with structural violence. So too do the words of one of Farmer's interlocutors from the central Haitian plateau, who summarizes traditional therapies as "shit medicine for poor people," and Farmer's own assertion in *Infections and Inequalities*: "If folk healing were so effective, the world's wealthy would be monopolizing it" (2001: 259). I am sympathetic to these social critiques and political sentiments.

However, from where I sit on the roof of the world, I *do* see such monopolization, even as health disparities persist in many Tibetan and Himalayan communities I've come to know, even as arbiters of Sowa Rigpa knowledge and practice struggle to defend and transform their traditions. Over the years this conversation has stayed with me. It has helped me to form a response, in the form of this book, to questions posed by one of Farmer's mentors, Arthur Kleinman (2006), when he asks what is at stake and what matters most during times of uncertainty and transition.

CENTRAL QUESTIONS, KEY CONCEPTS

In this multisited ethnography, I focus on the question of what it means to say a medicine works. My research on Tibetan medicine in Nepal and China suggests the issue of efficacy needs to be addressed in far broader terms than narrow experimental or clinical perspectives on "what works" allow. Two central inquiries frame this book: How is efficacy determined? What is at stake in these determinations? In sociocultural terms, efficacy is the capacity to produce desired outcomes. In biomedical terms, efficacy measures the degree to which therapeutic substances or treatments achieve desired results within controlled clinical circumstances. Yet, as medical anthropology teaches us, these two definitions are linked and these two fields of knowledge shape each other. They are further influenced by environmental, political-economic, historical, and epistemological conditions. Answers to these central questions—*What makes a medicine "work"? How are such assertions made, by whom, and to what ends?*—hinge on the varied social ecologies in which therapies are made and evaluated, practitioners are trained, and patients are treated.

My use of the term *social ecologies* here is multivalent. At one level, I am inspired by social ecology models and ecological systems theories as they are used in public health, epidemiology, and my own discipline, medical anthropology. Such conceptual frameworks acknowledge the interdependent and mutually constituted relationship between human beings and the environments they inhabit. Medical anthropology has demonstrated that the ways an illness is socially conceived can bear on how it is individually experienced and expressed (Kleinman 1988; Luhrman 2001; Biehl 2005). The discipline has further demonstrated that the "therapeutic process" (Csordas and Kleinman 1996) encompasses much more than a one-off interaction between doctor and patient; rather it is inclusive of micropolitics, affect, and the structures, at once socioeconomic and political, that define a therapeutic system. A social ecological approach adds to this an explicit focus on *environments*, broadly conceived. This approach strives to account for how factors influencing health and illness exist across nested registers of meaning and experience, from the level of an individual's behavior to influences of ideology, and much in between (Hawley 1950; Bronfenbrenner 1979). Whether used in the context of health promotion (Stokols 1996), the epidemiology of infectious disease (Mayer and Pizer 2007), or anthropological analyses of postsocialist reforms (Janes and Chuluundorj 2004), social ecological approaches demand we think holistically about how and why people fall sick, seek care, take medicines, experience the outcomes of these actions, and make sense of such events.

At another level I use the social ecologies concept as a way of acknowledging that the environmental challenges we face, including illness, are fundamentally social, political, and historical challenges, and that we would do well to think beyond an ethos of dominating nature(s) toward new forms of sustainability and cross-cultural collaboration (Bookchin 1996). Following the work of Gregory Bateson, I recognize that individuals, societies, and ecologies coexist in ways that foster both competition and interdependency. My ethnography bears out the idea Bateson puts forth in his *Steps to an Ecology of Mind* ([1972] 2000). Namely, that the *ideology* of science and the hubris it can allow—distinct from the curiosity, humility, and empiricism inherent in the *scientific method*—can contribute to a range of human problems, including foreshortened lives, depleted environments, ethnocentrism, and other forms of inequity.

As you will see in the chapters that follow, this multivalent approach to social ecology converges through narratives my interlocutors in Nepal and China tell about their diverse, complex, and at times contradictory efforts to legitimate and recontextualize Tibetan medicine. They do so through engagements with biomedicine and clinical research, conservation-development projects, national and international regimes of governance, commoditization, and the politics of Tibetanness in Nepal, China, and beyond. When it comes to the more intimate spaces between patients and healers in the context of culture (Kleinman 1980), thinking in terms of social ecologies allows me to envision medical pluralism—the coexistence of multiple medical realities in a given context—in new ways (Ernst 2002; Cant and Sharma 2005; Johannessen and Lazar 2006). The term *social ecologies* helps to capture the interrelationships among environmental, socioeconomic, biological, political, and cosmological sources of, or explanations for, health problems.

Furthermore social ecology seems an apt framework for analysis of a medicine whose theories of health and disease emphasize the porous boundaries between internal and external worlds, which produce sickness and provide remedy. Sowa Rigpa theory hinges on the relationship between the three "dynamics" or "faults" *(nyépa sum)* of wind *(lung)*, bile *(tripa)*, and phlegm *(béken)* and the five elements *(jungwa nga)* of earth *(sa)*, air *(lung)*, water *(chu)*, fire *(mé)*, and space *(namkha)*.[1] The three *nyépa* further correspond to the Three Mental Poisons (T. *duk sum*, Skt. *Klesa*) of desire/attachment, hatred/aversion, and ignorance. Within a Buddhist framework, these are the roots of all suffering; they become embodied as physical sickness through interactions with the five elements and other factors. Tibetan medicine pays attention to patterns of health and illness not only as they emerge in biological bodies *(lü)* and heart-minds *(sem)*, but also as expressions of what Scheper-Hughes and Lock (1987) call the "mindful body" located within individual, social, and political realms. Even more relevant for Sowa Rigpa is Elisabeth Hsu's (1999) addition of the "body ecologic" to Scheper-Hughes and Lock's "three bodies" model, and what Geoffrey Samuel (2001) calls Sowa Rigpa's "body-mind-world dynamic."

In Tibetan settings, patterns of illness and prospects for treatment can be linked to concepts such as karma *(lé)*, sin *(digpa)*, spiritual defilement *(drib)*, the work of nefarious spirits *(döndré)*, and deities who reside in specific ecologies such as water sources, mountains, streams, or earth (Millard 2006; Vargas 2011). People get sick because of their environment, but this sense of environment includes, perforce, *social* relationships with other human and nonhuman sentient beings in particular settings. According to Tibetan sensibilities, the phenomenon we like to abstract as "nature" establishes and maintains order between humans and divine forces that inhabit and enliven this animate earth. Likewise Tibetan therapeutic processes derive some of their efficacy from the locations in which they are performed, and Tibetans sometimes link the healing possibilities of *materia medica* to the places where they are gathered, how they are collected and compounded, and by whom.

In Tibetan the term most commonly translated as *efficacy* is *phenü*, a conjunction of the words *benefit (pentok)* and *potency (nüpa)*. This coupling of *that which is useful* with *that which is powerful* is relevant when one considers how the concept of efficacy has been approached in anthropology. One need only look as far as Evans-Pritchard's *Witchcraft, Oracles and Magic among the Azande* (1976) or Lévi-Strauss's insights in "The Sorcerer and His Magic" (1967) to understand that people experience efficacy in part through ritualized action. A more general concern with what is meant by efficacy across healing systems has produced an array of methodological and epistemological analyses, which have not only provided ethnographic examples of efficacious (or inefficacious) practices but have also asked what the value of cross-cultural comparisons of efficacy are, in theoretical and pragmatic terms (Ahern 1979; Etkin 1988; Anderson 1992; Waldram 2000; Barnes 2005). Some anthropologists have described typologies of efficacy. Waldram (2009), for example, distinguishes between restorative and transformative efficacy in the context of ethnography among Canadian First Nations and indigenous communities in Belize. Whyte, van der Geest, and Hardon (2002) argue for the importance of parsing social and pharmacological efficacy. However, they also note, "It is important to remember that the different forms of efficacy, though distinguishable analytically, are experienced simultaneously" (36).

I argue that efficacy is produced at the intersections of ritual action and pharmacology, within distinct social ecologies. Efficacy is a measurement of micropolitical power, biopsychosocial effects, and cultural affect. It is an inter-subjective phenomenon, by which I mean that one cannot really know whether a medicine or therapeutic approach is efficacious until a practitioner makes and/or prescribes it, a patient uses it, and then reacts to its use. I suggest we should pay close attention to the ways history and politics, language and culture imbue an herb, a clinical encounter, a training curriculum, or a research methodology with the capacity to produce a desired outcome. While I find some of these typologies of efficacy useful, they do not resolve the issue to which Whyte and colleagues point: that while we might be able to isolate a drug's bioavailability, an herb's active ingredients, or a healer's record of positive patient outcomes for analytic purposes, they are often *experienced* as a synthesis. Comparatively, failures of efficacy are often attributed to the analytics of statistical significance, the intentionality of a patient, or a healer's lack of technical skill. Yet one could also interpret moments when desired outcomes are *not* produced as the result of incommensurability or problems of translation. The standards, forms, and instruments used to measure outcomes are enmeshed in historical and political relations of power that value some ways of knowing over others and that often are not that well equipped to account for a multiplicity of meanings.

It is crucial to note that methodological and disciplinary dissonance surfaces between social science and biomedical definitions of the terms *efficacy* and *effectiveness*. As Witt (2009) points out, to a biomedical practitioner *efficacy* means the specific measurable effects of a drug or therapy under the controlled circumstances of an RCT; *effectiveness,* in contrast, refers to the observable and felt effects of a medicine or a therapeutic process in the context of a pragmatic or observational trial and in what we might also call "real life." For a social scientist, this distinction is often lost in translation, or the terms are used interchangeably. This important discrepancy notwithstanding, practitioners and producers of Tibetan formulas are increasingly aiming to prove the efficacy of their medicines through clinical research, in biomedical terms. Tibetan medicine is not alone in this trend. Indeed one can understand an increased concern for rendering legible nonbiomedical praxis within the framework of biomedicine and technoscience as a predictable outcome of a moment in the politics of global health that is shaped by multiculturalism, on the one hand, and neoliberalism, on the other.

Healing Elements: Efficacy and the Social Ecologies of Tibetan Medicine explores what it might mean to support Traditional Medicine (TM) in the twenty-first century.[2] In this book you will see how Tibetan medicines are both social and pharmacological things: how they move through diverse settings as commercial goods and gifts; how they are consumed as targeted therapies and anodynes for biophysical and psychosocial ills; and how they elucidate a larger biopolitics of traditional medicine. In this sense, my work helps to illustrate what Petryna and Kleinman (2006: 20) call the "pharmaceutical nexus," the ways medicines mediate the "sheer scale and complexity of our interconnected world and its uncertain social and biological outcomes in local and national settings." For, in addition to my central focus on the social ecological contexts in which efficacy is produced, I refer to the political-economic distinction between *use values* and *exchange values,*[3] as they inform Tibetan ways of conceptualizing the nature and the benefits of *materia medica.* I analyze the differential regimes of value (Myers 2001) that surface in the translation of science and medicine across cultures. I challenge views that would simply pit "traditional" against "modern" medicine, "underdeveloped" people or places against their "developed" counterparts, cultural belief against clinical evidence, moral economies against market economies.[4] Ethnography reveals the inherent limitations of such polarities, both in analytical terms and with respect to honoring the complex lives people live. I argue that it is possible, beneficial even, to engage with so-called traditional medicine(s), even as practices and practitioners change in response to the forces of globalization and modernity. This includes a commitment to critically evaluate the impacts of scaling up commercial production of traditional formulas and privileging RCTs as the "gold standard" for determining whether a therapy has the capacity to produce desired outcomes.

In her memoir *Finding Beauty in a Broken World,* Terry Tempest Williams writes, "A mosaic is a conversation between what is broken" (2008: 20). Her words provide me with a useful metaphor for contemplating the diverse, sometimes paradoxical ways Sowa Rigpa practitioners in Nepal and China are adapting to new medical and social landscapes, adopting novel modes of self-representation, and exploring pathways along which to protect and reimagine their practice. Likewise I think about how illnesses can shatter lives, senses of self, and household economies. Illness is a world broken. Finding a way out of illness can be thought of as piecing together a mosaic of medical pluralism. One might argue that local, indigenous ways are being irrevocably shattered in this fully, fiercely global world, and that the beauty and specificity of people and places are sacrificed in the process. Yet this denies culture's inherent dynamism and our human capacity to piece together shards into something newly whole: a pathway through sickness, a practice one can make peace with, a reinvention of what Volker Scheid (2007) has called the "currents" of medical tradition.

The French anthropologist Claude Lévi-Strauss (1908–2009) might have identified what Williams recognizes in the mosaic metaphor by the term *bricolage,* a process of making use of whatever materials or resources one has on hand. A Tibetan doctor working at a township clinic takes a patient's pulse, diagnoses a blood-bile disorder, and then prescribes a biomedical drug, for this is what he has left in his pharmacy. A nomad woman living in a yak-hair tent on the northern Tibetan Plateau takes down a precious pill *(rinchen rilbu)* from the altar and dissolves it in boiled water by the light of the full moon, hoping this medicine will ease the pains of her aging father. A Tibetan doctor in rural Nepal uses just a pinch of camphor in a formula that calls for about a gram, but to use more is beyond his means. In this book you will see patients and healers become *bricoleur,* engaging in the creative and resourceful practice of using whatever resources they have available, sometimes despite their initial or intended purpose, to effect change.

In what follows I frame the field sites in which I've worked and provide some background information on Sowa Rigpa history and the contexts in which Tibetan medicine exists in Nepal and China today. I then discuss my research methods, describe the positions I've occupied in relation to my interlocutors, and sketch the scope and structure of this book.

SHARED FOUNDATIONS AND MULTIPLE PRACTICES
ACROSS TWO FIELD SITES

Against the backdrop of a Himalayan valley, rimmed with mountains and dappled with barley and buckwheat fields, a middle-aged Nepali woman leans up against her whitewashed home. She speaks in her native Tibetan dialect.

"The harvest got the best of me," she tells the *amchi*, as practitioners of Sowa Rigpa are called here. "Pains in my chest and swelling in my legs." She lifts her skirt and pokes at the flesh around her knees. The *amchi* reaches for each hand, in turn. He listens to her pulse and diagnoses her with a wind and phlegm disorder. This exchange precedes the *amchi*'s meting out of handmade pills and powders, comprised in part of local ingredients. He is then plied with invitations to tea. The *amchi* deflects his patient's attempts to place a mottled 100 rupee note ($1.25)[5] in his hands. Even so, he struggles each year to meet the health care needs of his community and to pass on his knowledge to members of a younger generation who are torn between village life and the risky yet tantalizing proposition of becoming wage laborers in foreign lands—working construction in Seoul, babysitting on Long Island, farming shrimp in Dubai.

On the outskirts of Lhasa, an *amchi* sits in his office at a Tibetan medical factory, an opulent structure of concrete and tinted glass, filled with high-tech stainless steel contraptions that dry *materia medica*, grind herbs, and sort pills. The doctor was born a nomad and is a survivor of China's Great Leap Forward (1958–61) and Cultural Revolution (1966–76). During this time, when Tibetan medicine was labeled "superstitious" and seen as an affront to Maoist ideals, he became a barefoot doctor.[6] Now the physician contemplates a book of standard operating procedures, written in Mandarin. He is at the forefront of movements to transform Tibetan medicine according to technoscientific standards that represent radical departures from how he was trained to make medicines, but that also marks a chance to modernize and even profit from a core aspect of Tibetan culture. Like many people of his generation, this doctor is charged with recasting the language and logic of his tradition to produce medicines that conform to Chinese Drug Administration laws and comply with Good Manufacturing Practices (GMP). This factory produces newfangled Tibetan pharma, elaborately packaged for primarily high-end domestic and export markets. Most of the time he is glad that Tibetan medicine is becoming, in his words, "developed," but he sometimes questions the quality and potency of medicines he makes in this factory, and he misses treating patients.

The basic goal of Sowa Rigpa is to address causes and conditions of human suffering. Yet as these vignettes illustrate, Tibetan medicine is enmeshed within multiple social ecological realities, whether in Nepal, Tibetan areas of China, or beyond. Today forms of Sowa Rigpa are practiced in places as far afield as southern India and Scotland, Boston and Buryatia. This is a testament to the fact that Sowa Rigpa has never been exclusively a local tradition (Saxer 2010a). It retains influences, from *materia medica* to evaluative tools, that bespeak a long history of interaction with other medical systems since at least the seventh century, including those from South Asia, East Asia, and the Greco-Arab world (Beckwith 1979; Meyer 1995; Hsu 2008b; Saxer 2010b; Yangga 2010) as well as with forms of biomedicine since the nineteenth century (McKay 2007, 2010).

Sowa Rigpa practitioners across a range of social ecologies share a connection to Tibetan Buddhism. The Medicine Buddha, Sangye Menla, is viewed as a primordial source of medical teachings and the inspiration for the ethical conduct of Tibetan physicians. Many aspects of Sowa Rigpa curricula intermingle with Buddhist and Bön texts and traditions.[7] Oral transmissions of knowledge, including instructions on medicine making, are connected to ritual practice, indicating one of the many ways that Sowa Rigpa exists between science and religion (Adams, Schrempf, and Craig 2010). Yet not all practitioners identify strongly with or are active practitioners of Buddhism. In Tibetan areas of China overt references to religiosity can be politically problematic. In Nepal connection to Buddhist images and ideals might be more overt, but this too emerges from a particular cultural politics.

Throughout the book I use the term *Sowa Rigpa* as an imperfect synonym for *Tibetan medicine*. I make this methodological decision even as I recognize that to speak of Tibetan medicine in the singular is disingenuous, and that to speak of Tibetan *medicines* might be more apt (Pordié 2008c: 20). Other terms are at play as well. *Bödmen*, literally "Tibet[an] medicine," is common in China, while *amchi medicine* is used in Ladakh and Nepal. The Bhutanese reference Sowa Rigpa as *Buddhist medicine* and Mongolians speak of Sowa Rigpa as *Mongolian medicine*. Of course variants of Sowa Rigpa abound in these different locales, differences manifest through distinct lineages of teachers, textual traditions, *materia medica,* recipes, etc. Yet I argue there *is* something profoundly shared, or at least implied, in the fact that people across a vast territory actually use the term *Sowa Rigpa* to describe the theoretical principles that underlie their practice. There is also something shared in how speakers of Tibetan frame biomedicine: as foreign medicine *(chi men, gya men, or jer men),* medicine connected to India and China *(gya men),* or even medicine connected to the Communist Party *(tang men)* (Schrempf 2010: 165; Hofer 2011c: 26). Likewise, while I tend to privilege the term *amchi* as a way of describing Sowa Rigpa practitioners—in great part because this is a term used as a marker of social and political identity by colleagues in Nepal, and because it is at play in central Tibet—I acknowledge other terms as well. The term *menpa* is much more commonly used in eastern Tibet, and I refer to individuals in those contexts as such (cf. Schrempf 2007: 91). I also use the terms *Tibetan doctor* and *practitioner of Tibetan medicine.*

These diverse streams of knowledge coalesce around a shared set of texts. The *Gyüshi,* which I translate as *Fourfold Treatise* but which is also called the *Four Tantras,* outlines core components of Sowa Rigpa theory and guide practice. Parts of the *Gyüshi* are derived from texts of Indic origin, especially the *Astangahrdaya Samhita* by Vagbhata, a seventh-century physician. Though subject to debate, the *Gyüshi* was likely codified in the twelfth century. Full and partial translations exist today in a range of Asian and European languages, from Russian, German, and English to Mongolian and Japanese. The *Root Tantra* synopsizes Sowa Rigpa theory; the *Explanatory Tantra* covers topics about conceptions of the body, medical ethics, and an overview of diagnosis and treatment; the *Instructional Tantra,* the longest and most conceptual of the four texts, provides teaching on pathophysiology, symptoms, diagnosis, and treatment strategies for a range of disorders; finally, the *Subsequent Tantra* is a practical exegesis on diagnostics and treatment, outlining pulse diagnosis, urinalysis, tongue analysis, questioning the patient, and describing the indications for a range of ingestible and external therapies (Meyer 1995: 114). Written as something of a prose poem and highly metaphorical in nature, the *Gyüshi* requires guidance through oral instruction and further study of medical commentaries in order to put the knowledge it contains to use. Practitioners commit much of the *Gyüshi* to memory, even today.

Tibetan medical institutions have taken the form of large, state-supported schools and small, local institutions, often connected to patri-lineage, households,[8] specific medico-religious teachers, or monastic institutions. Chagpori, often called the first "college" of Tibetan medicine, was founded in 1696 in Lhasa. This process was overseen by Desi Sangye Gyatso (1653–1705), the regent of the "Great Fifth" Dalai Lama and an important figure in the history of science and medicine in Tibet on the cusp of modernity (Gyatso 2004). In a sense Chagpori was the institutional precursor to the Mentsikhang, literally the "house of medicine and astrology," which was founded in 1916 by an equally important monk-physician, Khyenrab Norbu (1883–1962) with support from the thirteenth Dalai Lama. Yet Mentsikhang differed in one very significant way from its predecessors. While Chagpori and related institutions such as the medical college at Labrang Monastery in Amdo were fundamentally linked to religious authority, Mentsikhang was not. Mentsikhang was emblematic of a reformist push within what Melvyn Goldstein (1989) has dubbed the Lamaist state. One could argue that it was this more secular orientation, combined with an early public health mandate, that allowed Mentsikhang to weather the tides of political upheaval since the 1950s (Janes 1995; McKay 2007). Mentsikhang still exists in Lhasa today, and its form and structure have been replicated in other Tibetan regions in China. This institution was also re-created in Dharamsala, the seat of the Tibetan government-in-exile, in 1961.[9] (For clarity, throughout this book I refer to the Lhasa-based institution as *Mentsikhang* and the Dharamsala-based institution as *Men-tsee-khang*.)

Until quite recently Tibetan medicines were made and circulated primarily within local and regional spheres. As articulated in key texts such as the *Fourfold Treatise* and a range of pharmacopeia and through oral transmission of medical knowledge, Tibetan medical theory provides a basis for ways *materia medica* should be harvested, prepared, and compounded, including elaborate guidelines for the purification and detoxification of substances that might otherwise be poisonous. A medicine's quality, efficacy, and value have often been determined within the constraints of local and regional economies, from the ability of practitioner-producers to access the plant, mineral, and animal products on which Tibetan pharmacy is based, to an ethics of medical practice that can actively discourage commoditization (Besch 2007; Blaikie in press). This is not to say, in either historical or contemporary terms, that everyone who desires Tibetan medicines can access them. Hierarchies of medicinal value and health care access have a long history in Tibet (Beckwith 1979; Janes 1995; Gyatso forthcoming).

Likewise theoretical "best practices" of production, as articulated in sources such as the *Seven Limb Procedure (yenlak dün)* within the *Fourfold Treatise,* can be adapted to local conditions; *materia medica* substitution is widely acknowledged. Over the past few decades mechanized production, especially the use of machines to grind raw materials, has become standard practice in many sites of Tibetan medicine production in China, India, and Nepal. In the most remote communities in which I've worked, however, *amchi* and their assistants often still pulverize herbs by hand, using a mortar and pestle or grinding stones. In contrast, many Tibetan medicines produced in China today are state-certified commodities that come in fancy packages and are sometimes reformulated into capsules, blister tablets, and the like. Some have become prohibitively expensive for Tibetans to buy, as formulas circulate through national and global exchange networks (Janes 2002; Pordié 2008c; Craig and Adams 2008; Saxer 2010a). This transformation has been as profound as it has been rapid and recent.

In some respects these changes reflect parallel histories of the industries that have grown up around Ayurveda (Bode 2006; Wujastyk and Smith 2008; Banerjee 2009; Halliburton 2009), Chinese medicines (Taylor 2005; Hsu 2009; Zhan 2009), and Asian medicines in general at a time of globalization (Høg and Hsu 2002; Alter 2005). In addition, contemporary Tibetan medicine is part of a much larger story that encompasses both disaffection with conventional biomedicine and the global health needs of the twenty-first century. Complementary and Alternative Medicine (CAM) practice, production, and consumption are on the rise around the world. As we will see, agencies such as the World Health Organization (WHO) and national institutes of health are paying attention to the roles such medicines play in therapeutic and commercial contexts (Bodeker et al. 2005).

But what of the specific historical and legal frameworks in which Sowa Rigpa exists in the two countries where I've conducted research for this book?

The *amchi* with whom I work in Nepal operate, by and large, on the literal and figurative fringes of the Nepali nation-state. They are not legally recognized as health care providers, despite more than a decade of active lobbying. Even so, private practitioners, NGO-supported schools and clinics, and health camps into which *amchi* are incorporated do exist and *amchi* are often at the front line of health care for many of Nepal's high mountain communities.

Biomedicine was first introduced to Nepal on a broad scale beginning in the 1950s, with capital and expertise provided by foreign aid organizations (Justice 1986). As such, Nepal's embrace of biomedicine and the creation of public health infrastructure cannot be decoupled from ideas and practices of "development" (Des Chene 2002). Nepal's so-called underdevelopment was (and in many ways still is) pathologized, whereas a "healthy" nation-state has come to be defined as one oriented toward biomedical norms (Harper and Maddox 2008). Technically, the Nepali government is to provide free or otherwise affordable health care to its citizens, including those who live in the high mountains along the country's border with Tibet and northern India. Practically, rural hospitals, health posts, and sub–health posts are rarely functional—a situation that has been further exacerbated by a decade of civil war (1996–2006) and continued political dysfunction emanating from the Kathmandu Valley (Justice 1986; Stone 1986; Pigg 1992; Sharma 2010). As is consistent with the country's history, many Nepalis need to muster private funds to pay for health care, supplemented at times by care they receive from a range of foreign philanthropic, health development organizations, and voluntourism ventures, large and small (Citrin 2010).

Following the ideals set forth at the 1978 WHO meeting at Alma Ata, traditional medicine has been identified by the Nepali government and its development agency interlocutors as a force to be harnessed, appropriated, and "integrated" into public health paradigms (Pigg 1996). With the Health Service Act of 1996, the Nepali government recognized biomedicine, Ayurveda, and homeopathy as official Nepali medical systems; naturopathy was recognized in 2000; acupuncture and acupressure are practiced in private clinics of people trained in Traditional Chinese Medicine (TCM) institutions in China or elsewhere and are also enfolded within some Ayurvedic hospitals; Unani medicine occupies a similar position;[10] yoga is associated with Ayurveda but is unregulated as a medical therapy; and *amchi* medicine is acknowledged to exist in Nepal but is not granted state recognition or support (Koirala 2007).

In Nepal, Sowa Rigpa is not only *not* officially recognized, but it is also bound up in a cultural politics of ethnicity and identity, in which being affiliated with a non-Hindu high mountain minority has carried the weight of marginalization in a nation-state that, although home to vibrant, complex ethnic politics (N. *janajati*) movements since the early 1990s and a secular republic since 2006, was founded as a Hindu monarchy. Historically *amchi* and the communities from which they hail were positioned within Nepal's caste hierarchy as "non-enslavable alcohol drinkers" (Höfer 1979). Although official discrimination associated with caste and ethnicity have been outlawed in Nepal for decades, and even after decades of active ethnic rights movements since Nepal's shift to a multiparty political system in 1990, *amchi* belong to the cultural and political margins. As border-dwellers, they inhabit distinct and important cultural, political, and economic positions in what has been dubbed the "Indo-Tibetan Interface" (Fisher 1978). Despite dynamics of marginalization, the communities in which *amchi* live and work are, arguably, crucial economic corridors and spaces of commerce in their own right—including conduits for the trade in medicinal plants (Saxer 2011); they are also key locations in which dynamics of ethnicity and citizenship in the greater Himalayan region are articulated, through lived experience as well as regimes of governance (Shneiderman forthcoming). Even so, as Nepal's political-economic alliances with China have grown increasingly strong, Sowa Rigpa's cultural associations with Tibet further complicate the positions *amchi* occupy in their quest for recognition and support.

Up on the Tibetan Plateau, governmental backing for Tibetan medicine has weathered the transition from the pre-1959 "old society" to the era of the People's Republic. Tibetan medicine in China is supported as one of a suite of "minority nationality medicines" (Ch. *minzu yi yiyao*). It is incorporated into clinical care from village to provincial levels, is taught in private schools and state-funded colleges, and its formulas are manufactured in state-certified factories that have been made to comply with new regulations involving massive infrastructure investment and have benefited from public-private partnerships and, in some cases, state subsidies. Yet this support is intertwined with Tibet's troubled political history and with complex processes of modernization, standardization, and marginality—core themes that emerge in this book as well as the work of other scholars (Janes 1995, 1999a, 2001; Adams 2001b; White 2001; Tibet Information Network 2004; Glover 2006; Saxer 2010a; Hofer 2011c).

Such state support has included integrating Tibetan medicine into the Cooperative Medical System (CMS), a model of providing rural health care first promulgated in the post-Mao reform era, beginning in the 1980s, after the dissolution of state-supported health care in the more overtly socialist era. The CMS model has included support for both Chinese-style biomedicine and minority nationality medicines, modeled on state-supported TCM, itself essentially an invention of the 1950s (Taylor 2005; Hsu 2008a). The CMS system has gone through cycles of critique and reform, including a recent wave of national reform in 2005 (Ho 1995; Bloom and Xingyuan 1999; Carrin et al. 1999; *China Daily* 2005). In my fieldwork experience these reforms took effect in many Tibetan areas by 2008–9. While most permanent urban populations in China now buy medical insurance, rural populations, including many Tibetans, struggle to afford the burden of health care fees. This is a result, in part, of the collapse of state-funded health care in the wake of China's economic reforms. The new CMS system requires a flat fee of 50 yuan ($7) per year, roughly a third of which is paid each by the central government, the provincial government, and the patient. Many Chinese citizens, including those about whom you will read in this book, have signed on, but the system is tiered, subject to limitations, and further stratified according to the type of coverage needed. Medical care can still be a burdensome out-of-pocket expense.

Tibetan medical institutions are directly affected by the push toward privatization, capital accumulation, and market-based approaches to health care that has taken hold in China since its experiment in market-based socialism began in the 1990s, and at an ever-increasing pace since its entrance into the World Trade Organization (WTO) in 2001. Tibetan formulas are being transformed from local medicines into "national heritage" drugs and "Chinese proprietary medicines" with regional and global appeal.[11] These changing forms of production raise questions with regard to intellectual property rights—concerns over who owns Tibetan formulas (Pordié 2008a; Saxer 2010a)—and reflect an emphasis on exchange value over use value in the context of neoliberal capitalism with Chinese characteristics. These political-economic transformations, along with the increasing mechanization of production since the 1980s, have involved shifts in the embodied practices involved in making medicines and practicing Sowa Rigpa.

Furthermore Tibetan medicine exists within fraught political spaces in the PRC. Tibetan medicine is framed as an indigenous science and part of China's heritage. It also allows for a valuation of Tibetanness within China's minority nationality/ethnic (Ch. *minzu*) policies in ways that at once allow for the possibility of cultural preservation and, paradoxically, challenge such efforts. In the wake of intense social unrest beginning in 2008 and continuing into the present, many ethnically Tibetan areas of China remain mired in de facto martial law or otherwise intense political scrutiny. Even so, the Tibetan medicine industry is a powerful domain in which Tibetan practitioners and entrepreneurs rival their Chinese counterparts within the People's Republic, in terms of the capital at their disposal to help build an industry. As this book goes to press, news of increasing self-immolations by Tibetan monks, hunger strikes, and other responses to political repression in China are matched by news articles announcing profits for Tibetan medicine companies in the millions of dollars and plans for some companies to make initial public offerings (IPOs) for their stock.

In summary, the historical underpinnings and contemporary political terrain on which Tibetan medicine is practiced, produced, and consumed in Nepal and China are at once distinct and interdependent: Plants sourced from Nepal help to facilitate the scaling up of Tibetan pharma production in China; the circulation of lineage-based teachings and other forms of legitimacy as well as ideas about clinical research flow from China (and India) into Nepal; patients and medicines move within and between these geopolitical entities. The fate of Tibetan medicine in each nation-state is implicated in the other.

ON METHODOLOGY AND POSITIONALITY

The mosaic metaphor alluded to earlier—the practice of making something new out of shards of experience or fragments of material—resonates with the process of writing, for ethnography is nothing if not piecing together observations, engagements, and reflections into something new and whole.

I first went to Nepal in 1993. I was nineteen at the time, an undergraduate study-abroad student intent on learning about the region's subsistence strategies, including the role of horses in the society, religion, and economy of Mustang District, Nepal (Craig 2008a). My initial interest in animals, and in how people in Mustang cared for their animals, led me to Tibetan medicine. Soon after my arrival in Mustang for a year's stay on a Fulbright fellowship (1995–96), I discovered that many people who were well-known for treating animals were actually *amchi* whose primary responsibility was treating people. This began what has become an abiding personal and scholarly interest in the struggles of Nepal's *amchi* to secure and revitalize their practice in the face of major socioeconomic, cultural, and political change. This work has included ongoing collaborative scholarship and applied research with the Kathmandu-based Himalayan Amchi Association (HAA) as well as continued fieldwork in Mustang and with people from Mustang now living elsewhere. This research has focused not only on *amchi* and Tibetan medicine, but also on experiences of migration and social change, women's health, development, and identity politics.

From 2002 to 2004 I lived in Lhasa and served as an anthropologist and research coordinator on a Maternal and Child Health (MCH) project supported by a grant from the U.S. National Institutes of Health (NIH) and the Gates Foundation, through their alliance in the Global Network for Women's and Children's Health Research. What began as a project focused on MCH care in rural Tibetan communities eventually splintered into two programs: a clinical research project described in chapter 7 and an NGO focused on Skilled Birth Attendant (SBA) training and the creation of a "network of safety" for Tibetan women and children (Craig 2011c). During this time I was also conducting doctoral research. My responsibilities on the clinical study included ethnographic research, helping to design research protocols, organizing trainings, and overseeing qualitative and quantitative data collection that preceded the actual RCT. I served as a linguistic and cultural liaison, working closely with U.S., Tibetan, and Chinese colleagues trained in Tibetan medicine and biomedicine, as well as other anthropologists, government cadres, and Tibetan and Euro-American staff and volunteers.

My engagement with Tibetan medicine has continued with more recent fieldwork in Yunnan (2007) and Qinghai (2010–present), at international workshops and conferences between 2001 and 2012, through ongoing trips to Nepal, and by hosting colleagues from China and Nepal in the United States. I have used a range of methods in conducting this research, including participant-observation, formal and informal interviews, surveys, textual analysis, translation, and action research (Greenwood and Levin 2006) approaches. In helping to interpret Tibetan medical theory for American obstetricians and midwives, writing funding proposals for Nepali *amchi,* assisting in the creation of the first Institutional Review Board (IRB) in Tibet, and volunteering my pregnant belly to rural SBA trainees in Lhasa Prefecture, I have both participated in and observed what Mei Zhan (2009) has called the "worlding" of Asian medicine. In her ethnography of contemporary TCM between China and the United States, Zhan describes her encounters in schools, clinics, and professional associations as spaces in which Chinese medicine is "co-imagined" (2). This idea of co-imagination speaks to me. I do not believe it is possible to transcend my complicated positionality vis-à-vis my interlocutors. Time spent in Nepal and China has enmeshed me in relations of reciprocity that extend well beyond the confines of an academic text, toward other forms of engagement. I have served as a grant writer, a translator, a fundraiser, a co-investigator, and a coauthor, among other roles. The choice to take on these responsibilities is personal and ethical. Many of the relationships described herein exist well beyond the distilled ethnographic instances that form the backbone of this book. But books must begin and end somewhere.

Postcolonial studies of science and history have taught me that strictly rationalist ways of knowing the world can neither do justice to the range of human experience nor produce scholarship that is wholly inclusive or reflexive. My views are limited, my vision is partial, and my ability to write this book implicates me in historical and disciplinary relations of power. This understanding informs the narrative strategy of this book. Quite often I render ethnography through dialogue. I draw practical tools and theoretical inspiration from methodologies that bridge those of anthropology and the literary arts (Narayan 1999, 2007). These choices raise issues about memory and representation, signature subjects of anthropology and critiques of the discipline, particularly since the "crisis of representation" era (Clifford and Marcus 1986). I heed such critiques. Indeed I have been schooled in and through them. However, I am convinced that, beyond a certain commitment to Geertzian thick description, the methods of creative nonfiction, among other genres, are useful to ethnography. They enliven narrative and enrich theory. My use of dialogue is an explicit, conscious choice—a way of writing theory through action and writing my own positionalities into the text.

To be clear, some dialogues recounted in this book are taken from taped transcriptions. They represent "natural language" that has been edited minimally for readability, after translation. Other dialogues are reconstructed from detailed notes taken during or immediately after an encounter. In all possible cases these notes were then back-translated and checked by interlocutors. Throughout the book I let the reader know in which language or languages a particular dialogue is occurring. When English or Chinese words are used in an otherwise Nepali or Tibetan sentence, I italicize them; the same is true when Nepali or Tibetan phrases are used in a code-switching manner in an otherwise English sentence. I use this strategy to render as accurately as possible the nature, expression, and intonation of a dialogue, but also because these patterns of code-switching provide avenues for analysis in their own right.

The issue of names—to provide anonymity, use pseudonyms, or not—reveals tensions between the need for greater transparency in anthropological practice and the ethical imperative, for researchers to protect their human subjects, as outlined by IRBs as well as by the social and political circumstances of some field sites. These tensions are highlighted in an era of increasingly collaborative research and a call to not hide "unnecessarily behind methodological artifice" (May 2010) but instead allow subjects to engage directly with the works in which their histories, words, and ideas are central. I have chosen a hybrid approach to addressing these ethical concerns. When introducing my research projects or starting to work in a new field site, I have always begun from the position that I will maintain confidentiality and, to the greatest extent possible, anonymity. In recording data (notes, interviews, etc.) I either de-identified individuals, used only initials, or assigned the person a pseudonym. I assured interlocutors they would not be identified by name or will be given a pseudonym in publications, unless they indicated that they would like to be identified. However, over years of work with people featured in this book, we have collaborated in many different ways, including coauthoring publications and presentations. Greater collaboration has brought about limits to the possibilities for anonymity. In order to address this, I have received permission from some individuals in this book to use their real names. Some interlocutors *actively sought* direct recognition of their names in this text. This is particularly true in the case of colleagues from Nepal. Political sensitivities in Tibetan areas of China have necessitated the use of pseudonyms in some cases or the exclusion of a name altogether. In a few cases, when I have not been able to directly contact an individual to ask for his or her preference, I have defaulted to the use of a pseudonym.

CHAPTER PRÉCIS

The first three chapters of this book focus mostly on practitioners and Tibetan medicine as a *process*. The middle chapter, chapter 4, focuses on therapeutic encounters, linking ethnography that highlights Tibetan medicine as *process* to Tibetan medicines as *products*. The last three chapters focus primarily on medicines and *materia medica,* their circulation as objects of sociocultural, medical, and economic value.

Chapters 1 and 2 are contemporary chronicles: one day spent in two main ethnographic sites featured in this book. They provide readers with a sense of the scope of this ethnography and introduce key characters. The narrative structure of these chapters follows the form of field notes or an ethnographic journal. That structure is *not* a conceit in that, with one exception,[12] all events recounted in these chapters took place on one day in 2008 and 2010, respectively. Chapter 1 tracks a day in the life of *amchi* from Mustang, Nepal. Chapter 2 is written about a day at Arura, a major Tibetan medical institution in Qinghai Province, China. This approach gives a sense of just how multifaceted the life of a Himalayan healer or Tibetan medical practitioner can be. As you move through these days with the doctors from rural Nepal and urban China, a simple vision of tradition versus modernity or local versus global becomes clearly inadequate to understand their lives. By witnessing a Mustangi *amchi* at home and at work, you can see how social ecology shapes experiences of efficacy and social life in an "out of the way place" (Tsing 1993). Gyatso and Tenzin, the *amchi* brothers from Mustang, travel only a handful of miles in the course of this day. They are intimately familiar with the landscapes in which they live and the people they encounter. Yet even in this rootedness, they traverse many worlds beyond the boundaries of this Himalayan community. Chapter 1 emphasizes the many responsibilities one rural *amchi* takes on in a national context where Tibetan medicine is not recognized by the government.

In chapter 2 we see a very different world of Tibetan medicine, operating in an urban Chinese context within distinct governance structures and possibilities for efficacious practice. Arura's hospital serves a large and diverse patient base. There are more obvious and daily translations occurring across medical systems—Tibetan medicine, Chinese medicine, biomedicine—here than in Nepal. You witness a certain level of standardization of practice and greater economic investments in Tibetan medicine here than in a rural community in the Nepal Himalaya. Whereas chapter 1 emphasizes themes of identity, knowledge transmission, and interactions with conservation-development agendas, chapter 2 illustrates engagement between Sowa Rigpa, the biomedical sciences, and commercial pharmaceutical production.

Taken together, these two chapters exemplify central arguments of this book: that efficacy is at once a biopsychosocial and political-economic idea, articulated in specific social ecologies, and that "traditional medicine" in the twenty-first century is inextricably tied to global regimes of governance, from conservation-development agendas to technoscience and the business of global pharma. Both chapters reveal the truth behind Pordié's assertion that it is best to speak of Tibetan *medicines* rather than Tibetan medicine in the singular. There is simply too much diversity in the practices and perspectives incorporated under this term to do otherwise. Yet the lives of people like Gyatso intersect with institutions such as Arura. Indeed one goal of these first two chapters is to show just how distinct yet interconnected these multisite realities are.

Chapter 3 uses the concepts of lineage and legitimacy to describe how forms of cultural and economic capital are produced through learning Tibetan medicine and through state support and recognition of this practice. I argue that standardized regulations of all sorts, from moral precepts about the behavior of healer-physicians to state-approved curricula to medical licenses, are rooted in particular histories and environments. Different social ecologies produce different ideas—at times complimentary and at times contentious—about what makes a good doctor.

In chapter 3 and 5 I explore how Traditional Medicine and Complementary and Alternative Medicine (CAM), as globalized frames of reference, shape Sowa Rigpa. How do labels such as these impact the ways practitioners of Tibetan medicine think of themselves? How do such categories shape a "politics of the possible" (Nichter 2008) for Tibetan medicine today, whether in Nepal or China? In this chapter I concentrate on the relationship between TM/CAM and more localized, vernacular understandings of legitimacy. What makes an *amchi* a legitimate healer in the context of a village or within a government-supported institution of Tibetan medicine? Are the sources of legitimacy the same? How important is lineage *(menpé gyü)* to garnering legitimacy? I examine what it means to seek government recognition in Nepal, where Tibetanness is associated with cultural "backwardness" and political sensitivity, and how this contrasts with Chinese health care policies that seek to capitalize on minority nationality medicines, and to subsume all nonbiomedical practices under the banner of state-supported TCM. Where does this suite of medical traditions—which we might unite under the banner of Sowa Rigpa but that is *not* easily or directly associated with *one* nation-state—fit within the WHO agenda to recognize Traditional Medicine, since this recognition hinges on developing regulatory structures *within sovereign countries and nation-states?*

In chapter 4 I draw primarily on fieldwork from Kathmandu, Mustang, and Qinghai Province.[13] I focus on what occurs in small, private clinics and how individuals narrate their experiences of illness. These illness narratives (Kleinman 1988) introduce you to an array of concerns regarding access and affordability of health care in culturally Tibetan areas. You see where Tibetan medicine fits into complex patterns of resort, issues of mistrust that surface with respect to biomedicine and state health care options, and the association between material and cosmological or spiritual understandings of illness causality and possibilities for treatment.

Next I outline the pathways people take through what Susan Sontag (2001: 3) has called the "kingdom of the sick." We see how social ecologies are at once maintained and transformed through migration and experiences of modernity, including the circulation of medicines between people from Nepal and China now living in the United States and their relatives back home. In the final section I explore how specific diseases and patterns of illness experience are linked to material, cosmological, and place-based understandings of the causes and conditions giving rise to health problems. We see that medicine is a dynamic engagement between the oft-polarized extremes of "science" and "religion."

In chapter 5 I present ethnography that spans nearly a decade, from 2002 to 2010, conducted in the TAR and Qinghai. I discuss the implementation of Good Manufacturing Practices and related regulations on the commercial production of Tibetan medicines. GMP are regimes of pharmaceutical governance that define the conditions under which raw materials are evaluated and processed and medicines are produced. When combined with Chinese Drug Administration regulations, including the practice of applying for registration numbers to produce Tibetan formulas, such regimes of governance bear on how products are marketed and sold, as well as at what price and to whom. GMP regulations can be traced to social, political, and scientific agendas that emerged at the turn of the twentieth century, of which the creation of the U.S. Food and Drug Administration is emblematic (Immel 2000).

In this chapter I argue that Chinese state implementation of GMP for commercial production of Tibetan medicines must be understood within the context of global pharmaceutical governance of Traditional Medicine, as the WHO defines it, and within expanding international markets for CAM therapies. Heavily value- and culture-laden terms such as *quality, safety,* and *efficacy* undergird the creation and implementation of GMP in China, even as they too are cultural products emerging from institutions such as the WHO and the U.S. FDA and, arguably more importantly, from Chinese institutions and laws. Especially for non-Tibetan consumers, these biomedically derived markers of standardization remain essential, even as they are attracted to aesthetic markers of "the traditional" that are employed by marketing the exotic elements of Tibet and what Saxer (2010a) and Kloos (2010) both describe as specific moral economies linked to, and fashioned from, "Tibetanness."

Chinese refigurations of international biomedically oriented regulations have specific cultural and political effects when connected to a minority nationality such as Tibetans in China. At stake are not only the parameters by which the quality, safety, and efficacy of Tibetan medicines are determined; so too is the future of Tibetan science and related issues of cultural identity and environmental stewardship, given the technical expertise and natural resources upon which Tibetan pharmacology depends. Tibetans involved in the industry are themselves divided about the impacts and meanings of regulations such as GMP and the larger process of commoditizing and standardizing Tibetan formulas. Even as GMP regulations may not, in themselves, prompt areas of practical incommensurability, their implementation has provoked contested discourse on what makes for "good" medicines.

In chapter 6 I examine how *amchi* interact with conservation-development practitioners, policies, and projects, drawing on fieldwork from Yunnan Province, China, in a region that is actually called "Shangri La," as well as ethnography from Nepal and Bhutan. Perhaps surprisingly, insights about the nature of health and illness, the social lives of medicines, and the political-economic possibilities and constraints for meeting global health needs only infrequently intersect with insights from political ecology.[14] Much of what exists in both academic and popular literature tends to focus on the interface between ethnobotany and biomedicine, specifically around bioprospecting or biopiracy: the search for "magic bullet" plants and the well-founded fears that indigenous knowledge will be appropriated and commodified without sufficient forethought or compensation to the bearers of that knowledge.[15] Some work has focused on the ways plant knowledge is also social knowledge, the sense that herbal remedies are "social artifacts," in the words of Hsu and Harris (2010), and that medicinal plants are what Pordié (2002) has called "biocultural objects." Other points of convergence have occurred around issues of environmental health and the biopsychosocial effects of conservation-induced displacement, natural disasters, or otherwise environmentally prompted migrations on local populations. As such, my goal for this chapter is to link medical anthropology and political ecology by examining connections between the commodification of nature and culture in the context of *amchi* involvement with conservation-development, looking at how this relates to their role as health care providers and transmitters of Sowa Rigpa knowledge in and of specific places.

In chapter 7 I recount the "social life" (Appadurai 1986; Whyte et al. 2002) of *zhijé* 11, a Tibetan formula, from its mythohistorical creation by a female adept of the *dharma* in the thirteenth century to its description in Tibetan medical texts in later centuries. I discuss how Tibetan women use this eleven-ingredient compound during childbirth, and how Mentsikhang obstetricians and other Tibetan doctors prescribe this medicine. I analyze what happens when this formula becomes one of two study drugs in the first hospital-based RCT in Tibet, in which the other study drug is a biochemical compound called misoprostol. Both medicines have multiple indications, but they are used in this instance to test which has the greater capacity to reduce blood loss after delivery, thereby helping to prevent Postpartum Hemorrhage, a complication of childbirth that kills scores of women worldwide *every day* (WHO 2008). As you will see, *zhijé* 11 comes to embody possibilities and constraints, the points of innovation and compromise, that occur when biomedicine, clinical research, and Tibetan medicine intersect. In this sense, the biography of *zhijé* 11 becomes a parable for all that is at once hopeful and unnerving, exciting and daunting about the future of Tibetan medicine(s) in Nepal, China, and beyond.

CHAPTER I

Portrait of a Himalayan Healer

We have weathered so many journeys, and so many forms of
love. Would it have been the same, we ask one another, had
we stayed still, in the mill with the water running under us.
There is no way of knowing.

—Alastair Reid, *Whereabouts: Notes on Being a Foreigner*

READING SIGNS

It is early September 2008. The high-altitude air is tinged with autumn.
I walk through the alleys of Lo Monthang, the largest settlement in
northern Mustang District, Nepal. This is the time before animals have
been let out to graze, before children have gone off to the new local day
care,[1] to school, or to help gather dung and tend animals. I pass whitewashed homes decorated with protective door hangings above the
threshold: colored yarn webs holding sheep skulls, repelling nefarious
spirits and gossip. I hear the muffled sounds of cymbals, bells, and the
resonant drone of Tibetan Buddhist monks calling forth another day.

As I make my way through Lo Monthang, I am conscious of borders.
This is Nepal's northern edge, where the Indian subcontinent is sub-
ducted under the Tibetan Plateau. Mustang lies in the Himalayan rain
shadow; it is mostly high-altitude desert, abutting the Tibet Autonomous
Region, China. Jomsom, the district's headquarters, is linked to Pokhara,
the nearest city, by flights from a small airport and by trails. No all-
season motor road connects the district to any urban center, although
this reality is changing swiftly. Seasonal unpaved roads have been constructed over the past decade and are passable with tractors, jeeps, and
motorcycles. Mustang is encompassed by the Annapurna Conservation
Area, Nepal's largest protected area.[2] The district is home to approximately 14,000 individuals (2001 Nepal census), whose households and

property are partitioned into sixteen village development committees. Upper Mustang, at the center of which sits Lo Monthang, is home to Tibetan speakers, *tsampa* eaters,[3] and practitioners of Buddhism and Bön, indigenous religious practices of the Tibetan plateau (Snellgrove 1981; Samuel 1993). These moral cosmologies lend structure and meaning to life here, along with what Charles Ramble (2008) calls a "civil religion," which prescribes social norms and governs natural resource use, further defining the region's cultural and natural landscape.

Mustang's Kali Gandaki River and settlements situated along its banks have been a locus of trans-Himalayan trade for centuries, including the exchange of lowland grains for Tibetan salt. The people of Mustang have relied on agriculture, animal husbandry, and trade to wrest survival and even prosperity from the area for centuries. Mustang was incorporated into the nation-state of Nepal in the eighteenth century, though the area has maintained cultural, economic, and political alliances with Tibet (Ramble 2008). The most significant and enduring of these connections is the lineage of kings, descendants of western Tibetan nobility who, since the fourteenth century, have wielded influence over the region, particularly in upper Mustang, or what is known as the Kingdom of Lo (Dhungel 2002). Jigme Palbar Bista, the twenty-fifth in the lineage of Lo kings (T. *gyalpo,* N. *raja*), still lives in a looming whitewashed palace at the heart of Lo Monthang. His wife, the queen (T. *gyalmo,* N. *rani*), hails from Shigatse, the second largest city in the TAR. Tibetan Resistance forces occupied Mustang from 1960 to 1974, as they waged guerrilla war against the Chinese People's Liberation Army (Knauss 1998; McGranahan 2010). A permanent Tibetan refugee settlement has existed in southern Mustang since the 1970s.

Due in part to this sensitive political history, foreign access to upper Mustang was prohibited until 1991. Travel to the region is now allowed on a restricted basis, requiring a permit that costs $50 per person, per day.[4] In contrast, villages in lower Mustang are part of the Annapurna trekking circuit and have been a mainstay of Nepal tourism since the late 1970s. Lower Mustang is also more accessible to roads and regional markets. These distinctions have real-world effects with respect to economic opportunities and the provision of government services, including health care. Many from the region spend the winters engaged in small business in northern India, Pokhara, or Kathmandu. During Nepal's decade-long (1996–2006) conflict between Maoist forces and the state's army and armed police, Mustang remained the only district in the country that did not see active combat. Yet this conflict—along with the chance to earn social and economic capital by working abroad—has propelled many people to leave Mustang (Craig 2002, 2004, 2011b).

On this crisp September morning, I round the corner past Thubchen, a fifteenth-century monastery that has been restored recently (Lo Bue 2011). I walk past a row of reliquaries (T. *chöten*, Skt. *stupa*) and stop before the wood-and–corrugated metal door leading to a school. A window, rimmed in black and red paint, rests above the door. Between window and door hangs a trilingual signboard. There is an arc of English— "Lo-Kunphen Traditional Herbal Medicine Clinic and School"—under which is written an approximation of the same, first in Tibetan and then in Nepali. The Tibetan reads *Lo Kunphen Mentsikhang Lobdra*. The Nepali reads *Lo Kunphen Aamchi Aaushadhyalaya Skul*. My friends and colleagues, Gyatso and Tenzin Bista, run this small institution.

Many elements of meaning are lost and gained across the two-dimensionality of this sign. As mentioned in the Introduction, the term *mentsikhang* means "house of medicine and astrology." In its generic sense, this is a place where Sowa Rigpa is practiced. It is also the name given to major state institutions of Tibetan medicine in China and India. It becomes, simply, "clinic" in English. In Nepali *aamchi aaushadhyalaya skul* is an amalgam of language and history. The first term is a Nepali approximation of *amchi*, itself a Mongolian word long ago loaned to Tibetan, which means "healer" or "doctor." *Aaushadhylaya* connotes a medical establishment. It is formal, Sanskritized, the type of word most people from Mustang—though citizens of Nepal—would have trouble using in common speech. The word might conjure memories of failed School Leaving Certificate (SLC) examinations, and it would probably feel more foreign than the English word *clinic*. Finally, *skul* is a Devanagari approximation of the English term *school*.

I have passed this sign many times. This morning it stops me short. I realize that, in Nepali, there is nothing *Tibetan* about this place. In Tibetan, centuries of interconnected history between Mustang and centers of Sowa Rigpa in Lhasa, Dharamsala, and beyond are implicit in the choice of names given to this institution. In English, the deceptively simple signifier "traditional herbal medicine" supplants regionally and culturally specific understandings of medicine and heath care.

Nestled between the arc of English, Tibetan, and Nepali are the words "Estd. 2056." This is a reference to the Nepali calendar. No Gregorian or Tibetan lunar year is given, though it would have been 1999–2000 or the cusp of the Iron Dragon year of 2126, respectively. This detail on a sign—a tableau of identification, where space is limited—speaks to the struggle for recognition and legitimacy in which Gyatso, Tenzin, and other *amchi* in Nepal have been engaged for nearly two decades. It is easy to imagine "Estd. 2056" stamped on registration papers Gyatso and Tenzin filed with district and national authorities to start this institution: a vermillion mark soaking into the thick, uneven warp and weft of Nepali *lokta* paper.

The only other element on the sign is, in a sense, its heart: a small rendering of Sangye Menla, the Medicine Buddha, his offering bowl brimming with *arura,* the fruit of the myrobalan tree and the "king of medicines." This sign is a mosaic, an assemblage of meaning. To understand only one of these languages is to miss the negotiations of culture and identity wrapped up in my interlocutors' efforts toward increasing the social efficacy of their practice in a new age. To see this sign simply as a handmade entrance to a marginal institution in far away place is to miss the point. Certainly this is a remote locale. But it is a place connected to regimes of value and patterns of social change that stretch out from the Himalaya and Tibetan Plateau, down the Indian subcontinent, across the world, and back again.

Filled with these thoughts about identity and belonging, language and culture, tradition and contemporary life, I walk through the door and enter the courtyard of Lo Kunphen. Several students cluster around a water spigot, brushing their teeth. Older students ready the simple dining hall for breakfast, after prayers and before classes. I greet them and head toward the back door of Lo Kunphen, which lets me out beyond Lo Monthang's city wall, in front of Gyatso and Tenzin's home, the lower floor of which is devoted to an herbarium and small Sowa Rigpa museum. I climb the stairs and call out a greeting. Gyatso's familiar voice answers, inviting me in.

MANTRAS, IVS, AND MORNING TEA: 7:30 A.M.

Gyatso is seated on low cushions in the main room, drinking salt-butter tea. The brothers' infirm mother directs morning traffic. Two generations of this family's women perform chores as seamlessly as if playing a symphony. Gyatso's wife loads the stove with sheep and goat dung, blows embers awake, pours water into a kettle, and sets it to boil. She then breaks grassy clumps of brick tea into this tepid water and metes out a pinch of Tibetan salt. Her eldest niece carves a slab of butter from a block with the swiftness of a potter slicing clay. She tosses it into the tea churner. These acts mark a day's beginning here: art, routine, discipline each in its own right. This place would not run without its women.

A stack of notebooks sits on a wooden table in the corner, nestled between divans laid with Tibetan carpets. Some of these books are tea-stained and once or twice soaked through by rain. Their pages contain all manner of notations, written mostly in Tibetan, at times in Nepali, or in approximations of English, sounded out. They bespeak these doctors' networks: prescription notes, names of tourists who might become school sponsors, lists of plants and other raw materials to buy in Etum Bahal or Indra Chowk, old Kathmandu neighborhoods where herb traders hawk and bargain. Beside these notebooks are religious texts wrapped in cloth, a Tibetan-English medical dictionary, and a binder whose plastic sheaves protect stacks of receipts for school expenses. These pieces of paper must be carried to Jomsom in saddlebags, then on to Kathmandu in Chinese-made totes embossed with NGO insignia, gifts from academic conferences and conservation-development workshops these brothers have attended. In Kathmandu these recollections of rupees spent are presented to a Nepali accountant who reconciles the books and sends them to British, German, and U.S. charities that help to support the school. This institution is an experiment in bridging the gaps between Gyatso and Tenzin's father's generation and the worlds their children will inherit.

Tenzin comes into the room carrying a glass bottle of a glucose and saline solution, a splice of IV tubing, and a still sterile hypodermic needle. The glucose is Nepali made, though nearly every other commercial item in this house was manufactured in China: thermoses, blankets, solar panels that charge their satellite telephone. Tenzin moves toward his mother. This woman has been unable to walk for years and has, in a sense, been waiting to die ever since her husband passed away, in 1996. For all her despondency, she is still the center of this home, the voice to which everyone defers.

Tenzin calls his niece, a senior student at Lo Kunphen. They prop up the old woman so she can receive this IV infusion. I ask Tenzin why he has chosen to give this biomedical treatment to his mother. "It gives her strength, since she struggles to eat," he responds. The old woman seems calm until Tenzin produces the needle. Then she wriggles, moans, covers her eyes. The niece struggles to still her grandmother.

Seeing the task will not be easy, Tenzin calls for Gyatso. These sons reassure their mother. Then, deftly, Gyatso pins down her forearm as

Tenzin inserts the needle past layers of weathered mountain skin into the river of a bluish vein. Tenzin tapes the needle in place, attaches it to the tubing, and hangs the glass bottle from a hook fitted to the ceiling above the old woman's perch. All the while one of the youngest members of the extended family looks on with fascination, nestled beside her great-grandmother, enfolded in layers of wool.

This simple act—needle into vein and the slow, steady infusion of sugars, salts, and water into this old woman—reminds me there are no easy ways to parse this world of healing. Neither the terms *tradition* and *modernity* nor a presumed ideological divide between Tibetan medicine and biomedicine makes much sense here (Samuel 2006). These Buddhist *amchi* have given a biomedical anodyne with tenderness to their ailing mother. They do so in great part because empiricism has brought them here. They know it works because their mother's cheeks flush after such infusions. Just the same, a different empiricism instructs them to conduct long-life rituals and wear protection amulets. Ultimately they will face their mother's death as part of sentient existence: one karmic turning of the wheel of life.

MASTERS OF THE GIFT: 9:00 A.M.

Gyatso, Tenzin, and I move into the school's chapel *(chökhang)* and library. The phrase "someone who wears many hats" works in both English and Tibetan. This is often how I feel about these brothers. In addition to his responsibility as principal of Lo Kunphen, Tenzin is also a senior monk at Chöde Monastery, a *sakya* Tibetan Buddhist institution in Lo Monthang. Yesterday he spent half the day performing a ritual in the household of someone who had recently died. Gyatso, like his father before him, is the householder-priest *(nakpa)* and doctor to the royal family of Lo. Since 2003 he has also been the chairman of the Himalayan Amchi Association.

Yesterday, despite our plans to review clinic records and write a funding proposal, Gyatso was called to the palace to greet officials from across the border in the TAR. They had driven to Lo Monthang in a Chinese land cruiser to discuss trade relations. The "road" they drove in on is relatively new, but cross-border exchange is at once an old and an increasingly common phenomenon. Many obstacles to such exchange occurred this year, 2008. Lhasa erupted in riots in March, followed by continued unrest and repression across Tibetan areas of the PRC. The

Beijing Olympics resulted in further clampdowns. The closure of Tibet to foreign tourists meant more had ventured to upper Mustang. However, geopolitical problems also curtailed the flow of goods between this part of Nepal and the TAR, commodities on which the people of Mustang have come to depend. And so, when the Tibetan officials arrived, Gyatso was called to serve his king, as this traditional leader negotiated the terms of cross-border trade. To some in Mustang, such visits are welcome. To others, they bespeak unwanted Chinese influence in Nepali territory.

As is often the case, Gyatso was asked to read the pulse of these TAR visitors and give them medicines. I could imagine him rolling up the sleeves of a Tibetan official's dusty polyester blazer, reaching for the right hand and then the left, and, reading pulsations both deep and shallow, auguring a bile-related disorder or a chest infection. These officials, like the Tibetan constituents they represent, rely on Gyatso and Tenzin's medicines as they did their father's before them, maintaining *netsang*, relations of fictive kin and trading partners, with people across the border. Geopolitical boundaries and social ecologies do not always align. In parts of the TAR it can be difficult to access locally made Tibetan medicines such as those Gyatso make here. Some of Gyatso's Tibetan patients have been eating medicines made by his family for years, and they prefer them to the more expensive manufactured formulas trucked in from Lhasa.

Yesterday's unexpected visit put off our work on the grant proposal until this morning. Gyatso and Tenzin begin by reiterating to me their need for money. They struggle to raise sufficient funds to maintain this school of thirty to forty students, along with their "factory" and small branch clinics. Our current task is to craft a proposal for a London-based foundation that has normally supported only Tibetan refugees. On occasion it will accept applications from "Tibetan border peoples" such as those from Mustang.

We begin to work. A familiar process of translation ensues. In eloquent Tibetan, Gyatso and Tenzin speak of the decline of Sowa Rigpa across the Himalayas, the role of *amchi* in providing health care to rural populations, the importance of teaching and practicing *amchi* medicine, and then the punch line: the need for funds to develop a more advanced course in Sowa Rigpa in Nepal, to be based in the small city of Pokhara, and the need to expand their clinical practice in Mustang so senior students might have employment to keep them in their rural communities and so that local populations might have access to a complete pharmacy of Tibetan formulas, even those the brothers cannot produce themselves.

We also work on reports to current donors, an effort to translate Gyatso and Tenzin's daily work to people with good intentions but somewhat limited understanding of life in Mustang. Most donors expect this institution to become "self-sustaining." I struggle with this term. What does it mean to expect financial sustainability from people with relatively few resources when those of us with so much more still, so often, fail to achieve such a balance? What does it mean to expect cash payment for medical services from villagers who may not have rupees to spare? Or to expect *amchi* to set a fixed price for clinic visits or homemade pills, even if their ethical training demands the opposite? I question the logic, common among development projects, that views the monetization of social and medical exchanges as a measurement of success.

On the other hand, though, why will villagers eke out funds to travel to Kathmandu for a gall bladder operation or a cesarean section but see the support of local *amchi,* in cash or in kind, as something less important today than it was a generation ago?[5] What makes them view not only biomedicine, but also medicine accessed *outside Mustang* as superior to local health care provision? What makes people nostalgic for the care they received from *amchi* who have died but wary sometimes to receive treatment from living *amchi?*

Gyatso and Tenzin's search for funding consumes enormous time and energy. It sometimes results in frustrated donors who expect something different from what the brothers can deliver or anxiety between the brothers as they struggle to pay teachers, and buy *dal* and rice. At the same time, their relative success in running Lo Kunphen can promote local gossip *(mi kha)* about whether the brothers are personally profiting from their foreign connections. Models of governance, of transparency and accountability across cultures, often clash in the spaces where a family vocation bleeds into a formal institution and then spills over into requests for "deliverables." Miscommunication can occur. Consider the following example. For the first few years that a British charity, Kids in Need of Education,[6] supported Lo Kunphen, the brothers thought the organization's acronym was actually the name of a person, a patron whose surname was "Kinoe."

Without significant government support for Sowa Rigpa in Nepal— indeed even if such support materializes in the coming years— nongovernmental sponsorship remains paramount. In Tibetan, *jindag* means "master of the gift." These days it is a term used to describe charitable foundations, individual sponsors, private patrons, and NGOs. Gyatso and Tenzin know me as a researcher, a translator, and a friend.

But they also know me as a *jindag*. My engagement with Lo Kunphen has included raising money for the clinics and school, in part through an NGO I helped to found (www.drokpa.org). Just because I understand the nuance of an enduring Tibetan form of social relations does not make our allegiance to each other simple, though.

This morning Gyatso echoes a familiar refrain. "*Jindag* are like the wind and the rain," he says. "They come and they go. We cannot predict from which direction. But we need them for these seeds we have planted to ripen." It is an honest assessment, if also an organic metaphor voiced by a person who knows so well this earth of which he speaks.

We hunch over annual budgets and student examination reports. As we work I think about a conversation I had over dinner in the posh European home of one Lo Kunphen donor. I came bearing reports and pictures from the school. "Isn't it sweet," the donor said, "to see the students looking proper, lined up in uniform? Remember what they used to look like? Snotty-nosed ragamuffins," he scoffed. "Now at least they are cleaner and becoming literate in their own language. But I still doubt these brothers can pull off making them all into doctors."

As if to answer this memory of mine, Tenzin speaks about this year's examination results. "Our students made some of the highest marks in Mustang District. Not everyone passed the SLC, but we have some very good students, especially in class 9." Tenzin pauses. "Not everyone can become an *amchi*, though. I think if we have *ten percent amchi*"—he uses English here—"that would be a good result. Some do not have right motivation. Others do not have intellect. Others have both, but their parents or their own desires will send them down the path to foreign places." Indeed this has already happened. The roster of current students reveals the attrition of young women and men of talent. Chime has gone to Korea. Karchung's parents are angling for a U.S. visa.

Within the eldest cohort of Lo Kunphen students, now studying for their first formal degree, called *kanjenpa,* only one passed the state-certified examinations this year. All did well on the part of the exam covering Tibetan medical curricula, but most did not score high enough on government-mandated subjects: Nepali, mathematics, and the rest. The inclusion of these subjects in this otherwise Tibetan medical curriculum was required in order for Lo Kunphen to earn recognition of its program by the Ministry of Education. But state certification and "SLC-pass" are approbations these students care about. They epitomize an "expectation of modernity," as Ferguson (1999) calls it. In some ways, passing the SLC is a more tangible marker of the school's social efficacy than a *kanjenpa* certificate, since Nepal does not officially recognize Tibetan medicine, unlike Bhutan, Mongolia, and China, where it is incorporated into state heath care.

This reality points to a double bind of institutionalization. These young people are coming of age in a world where certificates and licenses will be required of them in forms not known by previous generations. An aspiring *amchi*'s program of study must reflect not only local realities and theoretical principles, but also the state's conception of what a Nepali should know. Pedagogies can clash. Students struggle with questions of relevance—*Where will we put this knowledge to use? What will we remember? How will we support our families?*—even as they are quick to answer the anthropologist cum *jindag* that they are studying to be *amchi* to bring health care to their communities, to preserve their culture, to benefit sentient beings.

Gyatso, Tenzin, and I are interrupted by a knock on the chapel door. A mother arrives with her son. He fell off a horse two days ago and appears to have fractured his left forearm. The boy is no more than ten. Rivulets of tears trickle down his dusty cheeks. Gyatso takes the boy's pulse from his ear, as is standard for children, feeling along his shoulder and arm. Tenzin prepares an herbal ointment mixed with rapeseed oil. The boy cringes. Gyatso tells him not to cry. The brothers have established several small clinics in villages surrounding Lo Monthang, but the work of healing still often occurs in their home.

"He was taking care of our sheep and goat," the boy's mother explains. "He shouldn't have been on the horse anyway. He should have been walking, collecting dung. But he never listens!" This mother seems worried and exasperated. You see, she needs his labor. The cost of hiring lowland Nepalis (T. *rongba*) to herd or bring in the barley crop remains prohibitive for this family, like many others in Lo.

"Don't worry," says Gyatso. "The boy will be fine." Tenzin hands his brother the herbal mixture and two *kathag,* white silk offering scarves. Gyatso applies the ointment to the fractured bone and then bandages the boy's arm, creating a sling out of a blessing. Tenzin wraps up some of the powdery herbal mixture in a sheaf of paper. "Mix three spoonfuls of this with rapeseed oil. Change this dressing every day," he instructs. The woman pulls out a money purse that was pinned to the inside of her blouse. She attempts to hand Gyatso several hundred rupees ($2 to $3), but he exits the room, indicating that cash payment is not necessary. Instead the woman leaves a cotton satchel of dried cheese with Gyatso's elder sister, who accepts this gift.

As I watch this exchange, I struggle to square differential regimes of value. How might we reconcile the moral economy of *amchi* work and this in-kind payment of locally produced food with the political economy of becoming self-sustaining and the Excel spreadsheets over which we had just been laboring?

BIRTH OF THE CLINIC: 1:00 P.M.

After the young boy with the broken arm departs, Gyatso, Tenzin, and I set aside our paperwork. The proposal must wait. Tenzin heads off to teach a lesson from the *Explanatory Tantra*, one of four books that comprise the *Gyüshi*. Gyatso and I saddle two of the family's horses and prepare to visit the clinics north of Monthang. I am given Tenzin's horse, a lithe and lovely roan reputed to be the fastest in Mustang these days. The gelding once belonged to the king, but Tenzin succeeded in buying the animal after some negotiations. "The king can take his time getting from place to place," Gyatso explains, "but the *amchi* needs to move quickly when people call. This," he said, patting the horse's rump, "is Mustang *ambulance*." True enough. Just a few days before, a man from Namdo, a village near the Tibetan border, roused Tenzin from sleep with a message that his wife was severely ill. Tenzin and the husband set off in the predawn darkness. Tenzin treated the woman, left her with medicines, and rode the three hours home, only to see another patient in a nearby settlement later that day.

On this afternoon the horse lives up to its reputation. We fly over chalky paths, past verdant sedges and wildflowers that persist after Mustang's brief, bucolic summer. We arrive midday in the village of Thinker. The clinic sits above the village in the small mud-brick building that also serves as the government school, which on this weekday morning is markedly quiet. A lowland Nepali schoolmaster wanders out in his blue tracksuit, holding a stainless steel cup of sweet tea. I introduce myself in Nepali and ask where the children are. "Oh, since now is the harvest time, *no students much coming*," he replies. Gyatso whispers in quiet Tibetan, "He's lazy. A typical government teacher. Eats his salary and does no work!"

My friend opens the clinic, revealing the rudiments of health care in upper Mustang: a wooden cabinet filled with about fifty small bottles of neatly labeled Tibetan medicines, all produced by Gyatso and Tenzin, with help from senior students; a small table and bench, two chairs; a dusty but well-used clinic logbook in which the name, gender, and age of patients, a shorthand diagnosis, and prescriptions are recorded. This regime of accountability is as new as the clinics themselves, and not unrelated. Gyatso and Tenzin's father never kept such records as he traveled from neighbor to neighbor and received patients in his home. He had no clinic and no need for a written record of these therapeutic encounters. He was not accountable to foreign donors or to a nation-state. Now clinic records render the work of healing legible in new ways to people beyond this immediate social ecology. Reports generated from these logbooks can make the scope of *amchi* medicine visible to government functionaries—the district health officer, the Council on Technical Education and Vocational Training, the Department of Ayurveda at the Ministry of Health—and foreign donors. This information is intuitive for Gyatso and Tenzin, but not for their students. The data speak to a certain type of legitimacy upon which their reputations do not rest, but that will shape the trajectory of their pupils.

This record keeping is also part of Gyatso and Tenzin's hybrid pedagogy: part lineage-based local practice, part formalized institution. Senior students are required to spend time staffing the clinics. Logbooks hold them accountable to their own learning process and to patients because making records requires students to reflect, even briefly, on what they are diagnosing and prescribing. In addition, logbooks are windows onto which medicines are used most, what formulas need to be replenished, and what illnesses are most common in a given season. These rudimentary notes scribbled in Tibetan cursive with whatever writing implement happens to be nearby illustrate how Tibetan medicine is being made "legible" (Scott 1998) to the state and to nonstate actors like NGOs. The birth of the clinic, to invoke Michel Foucault (1973), marks the genesis of other shifts: new ways of relating to medicines and patients; new ways of experiencing the efficacy and the failures of *amchi* praxis; new ways of interpreting the science of healing.

Each year since the clinics opened, Gyatso or Tenzin have sent me copies of the logbooks or hand them to me in Kathmandu. With assistance from Lo Kunphen senior students and Dartmouth undergraduates, I have helped Gyatso and Tenzin transform these handwritten records into computer files capable of producing a new kind of authoritative knowledge: statistics. It is helpful to report that these clinics see an average of one thousand patient visits annually during the seven months their doors are open, and that this number has continued to rise each year since the clinics opened in 2004. Or that the median age of patients is forty-two, 46 percent of whom are male. Or that sandalwood- and saffron-based medicines are some of the most popularly prescribed, even though neither of these ingredients is local or affordable. Logbook analyses reveal that women suffer more from disorders of the channels *(tsa)* and of wind *(lung)*, and that men have more accidents.

And yet the more I delve into what these logbooks say, the more I notice what they do not say, or what they presume. What makes the prescription of an IV glucose drip the same general treatment category as golden needle acupuncture *(ser khab)?* Why does the arc of bile disorders peak in June? How do the graphic peaks and troughs of patients from across the border in Tibet reflect different local and regional geopolitics? Without having access to a great deal of information that exists outside the bounds of what these data reveal, the efficacy of the numbers themselves is limited. For example, I know that a Buddhist master came to Lo Monthang to give teachings in July 2007. There, graphically, is a spike in patients because his visit produced an upsurge in population; visitors from other parts of Nepal and the TAR sought out medical treatment while they camped out in Mustang, receiving teachings. Out-migration of young people for school or wage labor surfaces in the reality that the median age of patients is over forty. The lack of recorded women's diseases may speak to the ways male *amchi* have often distanced themselves from women's health. Alternately, women's disorders may be statistically hidden within other categories, such as blood and wind disorders.

There is a knock on the door. Normally this clinic is open only three days a week, staffed by a Lo Kunphen student who is also preparing for his SLC at the nearby high school. But word travels quickly when a senior *amchi* is in town. A local woman, middle-aged and moon-faced, stands at the door. She wears a woolen embroidered skullcap typical of upper Mustang's women of an older generation. She complains of sore, swollen knees. She lifts her frock and hitches up her petticoats to reveal fleshy, puckered skin, in marked contrast to her sun- and wind-beaten hands and face. Her knees are visibly inflamed. Gyatso directs the woman inside. She sits on the bench.

Contrary to what one might assume, this medical encounter does not begin with initial questions. Gyatso knows this woman and has treated her for years. Instead much of the therapeutic encounter flows forth from touch. Gyatso places his fingers along the woman's radial arteries, the gold and turquoise ring he inherited from his father glinting in the light. Pulse reading completed, he looks in her eyes and examines her tongue. Gyatso says the woman has a blood-wind disorder along with some infection. From here, stories of suffering spill out. "These keep me awake," she says, pointing at her knees with a look of accusation and annoyance, as if they were a barking dog. The woman asks if the disease is *nyingba,* literally "old," or if it is *drakpo,* a word that approximates "hard" or "recalcitrant." Gyatso reassures her that these pains can be addressed. He gives her two weeks' worth of medications, wrapped in pages torn from an old student notebook.

"Avoid eating too much salt, but poultice your knees with *bultog,*" he says, referencing sodium bicarbonate harvested locally. This harsh, demanding place provides at once the grounds for so much suffering and also, bountifully, the possibility of antidote.

OF SKY AND SOIL: 4:00 P.M.

Our visit to the Thinker clinic complete, Gyatso makes a few house calls before we head back to Lo. Tenzin's horse flies. I balance in the thick steel stirrups, perched above the wooden frame of a saddle, cushioned by carpets. I am bathed in sand, wind, and dust.

We slow to a walk and dismount on the far side of the river that separates the walled city of Lo Monthang from territory beyond. Gyatso leads our sweat-soaked horses across a tawny stretch of land, down the well-worn switchback to the river's edge, where poplars grow. We are tired, horses and humans both. We could have used a rest, but our time together is limited and the day has begun to wane. Instead we head off to Lo Kunphen's medicinal plant cultivation grounds.

The experimental cultivation of high-altitude medicinal plants is a relatively new phenomena in Nepal and has been brought forth by push-pull factors. Some species are being overharvested, in part driven by increasing demand for raw materials to service commercial production of both Ayurvedic and Tibetan formulas, as you will see in more detail later in the book; this trend has also been linked to increasing market prices for certain ingredients (Saxer 2011). Yet many such plants require specific soil conditions in which to grow. Some fail to germinate. Sometimes it becomes difficult to reconcile use values and exchange values when considering the lifecycle of a plant.

Interestingly, much of the cultivation of Tibetan medicines—at times combined with species distribution mapping and in-situ conservation—is being carried out by *amchi* on the fringes of the booming Asian medicine industries in China and India, rather than as part of a strategy for growth within these industries themselves. A lot of this work has been funded by conservation NGOs and bilateral research or development organizations. This cultivation project in Mustang is being funded by a grant from the United Nations Global Environmental Facility Small Grants Program, for which I helped the HAA write the proposal.

As Gyatso and I head toward the cultivation plots, I consider a refrain I have heard from *amchi* in Nepal: "Without plants, we are nothing. Without plants, we have no medicine. And an *amchi* with no medicine is like a bird without wings." This metaphor shifts at times—a car without gas, a teacher without students, a meal without salt, a trader without goods—yet the meaning remains constant. Without these medicinal plants, the future of Sowa Rigpa is jeopardized.

Even so, Sowa Rigpa maintains a long history of regional substitutions, as you will see in later chapters. Patterns of substitution can depend on local availability, the purchasing power of an *amchi,* trade partnerships, the pharmacological needs of a patient, and more. Sowa Rigpa is quite literally grounded in the distinct environments in which it is practiced, in part because this science of healing allows for pharmacological flexibility. As I stare across this "plain of aspiration," as Lo Monthang translates from the Tibetan, in the rain shadow of Earth's greatest, youngest mountains, I'm reminded of how the power of this medicine emerges, at least in part, from the soil in which it grows. And yet the bulk of ingredients used in Sowa Rigpa formulas come from tropical and subtropical environments. Cross-cultural borrowing of healing knowledge and trade in *materia medica* has always been essential to this practice.

Gyatso and I hitch our horses beside the cultivation fields. I follow my friend along the raised perimeters of barley, sweet pea, and buckwheat fields toward a large plot of land rimmed by a wall of adobe brick and stone. As we walk Gyatso explains that the cultivation project is renting this land from a local family, one of many in Lo who, for reasons related to out-migration and the prohibitive cost of hired labor, are growing less food these days. Instead they are relying on purchased staples, many of them from China.

"We pay a lease of 200,000 rupees—[approximately $2,800] for the project for three years. We have 3,000 square meters of farmland and have not used all of it. In the future we could cultivate more," my friend explains. "Water can be a problem, though. And we need to have a path to market. This will get easier when the road really comes to upper Mustang. At present it is difficult to make a profit when the price of transportation to Jomsom remains so high. But in the future, I think there will be opportunities for common people to make money by growing medicinal plants instead of only peas and barley."

My friend has had preliminary discussions with representatives of the Ayurvedic giant Dabur, whose Nepali affiliates are growing plants in lower Mustang District, as in other parts of Nepal and India.[7] They suggested that farmers in Monthang produce *akar kara (Anacyclus pyrethrum)* on contract. The plant, harvested for its essential oils and used as an anti-inflammatory, stimulant, and aphrodisiac in Ayurveda, seems to grow well here. Gyatso is taken by this idea, but he is also skeptical that local farmers can produce sufficient quantity to meet Dabur's tonnage requirements. Economies of scale advise otherwise. This *amchi* waxes eloquent about the possibility of growing a more local, though commercially viable crop called *zimbu (Allium przewalskianum),* a wild chive that is a staple spice in *dal,* Nepali lentils. "With *zimbu,* we would not have to worry about not producing enough. Whatever is grown we could use and sell between Jomsom and Pokhara."

Gyatso's economics are lucid. As he fiddles with the lock on the gate, he calculates the cost of water rights and labor per square meter of land, the current market price for a kilo of barley versus a kilo of the three species of plants they are now growing and the cost of transport by horseback to the district headquarters in Jomsom, through middlemen, and then on to other markets. The profit margin is there, but barely.

Pema, a local farmer in his late fifties, meets us at the gate. He is the head gardener of these plots, a job for which this project pays him 6,000 rupees a month (about $80). Pema's plaid shirt peaks out from under a thin jacket, stained by soil and grease. His cream-colored woolen cap covers thinning braided hair, kept long. A small nugget of turquoise hangs from his left ear and a thin plate of gold across one of his front teeth furnishes the aging man a dignified look. Pema leads me through his domain.

Neat rows of *manu (Inula racemosa)* and *chumtsa (Rheum palmatum)* stretch across the cultivation grounds. The *manu* grows tall, its spindly petals reaching toward the sky, broad leaves open like arms. It will be a year before the plant is ready for harvest. To wait two more years would be ideal, but this is where the plant's trajectory and the need for project outputs diverge, and where maximum potency might be sacrificed for expedience. The next third of the plot is devoted to more vulnerable species: *honglen (Lagotis* spp.) and *tianku (Dracocephlum tanguticum). Tianku* huddles in small, thyme-colored bunches, close to the ground. Gyatso explains that this type of *tianku* is uniquely suited

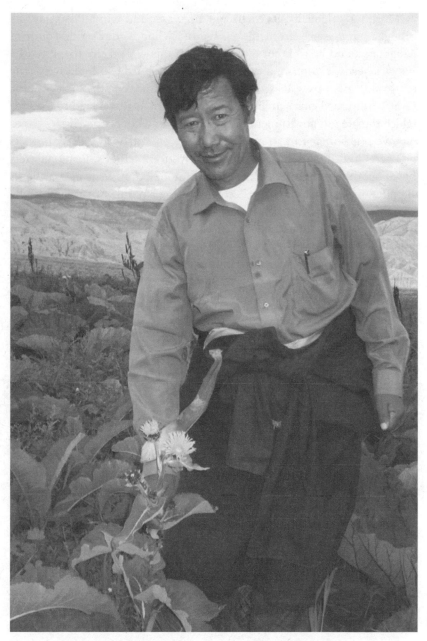

Amchi Gyatso Bista in the medicinal plant cultivation fields, Lo Monthang, Mustang District, Nepal, 2008. © Sienna Craig to Mustang's elements, its earth and air, water and wind. Pema says he brought *manu* seeds from the village of Geling, a day's ride south of Monthang, and he rode for a week west of this walled city to collect the *honglen* seeds. *Chumtsa,* a type of rhubarb, is sturdy and relatively easy to grow, Pema muses. Its seeds are resilient, adaptive in the high country. Gyatso admires Pema's ability to grow *honglen,* a threatened species for which the Nepali government has restricted wild collection.

"We use *honglen* in so many medicines," Gyatso says, describing its potencies and qualities. I ask about cultivation methods. Pema answers by complaining about wasted time and money that went into a workshop run by an NGO that has been cultivating a number of commercially valuable species in eastern Nepal. "They showed us how to make square plots, how to turn the soil and use compost, sand, and straw," he says. "But none of these methods worked for us here. I could have told him that they wouldn't, but we were supposed to try. I lost two months trying their techniques!" I ask more about why the methods failed. Gyatso and Pema offer an array of explanations: different soil quality, old seeds, temperatures that did not match in-situ conditions. Their answers also imply a critique of developmentalist assumptions about "replicability" (Sachs 1992). For all the good intentions that had gone into this workshop, the lofty goals of "capacity building" did not pan out.

Gyatso discusses *upal ngongbo* (*Meconopsis* spp.), the Himalayan blue poppy. "We have tried to get the plant to germinate," he says. "We collected seeds from up in the high pastures, north and west of Monthang, and planted them in our nursery. But the seeds become shy when they are taken down the mountain. Next year we will try again, also with *bongkar* [*Aconitum* spp.] and *pángtse* [*Pterocephalus hookeri*]. But this time we will make plots up in high pastures. Nomads watch sheep and yak. So why not have them watch plants?"

As I listen to Gyatso describe these plants that are difficult to cultivate, I am reminded that they are not only materials to use but also life forms to honor, things that by their very nature may defy cultivation, may resist scaling up. I also realize how much I do not know about this terra firma, the time it takes a plant to grow, the smells and tastes of medicine, at once bitter and sweet.

PRAYERS OF ASPIRATION: 8:00 P.M.

We leave the cultivation grounds. Horsetail clouds streak the sky, foretelling a day of rain. Gyatso and I walk slowly, clockwise as is expected, around the perimeter of the wall and back toward Lo Kunphen, horses in tow. We listen to the sounds of early evening in Mustang. Pressure cookers release steam. Donkeys bray. Children play hide-and-seek around rows of *chöten*. Tired-looking men and women return from harvest. Static-filled murmurs from satellite televisions diffuse into the cool air from the dark interiors of Monthang's few taverns.

Horses unsaddled and fed, we collapse on the same divans where we began this day. The room is bustling again. Gyatso's sister is cooking dinner. Tenzin arrives after his day of ritual attendance. Their mother orders her grandniece to give us tea and popcorn. There is not much left to do except to eat and rest, and we dive into both. I reach for more popcorn. Gyatso lets his chin droop to his chest. His eyes close. I watch him sink into sleep, letting the exhaustion of this man's life give way to a certain childlike surrender.

Then Tenzin sits down beside me with his laptop, fully charged. This is the problem of working with brothers. When one is resting, the other is ready to work. We have been discussing plans for Tenzin to visit the United States to fundraise for Lo Kunphen and see relatives in New York. I arranged a similar tour for Gyatso in 2003. The brothers alternate when it comes to foreign excursions; now it is Tenzin's turn. Tenzin's computer boots up. He loads a PowerPoint presentation, a process he has mastered, even though he speaks and reads virtually no English. As I wait for images to appear, I think of all the places these brothers have been: India, China, Bhutan, the United States, Britain, Germany, Japan, France, and Russia, including a stint as the resident doctors at a clinic in Tatarstan. This is difficult to square against the fact that about half of my own fellow U.S. citizens do not own a passport. In this sense "modernity" becomes a way of being in the world that lives within people who, according to stereotype, might seem the epitome of "traditional": a middle-aged monk with dirty robes and dirty hands, here on the edge of the world. In this sense Gyatso and Tenzin's life, and lifework, illustrate Bruce Knauft's (2001) point that there are many ways of being modern in the world today. To deny the complex local-global realities of people like these *amchi* is to silence key ways that ideologies and socioeconomic influences circulate and shape contemporary life, from the power to buy things to the power to represent oneself on a national or global stage.

"Sienna *la*," Tenzin says, with excitement, "let me show you pictures from England." Tenzin spent some time in the United Kingdom earlier this year and had occasion to lecture on the history of Mustang and the future of *amchi* practice at Oxford's Oriental Institute and the Wellcome

Trust for the History of Medicine in London. He had also been blessed by an audience with His Holiness the Dalai Lama. He describes his visit, aided by the digital images he took along the way. Tenzin in front of the Bodleian's ornate dome: "This library was built in the seventeenth century," he tells me, "when Mustang was also a great place." The next picture reveals Tenzin and Mingkyi, a person you will meet in chapter 3. This woman from Tibet is a Sowa Rigpa practitioner with whom I worked in Lhasa and to whom I introduced Tenzin some years ago. They smile beside the entrance to the Pitt Rivers Museum. "Did you know there are whole suits of armor inside?" Tenzin asks. This monk is most impressed by the material history of war and conquest. He advances through a series of images with His Holiness, resting on one of him bowed before the man Tibetans can refer to, profoundly, simply, as "Presence."

I ask him about this gift of time with the Dalai Lama. "I requested his advice about our school. How to move forward, what to do about the problems we face, how to keep working toward our goals," he answers.

"What did His Holiness say?"

Tenzin's reply turns toward prayer. He chants a long, low supplication. Is this Tenzin's answer to my question or His Holiness's answer to Tenzin? Really, both are true. After the prayer Tenzin tells me the advice the Dalai Lama bestowed on him: *Keep working with a pure heart. Keep making connections around the world. Keep finding points of shared interest and collaboration with other amchi. The path forward will reveal itself through this process.* The Dalai Lama then handed Tenzin several packets of *jinden,* ritually consecrated pills made each year in Dharamsala. Medicine from blessing born. This too is efficacious practice.

SUMMARY

This chapter illustrated how Sowa Rigpa operates in a rural community, in a particular social ecological context in Nepal. In spending time with Gyatso and Tenzin, you have come to see how Tibetan medicine fits into the subsistence lifestyles of Mustangi residents, but also how these remote people and places are connected to regional and global ideas, practices, goods, services, and values. You've seen the ways that one-dimensional descriptors such as "traditional" and "modern" are inadequate to understand the realities in which today's practitioners of Sowa Rigpa live and work.

This chapter has also given you a sense of the structural parameters—economic, cultural, political, geographic—that at once constrain and make meaningful the practice of Tibetan medicine locally. You've seen the ways that Sowa Rigpa operates within and beyond specific nation-states, languages, and cultures, and how this complicates the question of how best to train new generations of *amchi*. You've also seen some of the ways that competing, conflicting, or simply nontranslatable ideas are played out between the life of a local institution and the development and maintenance of an international network of support for that institution.

In the next chapter we scale up and move locations: from a small practice in the mountains of Nepal to a large, formalized institution in Qinghai Province, China.

CHAPTER 2

The Pulse of an Institution

This is not the way the world is. It is a possibility nonetheless
deeply seeded within the world. It is the way the world is
sometimes.

—Wendell Berry, *Leavings: Poems*

READING SIGNS REDUX

On an early morning in July 2010, I walk down a boulevard in Xining,
the capital of Qinghai Province, China. High-altitude sun inches over
the city. I pass high-rise apartment buildings and offices, some draped
in scaffolding. This is a city on the rise, a metropolis of more than two
million people on China's western frontier, in a region Tibetans call
Amdo. The hospital sits in a bustling, Muslim-dominated corner of this
city. Bakers wearing white cotton caps knead dough into leavened
disks. Butchers arrange slabs of pork and yak meat beside whirring
fans. Car repair stores are wedged beside noodles shops and China Mobile kiosks. A blue-and-white street sign comes into view. I do not read
Chinese, but Pinyin alerts me that I am approaching the Qinghai Zang Yi
Yuan, the Qinghai Tibetan Medical Hospital. *Zang yi,* the medicine of
Tibet, or Xizang, as it is called in Mandarin, fits within the general category of *yi,* a Chinese word for "medicine." *Zhong yi,* the phrase used to
describe Chinese medicine, literally means "medicine of the Middle Kingdom," itself a gloss for diverse currents of tradition (Scheid 2007) in
Chinese approaches to healing. Notably, *Zhong yi* contains no ethnic
master. It is the unnamed norm, connoting Han majority.

Chinese gives way to Tibetan on the sign marking the hospital's entrance. *Tso Ngon Zhing Bö Menkhang.*[1] Literally, "Blue Lake Province
House of Tibetan Medicine." Tibetans often refer to Qinghai Province as

Tso Ngon, after the blue lake whose waters have attracted visitors for centuries, from the courts of the Chinese emperors to the Mongolian khans, who called the expansive body of water Kokonor. Today Qinghai Lake attracts many tourists: it has even become a destination for weddings, music videos, and high-altitude bicycle rides. To those from Amdo, Tso Ngon marks cultural identity as much as geography. The term used on this sign to indicate Tibetan medicine is *bö menkhang*. *Bö* is what Tibetans call their world, a place that extends far beyond Qinghai but is inclusive of it. Ethnographers and historians refer to this as "ethnographic Tibet," inclusive of areas in the TAR and parts of Yunnan, Qinghai, Gansu, and Sichuan provinces, as opposed to "political Tibet," which has been delimited around the TAR only (Goldstein 1997).

As I walk in through the gates of the hospital, another Tibetan word comes to mind: *dzong*. These are citadels or fortresses that once marked sites of Tibetan imperial strength and regional authority. In Tibetan regions of China today, *dzong* has come to signify county-level government administration, while *chen* marks provinces and *zhing* indicates a prefecture's center, and *xian* indicates a county. Not far from the hospital are remnants of the adobe wall that once surrounded the *dzong* of Siling, as Xining is known in Tibetan.

Although not on the hospital's entrance sign, the word *dzong* feels appropriate for this medical compound. The inpatient wing has a looming staircase leading up to a structure designed with tapered walls, a signature of Tibetan architecture dating to the Tibetan Empire (seventh–ninth century C.E.) that was perfected in Lhasa's Potala Palace.[2] Here the *dzong*-shaped hospital represents another type of empire: the Arura Tibetan Medical Group, one of China's largest Tibetan medical enterprises. This group includes the Qinghai Tibetan Medical Hospital and Research Institute, as well as Qinghai's Tibetan Medical College, a Tibetan Medical Cultural Museum, and Arura Tibetan Medicine Co., Ltd. The Research Institute performs laboratory and clinical research on Tibetan formulas, publishes a journal, and is a repository for hundreds of extant Tibetan medical texts that a team of Sowa Rigpa experts from across China spent more than two decades amassing. These works are now being digitized, reprinted, and made accessible to new generations of practitioners and scholars.

Off-site, at the Qinghai Biotech Zone on the outskirts of Xining, the Arura Tibetan Medicine Co., Ltd. operates a for-profit pharmaceutical factory. The impressive museum is located nearby. As of 2006 the pharmaceutical company had assets totaling more than 500 million renminbi

($62.5 million), a net worth that continues to expand.[3] The cultural museum cost 120 million renminbi ($17.7 million) to build and covers 12,000 square meters, approximately double the cost of Arura's new GMP factory (*China Daily* 2006; Saxer 2010a: 215). In 2010 more than 100,000 visitors came to the museum, most Chinese,[4] and the institution has caught the attention of the Chinese press (China Tibet Information Center 2006a, 2006d, 2008a in Saxer 2010a). The museum houses a permanent collection of *materia medica*, more than 1,300 medical implements, and a full set of medical *thanka*, reproductions of the original scroll paintings commissioned in the seventeenth century by Desi Sangye Gyatso, regent of the "Great Fifth" Dalai Lama and a key figure in the history of Sowa Rigpa, to illustrate his medical text, *The Blue Beryl*. The museum also houses the longest Tibetan painting in the world, a maze of a canvas measuring more than 600 meters and depicting a history of Tibetan civilization. The Arura Group also supports the Tibetan Medical College of Qinghai University.[5]

Arura's chief executive, Dr. Ao Tsochen, is a Tibetan social entrepreneur and high-ranking official who has sought to promote quality Tibetan medical care and support Tibetan science and culture. His endeavors have garnered interest and market-based respect from China's governmental and private-sector elite. Points of compromise have undoubtedly marked the building of this institution, but so has foresight. Arura's pharmaceutical factory produces more than seventy-five commercial Tibetan medical products that hold national patents, twelve of which are classified as "nationally protected traditional Chinese medicines." Arura does not market its commercial medicines internationally, although future expansion to non-Chinese markets is a possibility.

When I first learned about Arura, I was tempted to "read" this institution as a preeminent example of the commodification of Tibetan culture and nature through the industrial production of medicines. Yet the strategic decisions Dr. Tsochen and others have made in structuring the Arura Group's multiple modes of activity defy such a simple reading. Certainly the company is a for-profit venture. It is invested in the melding of "cultural preservation" with economic development and, as such, is implicated in some of the paradoxes this implies. Yet Arura continues to creatively engage in a complex effort to at once legitimate and transform Sowa Rigpa today.

As we will see in chapter 5, the group navigates between national regimes of governance dictating how Tibetan medicines should be produced and the mandates of Tibetan medical theory and pharmacology, incorporating aspects of Sowa Rigpa unique to Amdo, eastern Tibet. While a certain vision of exoticized Tibetanness pervades aspects of its advertising campaigns, profits generated from Arura's high-end commercial products are funneled back into the hospital, which provides health care at affordable prices to thousands of patients each year. Furthermore the Group supports student scholarships, teacher salaries, and research at the medical college. Approximately three hundred people work at the hospital, and more than 1,500 students have graduated over the past decade from the medical college. As such, the Arura Group is a major employer of Tibetans in the region, a place where Tibetan language and cultural sensibilities are overtly valued and Tibetans earn a living wage during a time when interurban and urban-rural inequality between Tibetans and the Han majority continues to rise (Fischer 2005, 2008a). As the term *dzong* implies, Arura is a place of power and authority. It is also a place of strategic innovation.

MORNING RUSH: 9:00 A.M.

The lawn beside the outpatient building is already crowded with a multiethnic array of patients and their families: Tibetans, Uighurs, Hui and Salar Muslims, and Han. Some linger on the lawn, eating picnic breakfasts. Others walk slowly toward the patient wards. Nurses, doctors, and other workers arrive in street clothes, chatting on their cell phones before the morning rush begins.

Drolma, my research assistant, is a master's-degree student at Qinghai's Tibetan Medical College. Round-faced and affable, she meets me in the courtyard. "Demo," she calls, in Amdo greeting. We head toward the office of Dr. Namlha Khr. This Tibetan doctor specializes in gastrointestinal disorders and internal medicine, spending most of his time in the outpatient wards. He hails from Repgong (Ch. Tongren), a county known for its religious and medical institutions. Like Gyatso and Tenzin in Mustang, Dr. Namlha's father was a *nakpa,* a tantric householder priest. Unlike the doctors from Nepal, Dr. Namlha studied Tibetan medicine at the Repgong Health School, a county-level state institution that opened during China's Reform Era and served as a technical training school, within which medicine was one of several vocational tracks offered.

Drolma and I walk through the bustling entry hall of the outpatient unit, past the pharmacy, up to the second floor. The hospital has not been open thirty minutes, but this being a Monday, the place is already busy. We slip through the door and greet the doctor. He smiles, indicates that we can observe quietly, and suggests we sit on the stretcher along the wall. He returns to reading the pulse of a young man from Yushu Prefecture, a region of Qinghai that was devastated by an earthquake in April of this year (2010). I listen carefully to this still unfamiliar Amdo Tibetan dialect. Drolma whispers translations as the patient recounts his symptoms.

"I have stomach problems," the patient begins. "There is a lot of pain, especially when I eat. My urine is very yellow." The doctor presses firmly his right and left wrists. Dr. Namlha then looks at the man's complexion, examines his tongue.

"Will you take lab tests?" he asks. "Do you have funds for this?" The patient nods yes. "I think you have a gastric ulcer. This is a serious problem, but there is medicine to help."

"I am also worried about my lungs," the patient continues.

"There are no problems in your lungs," answers Dr. Namlha authoritatively. "The problems are in your liver, gall bladder, kidney, and stomach." The patient says he had been diagnosed some years earlier with a disorder that causes his liver to, as he put it, "shrink and become hard." He fears cancer. The doctor, firm but kind, reasserts the need for laboratory tests. Then he will prescribe medicines.

Two junior physicians assist Dr. Namlha. One reaches out to practice reading the patient's pulse, an act the patient hardly seems to notice. The other enters information about diagnosis and lab tests into the computer.

Two brothers and their father enter next. Both sons are in their early twenties. One is a monk.

"I have pain on this side," the lay brother begins as Dr. Namlha reads his pulse. The patient's father adds, "His stomach is swollen and has noises in it. After he eats cold food or drinks anything, the pain gets worse. He has not taken any tests, just some medicines from the local Tibetan hospital in our county."

Dr. Namlha listens more to the pulse than to the words of his patients, it seems, concentrating through his fingers, through touch. "The problem is in the intestine and stomach. You are not to eat cold, raw foods. I will give you a prescription now, to fill at the pharmacy. You are lucky! This is not serious. Your medicine will be cheap."

The monk sibling moves into the patient chair. Dressed in robes, he looks sunken, sallow. His kidneys hurt. His spine aches. The monk's father speaks these symptoms for him.

"I would like to be an inpatient," the monk says. "I would like tests. I need rest. If I am just an outpatient I will not be able to rest. I have applied for permission to be an inpatient from my monastery." *Permission to be sick,* I scribble in my field notebook. The monk reaches in to the folds of his robe and produces his government-issued medical insurance booklet. Dr. Namlha hands this bit of bureaucracy to his assistants and turns to the patient.

"The cause of the problem is not serious, but the outcome will depend on how you deal with the problems. I will see what I can do. Go to the inpatient ward." It may just be my rudimentary understanding of Amdo dialect, but Dr. Namlha's response, indeed the entire discussion with this patient, seems somewhat cryptic. I wonder if this monk has been involved in political unrest in the region, if he is using what medical sociologist Talcott Parsons (1964) called "the sick role" as a way of seeking political refuge. The monk's home region has been a hotbed of political unrest and state repression since 2008. Parsons' functionalist theory states that a sick person is exempt from normal social roles, that he is not responsible for his state, and that he has an obligation to try to get well. The "sick role" concept has been critiqued from many perspectives, mostly because it does not allow for sufficient balance between what an individual controls during an illness and the structural parameters in which sickness occurs. Yet as this monk speaks with Dr. Namlha, I can imagine him entering a space of "sanctioned deviance," in Parsons' terms—the hospital—as a way of removing himself from another context in which he might be politically suspect.

Another patient comes in waving lab results. He addresses the doctor. "The tests say I have hepatitis B and other liver problems, so I have to be admitted. Where should I go?" This is the first such interruption we witness, but the stream of patients is unrelenting. One of Dr. Namlha's assistants advises this person.

"We have another sick family member," interjects the father of the monk. "My mother has a liver parasite that was cured, but now her spine, which is normally straight, is curved."

Drolma leans over and whispers to me, in English, "This is very common practice. People come in for one problem, but they go home with medicines for everyone. This doctor, he has very good facility for making patients easy," I nod, charmed by her English usage as much as by her openness. As medical anthropologists at McGill University (Groleau et al. 2006) have noted, medical events can produce "chain complexes":

experiences of suffering that may be unrelated from a biological point of view but that exist for patients as a series of interconnected events wherein correlation morphs into a causal link between one health problem and another, or between a health problem and a life event that is pivotal for making sense of an illness.

A forty-eight-year-old Han woman enters next. Her slightly distended stomach pushes against her patterned polyester blouse, buttons misaligned. Her pants are frayed at the cuff. She looks poor.

"If my stomach is empty, it hurts. When I feel hungry, my stomach gets hard, like a stone." The patient hands Dr. Namlha a set of ultrasound images taken at another hospital. "I also feel acid in my throat and have headaches," she continues.

"Gall bladder," answers Dr. Namlha. "You are developing gallstones. You need to change your diet." The doctor instructs her to abstain from spicy food, including garlic and chilies. He writes prescriptions.

"Will you add some medicines to protect my liver?" the patient asks. The doctor asks the patient how much money she has brought along. As an answer, she pulls out one crisp 100-yuan note ($13). Dr. Namlha scribbles the names of medicines on his prescription pad. Drolma explains that sometimes doctors will ask patients to come back with enough money so they can actually prescribe good medicines, but when a doctor knows someone is poor, he adjusts the prescription accordingly. It is a delicate balance between providing quality care and, as Drolma puts it, "not making hardship" for people. The cost of medical care at this hospital is below the rates at Xining's biomedical facilities, where seeing a doctor might cost only 12 yuan, but laboratory tests and pharmaceuticals can cost patients thousands. Still, even here prescriptions add up.

A Tibetan woman enters with her seventeen-year-old daughter in tow. The mother does all the talking. "This girl has no appetite. She says her stomach hurts. When her stomach is empty she has pain." Dr. Namlha reads the young woman's pulse.

"Her problem is not serious. She has just been eating foods that do not agree with her. We need to increase her digestive heat."

"Don't we need machine tests?" asks the mother, anxious.

"No testing is needed. It is a simple problem."

"I would like her to have machine tests. She is preparing for college entrance exams. We do not want any worry. Can we see the inside of her stomach and her back?"

The doctor pauses, sighs, submits: "Okay, if you would like testing, I can order. But it is not necessary. I will give you a prescription."

"Thank you," says the mother. The daughter, still not having said a word, follows her mother out of the room. Drolma nudges me, "All mothers are the same—worried!" As a mother myself, I am sympathetic. As a medical anthropologist, though, I note the desire for technoscientific "proof" of a problem and the irresistible draw of accessing the interior world of the body not through listening and palpation but through concrete images (Adams 2002a; Adams and Li 2008). For the mother, efficacious practice requires this way of seeing. She will spare no expense, even though the doctor tells her that additional testing is unnecessary. In the end he acquiesces, making money for the hospital in the process.

The young man from Yushu returns, bearing an ultrasound. "They say I have an ulcer. I would also like to have a liver function test, to see if I have hepatitis."

"This is a good idea," concurs the doctor.

Drolma is serious. "I have seen cases like this before. He probably does have hepatitis B, along with his ulcer. This man is not well. He has lost many family members in the earthquake too. It is so sad," she says.

The poor Chinese woman returns, agitated. "I got the medicines," she tells Dr. Namlha, "but the notes on the bottle for one of them says things I do not like. Do I have to take this to have a good result?"

"Yes. You need to follow directions. Medicine is not like a banquet, where you get to choose what to eat," says Dr. Namlha, jovial but firm.

Drolma notes, "The hospital pharmacy must write all effects and problems that can happen with any medicines, even if it is very rare. Sometimes this makes people feel uneasy." This woman's sensibility about what we've learned to call "side effects" (Etkin 1992) is quite different from that of a pharmacy beholden to drug manufacturing requirements or concepts of risk and safety derived from bioethical paradigms and social ecologies that originated far away from this hospital in Qinghai.

In walks a Muslim couple. They speak flawless Amdo Tibetan, the dialect native to Dr. Namlha's hometown. Although significant Buddhist-Muslim tensions have existed in this region for years (Fischer 2008b), as I watch this elderly Hui couple and the doctor interact, the distance between them seems small. The woman suffers from chronic diarrhea.

Her husband explains that she has been to a TCM hospital in Sichuan Province. The problem resolved for some months but has now recurred. She also has gallstones, but she has not had an operation. The procedure is beyond their means, and she feels uncomfortable with the idea of surgery.

"We have heard Tibetan medicine is good to dissolve stones so you do not need to cut your body open," says the husband.

"Have you taken Tibetan medicines in the past?" Dr. Namlha asks.

"Yes, from the county hospital. They helped, but people say that medicines from this hospital are more powerful and doctors more knowledgeable," the husband continues, echoing a popular sentiment.

"What happens when you eat meat?"

"It is painful. I cannot control my bowels," answers the patient.

"Would it be good for her to eat snake meat?" interjects her husband.

Dr. Namlha seems surprised by this question. "I do not know of that remedy."

"Someone from our village had the same problem. After he ate snake meat he was cured." Dr. Namlha instructs the woman not to eat foods that are cold in nature, and meat. Here the doctor's orders do not refer to *nyépa* or other aspects of medical theory but rather a model of folk dietetics (Nichter 2008) that draws on hot-cold distinctions and injunctions that are easy to follow.

The husband turns to me. "What country are you from?" I answer that I'm from Ari, the standard Tibetan word for "America," which produces a puzzled look. "Mei guo," I then say, using the Chinese term. He flashes in recognition. "In your country, the leader George Bush was not kind to my people," he says, referring to Muslims, of course, not to Chinese. I reveal my left-leaning politics and the man gives me a thumbs-up sign before ushering his wife out the door. His comments remind me of another way of conceiving of social ecology, a world wherein religious belonging trumps national borders or ethnic sentiment, even though there is much that is distinctly Chinese, even distinctly *Tibetan*, about this couple.

In observing this morning of clinical encounters, I acknowledge the lack of privacy afforded patients here—standard practice in so much of the world outside Euro-American contexts. The diversity of patients is also notable, as well as how far some people have traveled to seek care. What holds my attention, though, is the sense that efficacious practice unfolds through negotiations between doctor and patient, against a backdrop of economic, cultural, and technoscientific possibility and constraint.

GOOD CLINICAL PRACTICE: 12:00 P.M.

After several hours with Dr. Namlha, Drolma and I are ready for a break. We've planned to meet Wangmo,[6] the head of the Good Clinical Practices (GCP) Division of Arura's research institute. GCP are regulations that state health services and international agencies use to govern clinical care. They are inclusive of bioethical standards regarding how clinical research should be conducted and define the roles and responsibilities of trial sponsors, investigators, and monitors. As a unit of social analysis and a tool for social regulation in medical settings, GCP draw links between clinical care, the business of medicine, and the global pharmaceutical industry, illustrating aspects of what Petryna and Kleinman (2006) call the "pharmaceutical nexus." This hospital is the only one in Qinghai with GCP status.

Wangmo meets us outside the pharmacy, looking somewhat flustered, clutching her cell phone. As we make introductions, her phone begins playing "When the Saints Come Marching In." She glances at the caller ID.

"*Excuse me,*" she says in English. "*Must take call.*" Wangmo looks to be in her midthirties. She speaks commanding, rapid Chinese into the phone. "*Sometimes there is too much work,*" she apologizes as she hangs up. Drolma threads her arm through Wangmo's and leads us down the hospital's driveway. We settle on a Sichuan-style restaurant beside the hospital and ask for a quiet table. Drolma orders spicy tofu, sautéed bok choy, and hot peppers with beef while Wangmo and I talk. Like nearly every such encounter I've had while doing research in China, she has already been briefed about me, but I tell her about my interest in clinical research on Tibetan medicine and the previous work I've done in the TAR.

We talk about the clinical research project with which I was involved in Lhasa, as you will read about in chapter 7. Wangmo is particularly interested in the ways we dealt with challenges related to informed consent, a standard of bioethics that requires researchers to explain the goals, risks, and benefits of research to potential subjects, to ensure patient confidentiality, and to let potential study participants know that they can withdraw from the study at any time without penalty. Such procedures often require subjects to sign a written consent form. But this act of signing a paper—and the entire informed consent process, in some ways—presents particular challenges in cross-cultural contexts, and also among populations who may not be literate (see Marshall

2007). This well-intentioned request is laden with cultural assumptions about ethical behavior and free will, as well as individual versus socio-centric ideas of the person and issues related to the dynamics of medical authority. While informed consent has become a globalized concept, and a lynchpin in the outsourcing of human subjects research, it is a powerful example of the uneven effects of globalization and the challenges of translating science across cultures, wherein the cultural norms behind the concept of bioethics are rarely challenged or analyzed (Fox and Swazy 2008).

"Informed consent is very important," says Wangmo, "but sometimes it is difficult to explain research. People get scared by being told all the things that can go wrong, and then they refuse to be in the trial." In Lhasa we spent a year creating an informed consent process (Adams et al. 2007; Miller et al. 2007a).

After a time I change the subject. "What units in Arura's hospital conduct clinical research?"

Wangmo unfolds her starched napkin, splits and files her chopsticks. "Three of our departments can do clinical research. Liver and gall bladder, heart diseases—*cardiology*—and herbal baths. That one is mostly for *osteoarthritis,*" she explains. The research institute has applied for permission to conduct clinical trials in five additional departments: skin disorders and dermatology, gynecology, gastroenterology and digestive disorders, internal medicine, and kidney disorders. The boundaries between Tibetan and biomedical understandings of physiology, anatomy, and etiology are fluid here, indicating that acts of translation are crucial to producing ideas of efficacious practice (Prost 2006; Czaja 2010; Gerke 2010). The work of healing is described in Tibetan, but the object of clinical inquiry is defined in biomedical terms. Spaces of incommensurability (Kuhn [1962] 1996; Pigg 2001) remain, sometimes revealed in hospital signage. One department is called, in English, "gastroenterology," but in Tibetan it is defined with reference to specific organs: the stomach and intestines. At other times Tibetan medical theory emerges as the organizing principle for hospital-based divisions, such that liver and gall bladder disorders have their own departments. "Internal medicine" is a catchall phrase for a department populated by senior doctors who may refuse biomedically oriented specialist designations.

"Are the clinical trials you conduct all for Tibetan medicines?" I ask.

"No," Wangmo answers. "Most trials have been for Western medicines or for TCM products." Her job extends well beyond this hospital.

Biomedical and TCM pharmaceutical companies and other hospitals hire her research unit to coordinate clinical research on their behalf. This generates revenue and prestige for Arura and the hospital. Even though Tibetan medicine has not (yet) been subject to the types of dynamics that characterize Big Pharma (Law 2006), wherein transnational pharmaceutical companies come to have direct impacts on the local cost of care, such connections do have parallels to the relationship between contract-based research, pharmaceutical companies' market interests, and the production of medical evidence (Healey 2006; Petryna 2009).

"We have an ethics committee," Wangmo goes on, hands wrapped around a cup of tea. "When a company approaches us about doing an RCT, we organize other hospitals in Xining to collect data. For example, if we need a hundred patients, we might only be able to recruit fifty from our hospital. If it is a Western or Chinese medicine we do not use, then the other hospital's ethics committee looks at protocol. If they agree it is okay, then we recruit patients at their hospital."

"Who designs the studies?"

"Sometimes company scientists have ideas about this, but mostly we design studies based on the type of government approval needed for a new medicine or product. We must follow GCP. This helps us know if we should do *one-arm* or *two-arm* study, and about placebos, blinding, randomization. Following international rules, we use *double blind* for new medicines. If it is a test of an older medicine—many Tibetan medicines are included here—these are different rules." Drolma struggles to translate this technical language, but Wangmo and I share a vocabulary for clinical research, which helps.

"No wonder your phone rings all the time!" I offer lightly. "You have much responsibility."

Wangmo smiles. "Sometimes it is difficult. Not many people know how to really do good clinical research. We have to teach many things. Sometimes people do not want to listen. They just want the certificates and good study results, even if their medicine is very similar to something that already has government approval."

I share with Wangmo the phrase "me-too drugs," medicines that are nearly identical to those that already exist on the market but that are clinically compared with placebos rather than existing formulas in RCTs. This is one way the pharmaceutical industry makes a profit. I tell Wangmo as best I can through translation about Adriana Petryna's (2009) ethnography of contract research organizations and how they figure into the globalization of human subjects, the commoditization of clinical trials, and the intermingling of market-based interests and medical practice.

"We have these problems in China too," she responds. "People thinking more about profit than about making good medicine. In our research unit we try to do our best, but sometimes doing clinical research makes *stress*." Wangmo tells me that a trial they oversaw this year for a TCM formula had very poor clinical efficacy, which they reported. The company that sponsored the trial was not pleased. They tried to dismiss the results, not on account of scientific process but by stirring up cultural biases. Tibetan medicine was inferior to TCM and biomedicine, unscientific, they argued, so how could a Tibetan medical institute run a good clinical trial? They said these things even though Tibetan medicine had nothing to do with the trial, and those like Wangmo were trained in biomedical sciences and conducted the trial at a TCM hospital.

"You have done some clinical trials of Tibetan medicines in this hospital, right?" I ask.

"Yes, but only with medicines used in this hospital, mostly old recipes." The hospital research institute conducted two RCTs between 2005 and 2008. One focused on *zhijé* 6, a medicine used for digestive disorders that is akin to the study drug described in chapter 7. The other focused on *samphel norbu,* a class of Tibetan "precious pill" *(rinchen rilbu).* This work predated Wangmo's time as GCP director.

"The problem of doing research on Tibetan medicine is that in our system, we follow the *Fourfold Treatise,* we look at a medicine's *nüpa,* its potency. We know medicines are effective, but we do not have good methods to measure how and why of measurement—to support an understanding of how and why the medicine works."

This comment cuts to the core of a central argument in this book. The standards by which Tibetan medicines are evaluated are often constrained when positioned within evaluative models that do not necessarily account for Tibetan medical theory or production practices. As we will see in chapter 5, sometimes such practices need not be incommensurate but instead exist side by side. People involved in this work have a desire—and feel the need—to translate their scientific principles, putting them into dialogue with biomedical ideas. Yet translating Tibetan notions of safety and efficacy, including the balance of the *nyépa* and five elements *(jungwa nga),* into the vocabularies of biomedical mechanisms and biochemical compounds remains difficult. Parallel types of translations occur quite often in clinical practice, so often that they can even go unnoted. In the formalized settings of clinical research, however, the stakes are higher and more clearly articulated around standardized outcome measures.

"There are problems about how to understand results," Wangmo continues. "There are also clinical problems. Tibetan medicine has many different ways to diagnose, many ingredients in our medicines. If we begin with a Western medical disease name, but we want to treat with Tibetan medicine only, this is one problem."

In response I mention Whole Systems Research (WSR), an innovative suite of methodologies that allows for diversity of diagnosis categories and complex treatment interventions in clinical research, and that is becoming popular as a method of evaluating both CAM and conventional biomedicine in Euro-American contexts (Ritenbaugh et al. 2003; Institute of Medicine 2005; Verhoef et al. 2005). WSR aims to reimagine the structure, purpose, design, and analytical tools used for clinical medical research. Its premise is that medical research can more effectively bridge the gap between efficacy as defined clinically and the social, medical, and biological interactions that can render a health intervention effective. In some ways WSR is a reaction to the narrowly defined "gold standard" of the Randomized Controlled Trial (RCT) (Kaptchuk 1998, 2001), which is really most appropriate for testing drugs aimed at mass prescription in hospital settings. WSR is a mosaic of approaches rather than one streamlined "method." The brilliance of WSR is that it begins with the premise that much clinical medicine, whether conventional or CAM in orientation, must be considered more holistically than is possible within the constraints of a traditional RCT. WSR emphasizes treating patients over treating patient *groups*. WSR researchers consider the relationship between patients and their providers an important component of understanding clinical outcomes. Its proponents also argue that biomedical systems are *by their very nature* dynamic and should be treated as such in research design. It values both qualitative and quantitative methods. For these and other reasons, it seems an appropriate possibility to explore in the context of Tibetan medicine.

"I would like to learn more about this, and also research ethics." We brainstorm about planning a WSR workshop together at Arura. While we both understand that such novel approaches will not resolve all points of incommensurability in the confluence of these currents of tradition, it might be a start—a way to further examine what it means to say that Tibetan medicine works.

We wrap up the remains of lunch, scuffle over who will pay the bill, and head back to the hospital.

SEASON, SOAKS, AND SICKNESS: 2:00 P.M.

As Drolma and I walk into the medicinal baths division of the hospital, the moist, pungent smell of steeping herbs wafts over us. The building is oriented around on a high-ceilinged rotunda threaded with an elaborate network of pipes. A digital display hangs above the nurses' station, informing workers about which patient rooms are filled. Medicinal baths and their more naturalistic equivalent, medicinal hot springs, are part of Sowa Rigpa's repertoire of external therapies. I've noticed that medicinal baths are not as popular in central and western Tibet as they are in the east. The medicinal baths department at this hospital attracts patients from around the world.

Dr. Ma greets us on the second floor. He is tall, with long, delicate fingers and a full head of graying hair. Dr. Ma is a Tibetan Muslim who ran this division until last year. He resigned, Drolma explains, "because he wanted to see patients." The demands of administration left him with limited time for clinical practice.

"How old are most of the patients you see in this division?" I ask. "Are there more women or men? What are the most common conditions you treat with medicinal baths?" The physician says the most common ailments treated by medicinal baths are *drumbu,* a type of joint disorder often equated with rheumatoid arthritis; *khäldram,* a kidney-related disorder connected to lower back pain; *lung* and *tsa* disorders, imbalances related to wind, circulation, and neurological problems; and noncommunicable skin diseases.

"Most people who come here are about fifty years old. Herbal baths are not for everyone," answers Dr. Ma. "Very old people cannot tolerate such heat. The baths can be forty degrees centigrade, sometimes hotter. If you are old, the heat can make a disease stronger. Also those with fevers of the lungs, infections, or heart problems should not use baths."

Dr. Ma explains that this treatment is seasonal. They close the department during the hottest months of summer and are very busy all winter. "If you came to talk with me when the snows are on the mountains, I would not have time!" In winter they treat many chronic diseases because "in winter energy stays in the body and it is easier to treat, but in spring and summer energy is released from the body and treating old problems is more difficult," he says. The doctor also explains that they treat more patients in the morning than in the afternoon. Therapy varies not only by season but also by time of day. Timing is paramount: what might be a beneficial treatment at one time in the year or day can be iatrogenic at others. Here too we see how social ecologies influence efficacy.

Dr. Ma leads us to a patient room equipped with a bed and a bathroom. The bathtub is lined with plastic and brims with an herbal mixture, viscous and muddy. A laminated Chinese-language chart is tacked to the wall, instructing nurses about the patient's condition, the ideal water temperature, and how long to keep the patient in the bath. I ask why the chart is in Chinese instead of Tibetan. I'm told that many of the nurses on this unit are Chinese, that GCP requirements are written in Mandarin, and that Tibetan, in this context, is more of a "specialty language," as Drolma puts it.

In the adjacent bedroom five Salar women pack up clothes and tidy the space. Only one of these women is the patient, but a network of female support, most of them relatives, surrounds her. The woman has been an inpatient for eleven days. She is now heading home. The patient looks to be in her forties. When she first came here she could not walk; her joint pain was that severe. Before coming to the hospital she went to a biomedical hospital and received some treatment, which only helped alleviate her symptoms so she could sleep. By morning she ached all over again. "When I first came here, my pain was very bad," she says. "Now it is much better."

We leave the woman to her packing. "Come, I will show you where we cook the herbs," says Dr. Ma. We follow him up the stairs to a tiled room filled with two rows of stainless steel vats and long tables stacked with bundles of herbs. The room is humid and hot. Rivulets of sweat run down my back. I inhale the rich, bittersweet smell.

"What herbs do you use? Where do they come from?" I ask.

"The main hospital production unit," Dr. Ma answers. Perhaps it is just a matter of translation, but this response is telling. He mentions not the regions where the plants come from, but rather the institutional "home" of these resources—sort of like saying that milk comes from the grocery store. It speaks to a certain level of alienation that occurs as Sowa Rigpa is scaled up. In contrast, I recall Gyatso telling his patient in Mustang to go collect bicarbonate from the cliffs behind her village.

The on-site facility Dr. Ma mentions is where all non-GMP-certified medicines are made and is distinct from the for-profit pharmaceutical factory where Arura produces high-end consumer formulas.

"We use five main herbs as the base of all treatments," Dr. Ma continues. "Sometimes, depending on the problem of the patient, we add others. For example, if a person has a *lung* problem, we will add herbs like *akar kara* to keep the balance."

The doctor gestures toward burlap bundles the size of a small load of laundry. "Today some of these plants are difficult to find." When I ask him why some of the plants needed for medicinal baths are becoming rare, he says, *"Global warming."* Indeed one of the least understood but most pervasive threats to Tibetan medicine is climate change. Here on the Tibetan Plateau, glacial melt is visceral, observable with the naked eye. Profound ecological transitions surface dramatically, as in the floods that would sweep away thousands of Tibetan lives and homes in August 2010, and quietly, as in the diminishing snow lotuses found in craggy spaces high above Tibetan grasslands. Dr. Ma does not mention overharvesting and the commercialization of Tibetan medicine as a cause of such scarcity.

"How are people diagnosed in this division?" I ask.

"This department is very popular. Most people come here based on the advice of other patients. Sometimes people are referred by other divisions." I learn that about 50 percent of the patients in this division hail from outside Qinghai. A full 15 percent or more travel here from foreign countries, especially Japan, Korea, and Russia. "Cold places," says Dr. Ma.

"How do people learn about Tibetan medicinal baths in other countries?" I ask.

"Some Arura doctors have been to Japan. We have a formal connection with a group there. In Korea there was a television show about Arura. The world is small." Dr. Ma smiles.

"When people from other countries come here, how do they communicate with the doctors?"

"Several of our doctors speak English, Japanese, Russian. Sometimes people bring a translator or hire a local tour guide to help," answers Dr. Ma. "The Koreans used a Chinese businessman who knows Korean. There is also a Korean travel agency that takes people to Xinjiang. Since our treatments are well known in Xinjiang, they make connections. The problem is that people may know a language, but they do not know medical terms. Communication can be difficult, but people still benefit from our medicine." The real key, I think, is having money for travel and treatment.

On this theme I ask more about the socioeconomic status of patients. The government instituted new Cooperative Medical System health insurance policies in 2008, which, here in Qinghai, includes coverage for Tibetan therapies. "Since then, nomads, farmers, many people are coming more often," explains Dr. Ma. A treatment that once cost a patient 1,000 renminbi ($130) in out-of-pocket expenses is now 50 percent subsidized. Dr. Ma also attributes the rise in patients to Arura's growing reputation, even its chain stores in major Chinese cities. "In the past, if you went to another province for medical treatment, your home medical province would not pay," the doctor explains. "Now there are collaborative agreements between Qinghai and our neighbors. If a patient shows his medical records from here back to their home health bureau he can get reimbursed." I appreciate this information, even though I recognize it as a rather rosy treatment of changes in the Chinese health care system that have also included trends toward privatization and new burdens of medical debt on many families, Tibetan or otherwise.

As we chat, Dr. Ma opines that another reason people end up here is disaffection with biomedicine and Chinese medicine. "Some people try all sorts of treatments before coming here. Suffering does this to people. Tibetan medicine works well. When they see good results but they realize [they] need long-term treatment, this can become a problem for poor people. At the beginning, the government will help pay. If a person is wealthy he can get good care and take time to be treated. If a person is poor, even if he gets some treatment, he will continue to suffer because he must return quickly to work."

The majority of patients who come to the baths division are women. When I ask about this gender imbalance, Dr. Ma responds, "A woman's body is not as good or as strong as a man's." Drolma and I shoot each other looks, but Dr. Ma qualifies this statement. "After births or miscarriages, or even during a menstrual period, a woman's body is weak and can benefit from this type of care. This is also a cultural problem," he continues. "Women are not given time to rest after they give birth. They are soon back to work. This gives them problems of the kidney, back, and joints as they age. Women are always working harder than men! Social conditions influence disease. Social conditions produce suffering." Medical anthropology perspectives such as those espoused by Baer, Singer, and Susser (2002) that locate the "upstream" political-economic causes of suffering seem intuitive to Dr. Ma, who pinpoints crucial relations between culture, political economy, and health. Specific social ecologies can produce or perpetuate illness, just as certain spaces of healing can produce something like a cure.

LIVING TREASURE: 4:00 P.M.

Drolma and I continue to explore the outpatient division. We pass rooms devoted to moxibustion, cauterization, acupuncture, massage, and cupping. We pass the room in which herbal poultices mixed with hot oil are applied externally for joint and musculoskeletal problems. The sign on the door reads "Grease Electric Barbeque."

The walls of another room are lined with anatomy and acupoint charts, labeled in Tibetan and Chinese. For all the ways it is tempting to view Tibetan medicine as something distinct from either biomedicine or Chinese medicine, it is often a mosaic of strategies for understanding the body and making sense of patterns of suffering in practice.

"I think Aku Nyima is in today," Drolma says as we walk down the hall. "Would you like to meet him?"

"Yes, if you think it would be okay. I don't want to disturb him." I answer. *Aku,* or "Uncle," Nyima (his full name is Lobsang Nyima) is a senior Tibetan doctor at Arura and one of the most influential living Tibetan medicine practitioners in China. Aku Nyima is a master of clinical practice, also renowned for his knowledge of medicinal plants and production techniques. In this age of specialization Aku Nyima practices with a virtuoso holism. He is about eighty. Born and raised in a nomad community on the shores of Qinghai Lake, he weathered the Cultural Revolution and subsequent waves of political and socioeconomic transitions across this Tibetan area of China, and continues to practice.

As this globalized world would have it, I first met Aku Nyima in the United States. In fall 2009 he traveled to western Massachusetts, not far from my home in Vermont, to give a lecture on the practice of psychology in Tibetan medicine and to honor the first group of American students who had just completed a four-year course in Tibetan medicine, offered through the Shang Shung Institute. Many of these American students of Sowa Rigpa had spent the previous summer here in Qinghai, completing a three-month internship as the capstone experience of their training. I attended the lecture and listened with pleasure as this balding, spritely man spoke about the distinctive relationship between mind and body, the causes and conditions that give rise to mental suffering. Now, half a world away, I am about to walk into his practice.

Drolma knocks on the door. *"Gen,"* she says, referring to the senior doctor simply as "teacher," "I am here with an American researcher who has met you before. May we come in?" Aku Nyima motions for us

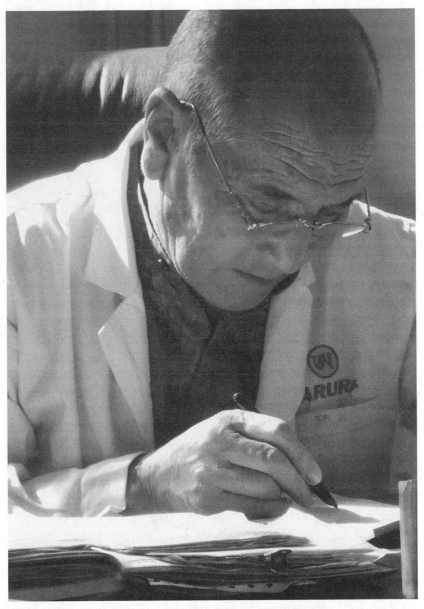

"Aku" Lobsang Nyima, one of the most senior practitioners of Tibetan medicine in Qinghai Province, in his office at Arura, Tibetan Medical Hospital, Xining, Qinghai Province, China, 2010. © Sienna Craig to sit down. He is writing a prescription. For an elderly man who has spent the day seeing patients, Aku Nyima seems lively. His balding head is haloed by afternoon light. Green suspenders peek out from under his Arura-embossed lab coat and grip the waist of brown trousers. His fedora and blazer hang on a coat rack in the corner. A small pillow covered in white silk rests on his desk. Frayed at the edges, the cushion represents a meeting point between doctor and patient, the place where pulse is read. Two assistants are busily typing his patients' diagnoses and prescriptions into a computer. Patients cluster on a bench outside his office.

Although I am glad to see this doctor, a man referred to as a "living treasure" by most who study with him, I am at a loss for words. Drolma nudges me. "It is okay. You can ask a few questions. You can speak Lhasa dialect. He will understand."

"Okay," I say. Someone who cannot swim diving into an ocean of wisdom, Tibetans might say. I ask Aku Nyima what types of illnesses he sees and treats.

"All diseases," he answers flatly.

"Is there anything you specialize in? Problems for which people often come to you?"

"Liver, gall bladder, and *lung* problems. Internal medicine."

"How do you spend your time? Is it mostly seeing patients?"

"Patients, yes. There are many. Also teaching."

Drolma pipes up, "Every Tuesday and Thursday when he is in Xining he does rounds in the inpatient division. Students come with him for this. It is a good opportunity to learn."

Aku Nyima adds, "When I go to inpatient with students, I correct their diagnosis and help doctors over there. Sometimes if a problem is not clear, I also help." The doctor calls in his next patient, indicating we can stay.

Three young Tibetan men usher in a middle-aged woman, presumably their mother or another female relative. Her face is burnished by sun and wind. She wears navy blue slacks that fall well short of her ankles, her quivering torso sheathed in a down jacket, even though it is warm. A sun hat adorned with plastic flowers hides a bun. The woman speaks. Her voice rings high and halting. "I am in pain," she says. "It is difficult to walk." The woman is helped into the chair beside Aku Nyima, who takes her hand in his. The doctor feels across her palm, down to her wrist, beginning the work of diagnosis. His eyes half close. Senses recalibrate.

"I have been in this state one week, Doctor. I have no energy," the woman continues as Aku Nyima reads her pulse. "The pain makes a circle around my kidneys."

"We cannot even touch her there," one male relative offers.

As the patient talks and Aku Nyima contemplates her pulse, one of his assistants enters diagnostic codes into the computerized electronic medical system, itself a new invention that allows input in Chinese and Tibetan. Diagnoses and specific indications of medicines are written in Tibetan, while prescriptions, lab tests, and costs associated with these are recorded in Chinese. This computer programming allows a space for Tibetan medical theory, even as it is accountable to parallel realities of state insurance schemes, standardized formularies, and the costs of health care. This novel system counts the amount and kinds of medicines dispensed each day, the daily gross income of the hospital, the number of patients seen. Fields for patient history and results of treatment are notated in Chinese, even as doctors keep separate, handwritten notes on patients.

In later conversations with the chief programmer of this computer system, I learn that while many at Arura view the conversion of medical records into this electronic format as a vast improvement over the burden of paperwork, challenges have surfaced. Junior doctors such as those assisting Aku Nyima have come to rely on the computer to define, in a sense, the limits of diagnostic possibilities based on the types of problems have been coded in the system and which are legible within the state system of health care subsidies and reimbursements, rather than assigning primacy to a patient's medical history and the individual complexities of illness. Of course, this is not unique to Tibetan medicine— similar dynamics have been noted recently in the United States as hospitals shift to electronic medical records—but it is a very new phenomenon here in Tibetan areas of China.

When I ask Aku Nyima about this new system he says young doctors' memories are getting worse. They are relying more on computers than mnemonic techniques for recounting diagnosis and treatment patterns, as taught in the *Gyüshi*. Technoscience is changing pedagogy and praxis of healing in this hospital, especially among the upcoming generations of doctors. Like the insertion of clinic logbooks into medical practice in Lo Monthang, this is a new method for standardizing, tracking, and generating authoritative knowledge about patients, as well as for tracking the money the hospital makes. It is also a new form of biological citizenship (Petryna 2002; Rose and Novas 2005), a way of linking biology and subjectivity on the one hand and making collective welfare claims of a state on the other. In this case, biological citizenship emerges not only by accessing Tibetan medicines, as both a medical and a sociocultural choice, but also through the possibilities for tracking citizens as they access health care and have such encounters recorded digitally, in ways that raise issues with respect to privacy. During our conversation, the computer programmer mentioned—with a sense of hope rather than irony—that soon the government would be able to "know all the health problems of all its citizens and to share this with pharmaceutical companies."

For people like Aku Nyima, the computer remains an auxiliary appendage. He writes diagnosis and prescription notes in quick Tibetan and hands these to his assistants. He also writes a prescription for patients to take to the pharmacy. At first this process seems duplicative. But Drolma explains: each medicine coded in the computer system is approved by health insurance; sometimes other prescriptions are actually filled, based on handwritten notations by doctors, even though what is charged to insurance reflects those limited reimbursable medicines. The computer records are for hospital statistics and reporting, while the other papers leave patients with a record of their care. This is in part to facilitate refilling prescriptions remotely, since so many patients travel quite far to be diagnosed at this hospital and cannot always return to access more medicines or receive checkups and recalibrations to their prescriptions.

"The problem is in your joints," Aku Nyima says finally, after releasing his grasp on the woman's wrist. "Kidneys also. Have you had blood tests?"

"No. My stomach has also been in pain. I took Western medicines for this, but it did not help."

"I advise you to be admitted," Aku Nyima responds. "You need blood tests and time to rest. The joint problems—these are clear. But the other pain and suffering you describe . . . I need to see you for more than this moment to know more." Aku Nyima looks the woman in the eyes as he speaks. His voice is slow, steady. The patient and her family members take this advice. The woman rises slowly, moving as if each step, each gesture sears her.

"Where is your home village?" Aku Nyima asks, perhaps on a hunch, perhaps because of her accent. It turns out she is from the same county as Arura's chief executive. In the choice of hospital and physician, efficacious practice emerges from enduring social relationships and a shared allegiance to place.

ENGLISH CLASS AND EARTHQUAKES: 6:00 P.M.

By early evening in Xining long shadows drape across the city. Drolma and I sit on the steps of the hospital, sipping water and munching sesame biscuits. We have been working hard, but there is still one more episode in this day of fieldwork: English class. The hospital runs an English tutorial three times a week for staff and students. I have offered to teach the class tonight.

I returned recently from the earthquake-devastated capital of Yushu Tibetan Autonomous Prefecture, down near the border with Sichuan. On April 14, 2010, an earthquake measuring between 6.8 and 7.1 on the Richter scale rocked the center of Yushu. The population of Jyekundo, Yushu's prefectural capital, was estimated at 80,000 to 100,000 prior to the quake, mostly Tibetans. The official dead numbered about 2,500, while unofficial reports put the death toll as high as 10,000. In contemplating this statistical dissonance, I am reminded of a saying a Tibetan friend once told me: *If a Chinese statistic is good, divide by four; if it is bad, multiply by four.* The natural disaster devastated an area that throughout history has been a hub for Tibetan entrepreneurship, medicine, ritual economies, and religious instruction.

Drolma had suggested that her fellow students would be interested in hearing about the public health situation in Yushu, including the status of the Tibetan medical hospital. She and several of her classmates volunteered in Yushu after the quake. Others were unable to go. Some students from Yushu lost relatives in this quake. Drolma thought they would be keen to learn about what I'd seen and heard on the ground. I had taken this trip to Yushu as part of my involvement with a maternal-child health organization with whom I've worked in the TAR.[7] The thought of talking with the students about Yushu and what I saw there made me wary initially. I was worried about politics.

This evening Drolma and I take the elevator to the top floor of the inpatient division, where we are greeted in the seminar room by the eager, kind faces of seventeen students. We make a circle out of desks and tables.

"Good evening," I say, ready to begin.

"Good evening," they echo. I introduce myself and ask the students do the same. A Canadian graduate student who will teach English to this group on a regular basis also joins the discussion. Eight of seventeen students are women. Two students are from Yushu. One is a monk who goes by the English name of Peter. The other is a young man with a grasp of English superior to many of his peers, and who talks about his desire to pursue research in public health.

At first we do not discuss the earthquake directly. I tell the students a bit about my career path, my home in the United States, the college where I teach. They ask questions: Where did I get my Ph.D.? Why am I interested in Tibetan medicine? What is medical anthropology? Students copy words I have printed on the board during the course of my introduction: *ethnography, epidemiology, indigenous, medical pluralism, maternal child health,* and *Skilled Birth Attendant.* I draw a rough approximation of a map of Nepal and of the United States, on which I locate Mustang and Hanover, New Hampshire. The white board renders an odd, if legible map of my trajectories.

Eventually I turn to the subject of Yushu. "Some of you have seen pictures of Yushu. Some of you have been there too. I just returned from a visit. The health situation is very bad. The Tibetan medicine hospital has been mostly destroyed, and so have many other hospitals."

I struggle to describe the landscape. The term *postapocalyptic* comes to mind, but I do not use this in the English class. On the ride from the airport into town, herds of yak gave way to rubble: piles of cheap cement bricks, crushed adobe, teepees of salvaged beams. In a land of few trees, even battered beams are gold. Moving closer to the city, a "model" rebuilt settlement came into view. The new constructions, eight-by-eight meter concrete blocks huddled close together in eerie symmetry, were supposedly better for earthquake zones. Their gray monotony, their dearth of windows, depressed me.

"Rebuilding has begun in some places," I say. "There were many businessmen on the airplanes. Now there are direct flights from Beijing to Yushu every week. I saw several private construction companies setting up operations beside the camps of soldiers, who are clearing away destroyed buildings and helping people." The presence of the state was strong in these quarters, and the money to be made on reconstruction by private contractors and public works agencies was palpable. It reminded me of New Orleans after Hurricane Katrina.

The first shells of structures on the outskirts of town had a surreal beauty to them, reflecting the raw power of the Earth. It has been estimated that more than 90 percent of the buildings were destroyed or will need to be demolished. Blue government-issued relief tents colonized the landscape, augmented by prefab buildings made of plywood and Styrofoam. Children in dusty school uniforms kicked dented Red Bull cans down side alleys littered with concrete and steel. A woman carried an IV for her husband as he ducked behind an Oxfam relief vehicle to pee. At a time of disorder the human propensity for order turns people into sorters, pickers-through of things. Stacks of wood and metal, piles of window frames, scraps of old clothes emerged, like islands rising up from a sea of destruction in this broken city. Shops had been re-created on sidewalks, in tents.

"Even though so much was destroyed, business is continuing in Yushu. People are selling yogurt and *yartsa gunbu* on the street corners," I tell the English class, referring to the medicinal caterpillar fungus *(Ophiocordyceps sinensis)*, literally worth more than its weight in gold and a key part of the Tibetan economy.

"I have heard that the price for one piece of *yartsa gunbu* is forty or fifty renminbi [six dollars] this year," one of the students comments. "This is better than last year. This money will help local people to recover."

A young woman raises her hand. "Please, may you tell us about hospitals. Are there doctors? Do peoples have . . . ," she searches for a word, "sufficient medicines?"

"The hospitals are working out of tents," I answer. "The military brought in mobile surgical units, vans in which to do surgery. Each hospital has between one hundred and two hundred beds. Some doctors and nurses from each hospital died. People are working very hard. There are not enough doctors." The two prefecture-level hospitals received donations of medical supplies and equipment from governmental sources and nongovernmental humanitarian aid organizations in Beijing, Shanghai, and Hong Kong. Foreign aid has been more difficult to channel, although much was raised through a coalition of local Tibetan NGOs. Provincial-level doctors from Xining were assigned to work in Yushu for the coming months, possibly up to a year or more. The county hospital was being run by the military since all their equipment was destroyed. The needs are huge. Despite this adversity, and losses of human capital, the hospitals were functioning, collectively serving thousands of patients daily.

"The Yushu Tibetan Medicine Hospital lost all but one of its buildings," I continue. "Arura sent medicines. The Tibetan medical hospitals in Dartsendo and Derge also sent medicines," I say, referring to Tibetan regions in Sichuan Province, not far from Jyekundo. "But the numbers and kinds of Tibetan medicines have been reduced. There are not enough supplies. The glass bottles in which medicines were stored broke." I think about the loss not only in terms of human capacity to address suffering, but also with respect to the natural resources that went into making those medicines. "Right now the Tibetan medicine hospital can see only outpatients. But hundreds of people come each day." This raises issues about the state's prioritization of healing modalities when the proverbial chips, and the buildings, are down. Perhaps they decided to triage around emergency services and acute disorders, but it was notable that inpatient facilities were not viewed as essential to re-create, even in tent form, for the Tibetan medical hospital.

"What about remaking hospitals?" another student asks. "How long to take?"

"It is not clear. Some say one year. Others say three. The Tibetan medicine hospital may be moved to a new location, away from the center of town, to out near the horse racing stadium on the edge of town."

"This will cause hardship for patients," a young monk offers.

"Yes," I answer. Where will Tibetan medicine find a place in Yushu's reconstructed landscape? The detail illustrates the politics of reconstruction. Rebuilding contracts offer high stakes for local and regional officials, military and private contractors. Billboards along the rubble-filled roads of Jyekundo, Yushu's prefectural capital, depict fields of tulips and shimmering Himalayan peaks, bespeaking hope in Tibetan and Chinese: *The New Yushu will be a glimmering jewel of Qinghai* and *With dedication we will rebuild the city.*

During my visit, two months after the quake, hospitals were no longer filled only with quake victims. Now these makeshift institutions were simply trying to meet the health needs of survivors and those who regularly rely on services in Jyekundo.

A young man raises his hand. "Please, about the sanitation. Will there be problems of infectious disease?"

"Yes," I answer. "I think this could be a big problem. There is water for people to drink, but not for people to bathe or wash clothes—only in the river. The toilet situation is very bad." In the tent city that cropped up in People's Park, where I stayed, local women with colorful face masks hunkered down against relentless dust as they prepared food or washed necessities with water they'd hauled from the river. The sanitation situation was abysmal. Plots of parkland had been given over to shallow latrines, already overflowing and surrounded by minefields of human excrement. The conditions would likely deteriorate through summer, as intense rains were followed by autumn hail and wind, and then winter. The garbage piles were already intense. I wondered if people would move farther out, push up more against the mountains, where they have buried their dead.

"What about dogs?" a student asks. Yushu is known for its Tibetan mastiffs, which, along with the swift sale in *yartsa gunbu,* provide locals with significant income. A Chinese businessman had recently paid more than $1 million for a prized pup.

"Many dogs were loose," I answer. "Maybe some of their owners had died. Other dogs were kept beside tents, but this is a problem. Do you know 'rabies'?" I ask. Some students nod yes. We spend a few minutes discussing this disease, as well as the problems of having hungry dogs living in close proximity to families with young children.

Another young man raises his hand. "How are the minds of people? It is much sadness?"

This question is difficult for me to answer. All I can think to do is report what I saw at the cremation grounds. The grounds amounted to two long ditches separated by a mound of earth, over which was placed salvaged rebar and under which were tires and kilos of butter. Corpses had been laid here and burned—more than one thousand people the first day, according to locals with whom I spoke. My first thought on seeing this place was that it was ingenious. Imagine the mindfulness it must have taken to engineer this space, in the midst of it all, the chaos and the wails.

"The monks are working very hard," I begin. "They are doing many rituals. The lines for having a monk come to your house to do a ritual for your relatives are long. Sometimes people have to wait weeks." Monks from one local monastery told me they were collecting the bones of the deceased, and local women were then crafting these remains into *tsa tsa,* offering sculptures. The monks would then release these offerings into the confluence of the rivers running through Jyekundo on an astrologically auspicious day.

Plastic flowers and piles of stones marked with the *kalachakra,* the "wheel of time" symbol, created an ad hoc cemetery beside the open-air crematorium. I watched as two people sat in silence, staring at the funeral pyre, now cool, and thumbing prayer beads. On the way down the mountain I met a nun. She was digging through rubble one stone at a time. She had lost someone here whose body had not been found. The area below the cremation grounds was an odd no-man's-land between destruction and creation: blue hard hats, metal doors, and bags of concrete where there had once been homes. That, and bulldozers and earth: a social ecology of suffering, laid bare, turned over, plowed through.

"Some people from China came after the earthquake to help people with their sadness," I say. The phrasing is awkward, but I'm not sure how else to render the term *grieving therapy* in simple English words. These well-intentioned individuals soon realized they had no business here. Grieving therapy, such as it is, is the domain of monks and family members. This is not to say, though, that many in Yushu might not have been suffering from what biomedical psychiatry calls posttraumatic stress disorder, a category that can have cross-cultural salience (Osterman and de Jong 2007). Monks, strong but for their nightmares. Mothers made anxious by the rumbling of a truck. But the efficacy of a diagnostic label from one cultural context can fail the test of meaning in another, at the level of practice.

"I heard about such people from my relatives," a man from Yushu mentions. "But for Tibetan people . . . this sadness help cannot come from outside. This is Buddhism works." I appreciate his double entendre, unintended though it may have been. For in this case, Buddhism does indeed work. It is potent. One of the local NGOs used some earthquake relief funds to sponsor a shelter for monks for the forty-nine-day period during which the dead travel through the *bardo,* the realm between death and rebirth. The thought of thousands of people mourning so intensely, on the same days each week, remains with me, as does the beautiful irony that this NGO was asked to fill this particular role because the government could not officially minister to this civil need, and the monastery, itself damaged in structure and substance, did not have the resources to fund the ritual themselves.

My time with the English class nearly complete, the students take a break and I prepare to leave. A young man from Yushu approaches me. "It is difficult to hear such things," he says, grasping my hand. "But to be good doctors we need to face the suffering. Just like the monks, but with different medicines." These comments remind me of how efficacy also emerges through people's abilities to deal with compassionate precision in the face of death, injury, and grief. Furthermore, after a day spent in a vibrant and powerful institution, a place where Tibetan medicine is alive and well, the limits of human action, of all that we cannot control, resonate.

SUMMARY

In this chapter you've glimpsed the ways that Tibetan medicine is practiced, produced, and consumed within one thriving institution in China. Between this and the first chapter, focused on Nepal, you now have a sense of just how diverse the practices that fall under the category

"Sowa Rigpa" or "Tibetan medicine" can be. The relative power and scale of Arura, when compared with Lo Kunphen, further illustrates this diversity.

You've seen how particular political economies shape the capacity for doctors and patients to arrive at desired health outcomes. This theme is explored in more detail in chapter 4. This chapter has also revealed the scope and impacts of governmental support for Tibetan medicine in China. It has shown how Tibetan medicine is at once part of China's health care system and, increasingly, part of a growing national and international effort to conduct clinical research on and market "traditional" therapies. You've also glimpsed some of the challenges facing Tibetan medicine as it is made to comply with regimes of clinical practice and medical production, themes that are explored in more detail in chapters 5, 6, and 7.

In the next chapter we turn to the issue of lineage and the source—forces that give practitioners of Sowa Rigpa a sense of legitimacy, whether they practice in their rural homes or in bustling urban hospitals.

CHAPTER 3

Lineage and Legitimacy

Taste all, and hand the knowledge down.
—Gary Snyder, *No Nature: New and Selected Poems*

THE MANY MEANINGS OF "TRADITIONAL" MEDICINE

On the day of our visit to the homeopathic hospital at Harihar Bhawan, Gyatso and I make it as far as the Bagmati Bridge before our taxi is forced to pull over. It is March 2007. The sky above the Kathmandu Valley is clear, but the streets are filled with unrest. Recent political agitation by *madhesi* groups along Nepal's southern border has left Kathmandu in a state of perpetual shortage.[1] Strikes and road blockades have stopped the flow of petrol, cooking gas, and other essentials into the valley. Although Nepal's second People's Movement that reached its apex in April 2006 put an end to the Nepali monarchy and a decade of civil war, political violence has continued to interfere with daily life. Today a *bandh,* or strike, is in effect, instigated by the Maoists, a branch of the Communist Party of Nepal that had been at the forefront of the civil war and has now taken up a leadership position in *naya* or "new" Nepal.

We step out of the taxi as a wave of protestors approach, flags waving, tires burning. Gyatso reaches for his mobile and calls the homeopath who serves as chairman of the Nepal Alternative Health Council (NAHC), the man we are attempting to meet. This body has been established more recently than the Nepal Ayurvedic Medical Council and the Nepal Health Professionals Council, both of which have been charged with regulating and registering the country's diverse array of medical practitioners since the 1990s (Koriala 2007). In fluent Nepali, Gyatso confirms that Dr. Khan is expecting us. We head up Pulchowk Hill, dodging smoldering bits of rubber and shielding our faces from acrid smoke, until we slip up a side street that takes us to the quiet neighborhood where the hospital is located. This white and blue concrete building, surrounded by stands of bamboo, is serene. Patients linger in cool corridors.

Homeopathy has been practiced in Nepal since the 1920s, when a member of the ruling Rana family recruited an Indian homeopath to address a cholera epidemic. The homeopathic tradition in Nepal continued through private practice until 1953, when one of Nepal's leading homeopaths petitioned King Tribhuvan to establish this hospital. Support for homeopathy came at a moment when biomedicine was being introduced to the country on a broad scale, with capital and expertise provided by foreign aid organizations (Justice 1986). Homeopathy still occupies an ancillary place in the health care hierarchy when compared with biomedicine and Ayurveda, but it has been recognized by the state for the past five decades.[2] Given this history, Nepal's homeopaths are in a unique position to lobby for the rights of other nonorthodox medical practices. And so it is that a German medical tradition, filtered through lineages of Indian practitioners, has provided an entrée for Nepali *amchi* to gain governmental legitimacy. The homeopath at the helm of the NAHC is a Nepali Muslim who has also studied Unani, a traditional medical system associated with Muslim South Asia.

Gyatso and I enter Dr. Khan's office and take a seat on his couch, behind a line of patients. While we wait for him to finish seeing patients, we chat in Tibetan.

"This hospital helps many people," Gyatso begins. "I have heard of good results from Dr. Khan's medicines."

"Do you know about homeopathy?" I ask. Gyatso is familiar with Ayurveda and he has been introduced to Chinese herbalism and acupuncture. But I wonder what he knows about homeopathy, a medical tradition founded in Europe in the eighteenth century, grounded in the "law of similars" with roots in a vitalist philosophy of healing.

"I do not know much about this medicine, but it came from the West, right?"

"Yes," I respond, "from Germany."

"Dr. Khan told me that homeopathic doctors do not usually treat with compound medicines, like we do. And they treat illnesses with medicines that have the same nature as the illness. So they are different from *amchi* medicine." We watch Dr. Khan prescribe a formula for a woman suffering from irregular menstrual cycles and another one for a colicky infant. Gyatso then turns to me and asks, "What does this word *alternative* mean?" The English term pierces an otherwise Tibetan sentence. Even though Gyatso is a member of the Nepal Alternative Health Council, he does not understand the meaning of this term, in either English or the Sanskritized Nepali equivalent written on the organization's charter.

"In general," I answer, "this word means a choice, an option. It can also mean something that is not the main way of doing things, but another path. When people talk about *alternative medicine,* it usually means *not* biomedicine," I say, using the phrase *nub chog gyi mén,* "medicine from the West."

"So, in English, the meaning of *alternative medicine* is like what people call *tradition medicine?*"

"Yes," I respond. Gyatso's use of English is sweet, but I am acutely aware of the relations of power at work in such designations. Don Bates (2002) has argued that we should really call biomedicine the true "alternative" medicine, for, despite its rise to global dominance, biomedicine as practiced since the mid-twentieth century remains the anomaly when one takes the long view on global histories of science and medicine. But Gyatso's question is pragmatic. The designation *traditional* or *alternative* means little to him in terms of how he heals. However, he sees the social and political value inherent in being able to use these buzzwords and to think strategically about how to classify Sowa Rigpa to an array of "outsiders," be they colleagues such as Dr. Khan, Nepali government authorities, or foreigners interested in CAM and Tibetan culture generally.

Dr. Khan takes a break from seeing patients to update Gyatso on the government ratification process of the NAHC's constitution and the proposed Alternative Health Act. These documents were drafted the previous year, in a meeting chaired by the general secretary of the Ministry of Health and Population. Overt political instability and perhaps a more implicit desire to hold fast to biomedical hegemony have kept approval at bay. "The Ministry of Health makes obstacles," says Dr. Khan. I ask him about the benefit of the proposed legislation.

"Until now, we have been going to the government one by one," he answers. "But we need to work together." Dr. Khan explains that people representing heterodox medical traditions need to draft legislation that will help ensure their rights to teach and practice. This requires that such medical systems become "legible" in the eyes of the state: visible, quantifiable, and possible to track (Scott 1998). Yet unlike the "legibility" James Scott describes in relation to sedentarizing mobile populations so as to more easily conscript, tax, or otherwise control them or natural resources such as forests. In Scott's examples from this and other works, the legibility occurs around the need to render heterodox knowledge in forms that make sense to the state and its functionaries, so that it can be legitimated and, in the process, tamed—or even capitalized on. The subtitle of Scott's *Seeing Like a State* is "how certain schemes to improve the human condition have failed." It is precisely this possibility of failure, coupled with the hope that one's government will be at once benevolent and supportive of the human condition, that at once keep Nepal's *amchi* lobbying for state legitimacy and yet ambivalent about what such recognition might do, or bring, to their practice.

To think about this question of legitimacy and legibility in a different way, the NAHC is consciously engaging the structures and practices of what Michel Foucault (1991) calls "governmentality," the organized practices by which citizens are subject to particular forms of power, which in turn shape their subjectivity. Such work requires compromise, but Dr. Kahn and other NAHC members feel the benefits of state recognition are worth the risks. Despite their engagement with the Ministry of Health and Population, the Council has seen no progress for months. "The document is gathering dust in the Ayurveda and Alternative Medicine section of the Ministry," says Dr. Kahn.

Gyatso checks the Nepali-language verbiage within the NAHC documents describing Himalayan *amchi* medicine. The text testifies to Sowa Rigpa's historical roots in Nepal and the greater Himalayan-Tibetan Plateau and its connections to Buddhism. It describes Himalaya *amchi* medicine as at once uniquely Nepali, part of the nation's cultural heritage, and more broadly representative of Traditional Medicine, as defined by the WHO. Significantly the text makes no mention of Tibet. To do so might compromise the efforts of *amchi* in Nepal to gain state support in a political era in which Nepal is aligning more and more closely with China, often at the expense of exile Tibetans who have taken refuge in Nepal.[3] This statement also illustrates how global discourses about the place of Traditional Medicine in health-development work are shaping local narratives about the value, history, and efficacy of Sowa Rigpa, even as such engagements are changing what it means to be an *amchi* today.

Furthermore this proposed legislation responds to a commonly held stereotype within the Ministry of Health that *amchi* practice falls outside the bounds of what is even *possible* to recognize as a legitimate Nepali medical system, due to a lack of textual sources written *in Nepali* about this tradition, and the lack of precedent for levels of certification compara- rable with existing state health and education certification requirements. In response the NAHC document outlines four distinct "grades" of *am-chi* in Nepal, based on a standardized curriculum that the HAA developed with help from the Council on Technical Education and Vocational Training (CTEVT), itself part of the Ministry of Education and Sports.[4]

A-grade *amchi* are practitioners who have passed *kachupa*-level examinations (a five-and-a-half-year course equivalent to a Bachelors of Medicine and Surgery [MBBS] degree).[5] Notably, few Nepali citizens fall into this category; those who qualify for this A grade must have graduated from a Tibetan medical institution in India or China. B-grade *amchi* are those who pass *durapa* examinations (a three-year course, equivalent to a health assistant degree). Currently no *durapa* courses are offered in Nepal, but Lo Kunphen is in the process of developing such a curriculum. C-grade *amchi* designate those who pass *kanjenpa* examinations (a one-and-a-half-year course equivalent to a Technical School Leaving Certificate and a community medical assistant degree). This is the only official recognition now granted *amchi* in Nepal.

Finally, D-grade *amchi* comprise the majority of HAA's membership: male doctors (monks, *nakpa,* and laymen) who were taught medicine through family-based lineage practice *(menpé gyü)* and whose legitimacy can be attested to by a panel of peers, but who the state does not consider suitable to teach above the *kanjenpa* level. This classification system not only creates parallel structures with Nepal's hierarchy of biomedical certification; it also mirrors the ranks assigned to practitioners in Indian and Chinese institutions. For D-grade *amchi* in Nepal, these shifting models of legitimation can translate into a newfound sense of self-consciousness about *what* they know, *how* they know it, and *where* they learned it.[6] These dynamics play out in distinct ways within Nepal and China, in further dialogue with centers of the exile Tibetan medical authority in India. Sometimes the social efficacy of one form of legitimation—a government-issued license or a degree from the Tibetan Medical College in Lhasa or the Dharamsala Men-tsee-khang—is further validated with reference to root teachers or patrilineages. At other times even fellow practitioners from India and China sideline these lineage practitioners.

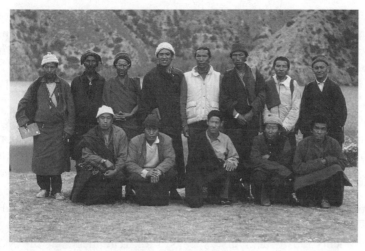

Members of the Himalayan Amchi Association from Mustang and Dolpo, on a medicinal plant collection, identification, and research expedition in Shey Phoksumdo National Park, Dolpa District, Nepal, 2000. Amchi Tshampa Ngawang, pictured on the cover of this book and featured in chapter 4, is in the back row, fourth from the right. Amchi Gyatso Bista is just below him, in the front row, third from the right. All of these *amchi* would be considered D-grade practitioners. © Thomas Kelly

Gyatso reads the Nepali text one more time before signing his name to this document. We bid Dr. Khan goodbye and head out into the smoldering city.

Our next appointment is with Dr. Joshi,[7] the director of the Ayurveda and Alternative Medicine section of the Ministry of Health and Population. This organization implements the National Ayurveda Health Policy, first promulgated in 1996 and amended in 2001 (Koriala 2007). We walk across the Bagmati Bridge, down to the Ministry, a beleaguered brick building at the far end of Ramshah Path. The bilingual Nepali-English nameplate outside Dr. Joshi's office indicates the doctor is in.

"Hello, Sir," calls Gyatso, knocking softly.

"*Amchi ji?* Come in," comes the reply. I follow Gyatso inside. Sunlight filters through a dingy window, throwing Dr. Joshi into silhouette. Gyatso introduces me and tells the doctor we have just seen Dr. Khan to review the NAHC documents. I notice my friend's bowed head, his deference.

"I would like to know, Sir, if there is anything else we need to do to approve the new Council constitution."

"No. But this approval is not easy. It will take maybe two, three months, if things go well. Making rules for your kinds of medicine is difficult," Dr. Joshi answers. "After these papers are filed, you will need to translate the history of your *amchi* medicine. You say you have many books, but what am I going to do with all these things written in *Bhote bhasa?*" he asks, referring, disparagingly, in Nepali to the classical Tibetan of medical texts as the language of unrefined beef-eating, beer-drinking Buddhists from the boondocks.

Gyatso does not respond to this affront. Instead he says, "We are making a new *curriculum* of *amchi* medicine with CTEVT. Our new *textbook* is based on our important books. We cannot translate these books into Nepali. There are too many problems of translation. But we have summarized the lessons and made a table of contents in Nepali." Gyatso continues, "Sir, our goal is to join with government health posts in the future. To make the health of our villages better and to give our students jobs." As Gyatso speaks, I am reminded that the Nepali Ministry of Health is heavily dependent on foreign aid for its operation and programs. Biases regarding what is a legitimate or knowable practice in the eyes of the state are not simply a reflection of ethnicity or nationalistic politics. They also reflect donor agendas and normative assumptions about the universal applicability of biomedicine (Lock and Nguyen 2010).

Dr. Joshi scoffs. "You will need to fight hard for a place in the system. Now there is only room for Ayurveda and Western medicine, and a little corner for homeopathy. We know these medicines work. We see their benefit. People say your *amchi* medicine is good, but how can we prove this? How can we know that someone who calls himself an *amchi* is really qualified, not a fake?" Dr. Joshi speaks to assumptions about efficacy and its inverse, which would pitch Sowa Rigpa as nothing more than quackery and charlatanism (see Langford 1999). While members of the HAA have internally debated the question of who should qualify as an *amchi* (Craig 2008b), they share an implicit empirical understanding that Tibetan medicine *does* work, that its theoretical basis undergirding clinical practice is sound.

Gyatso takes a different tack in responding. "*Amchi* treat sick people in areas where government health workers just eat their salaries and leave their posts. They sell medicines illegally. They do not practice with care. They do not speak our language. They do not like living in our villages." He sheds some of his deferential demeanor. "The WHO says health care is a basic right for all people, but our government does not provide this. Supporting *amchi* medicine does not cost much money. We do not need fancy machines. Our medicines are affordable." My colleague becomes more emboldened as he speaks. He explains that, while *amchi* in Nepal have some support from foreign donors, this cannot replace governmental backing. In explaining why the Nepali government is failing its high mountain populations, Gyatso also implicitly criticizes an approach to health development that is driven by aid organizations and NGOs as a proxy for a strong public sector. His use of the WHO framework and universalist approaches to the notion of health as a human right to create leverage in this conversation is remarkable in that it shows the impacts of global discourse on national politics and on shaping the subjectivities of marginalized groups.

"If you want *amchi* to be part of the government health care system," answers Dr. Joshi, "then *amchi* need to be trained within that system." He then turns to a military metaphor to describe the process by which *amchi* will need to engage the state to gain its support. "The Maoists recently succeeded in capturing the houses of government in Kathmandu," Dr. Joshi explains. "They know the weaknesses of the existing system." So too, he says, with medical systems intent on "infiltrating" the Ministry of Health. Yet unlike the "weak government and greedy politicians" that dominate Kathmandu's political scene, biomedicine and Nepali Ayurveda are powerful forces to reckon with. "Our houses are well guarded," says Dr. Joshi.

"Besides," the Nepali government functionary goes on, "there are many underemployed health workers who have received authentic medical training. Convincing the Ministry to take money away from such people in favor of *amchi* is unlikely. We cannot just hand out government salaries for the work you say you do. *Amchi* must be trained in a program that we have control over." This exchange reveals aspects of what Foucault (2007) and others have dubbed "biopolitics": styles of government that regulate populations by infusing political power into and through forms of human life. In this case, the Nepali state, "weak" though it may be, will continue to exert pressure on the ways *amchi* make and practice medicine until this process resembles something that is knowable, familiar, tamed. It is important to remember we are not just talking about curriculum in the abstract, as disembodied, bookish knowledge, but rather a particular way of using one's body and mind to affect healing and transmit knowledge within a particular social ecology, and to do so with reference to specific texts and oral tradition.

"The work you have done with CTEVT is a first step," Dr. Joshi continues, kinder now. "But we are doctors. *Amchi* are not, at least not in the same way. We need to know more about the ways you practice."

"I see, Sir," Gyatso responds, his face revealing frustration and resignation by turns. "Dr. Khan will contact you soon."

As we walk out of the Ministry into the flood of foot traffic, Gyatso says, "I worry all this effort will not bear fruit." Gyatso and other HAA members have felt compelled to engage the government, despite obstacles, not so much for their own future as for the future of their students and children.

"Sometimes I wish I did not need to come to *phayul* at all," Gyatso continues. This sentence is revealing. *Phayul* is a common Tibetan term for Kathmandu, but it also can mean, simply, Nepal. In other words, to travel to Kathmandu *is* to come to the nation-state of Nepal, even as the border zones from which *amchi* hail comprise a crucial space through which the nation-state of Nepal is imagined and defined (Shneiderman forthcoming). For *amchi* like Gyatso, the bounds of Nepali citizenship exist most clearly within the social ecology of the capital. With distance from Kathmandu, Gyatso's identification as a Nepali citizen shifts in favor of alliances that are at once more local and more transnational (Ramble 1997).

The events of the morning remind me of a conversation Gyatso and I had in December 2001. We had been participating in a workshop on medicinal plant use and conservation in Kathmandu. In their presentations many of the social and natural scientists used the acronym TMP, Traditional Medicine Practitioners, to refer to people with whom they interacted to document species and craft conservation guidelines. At one point during the meeting, Gyatso whispered to me, "What does 'TMP' mean?" I explained. Gyatso beamed in response. "TMP. This could be 'traditional medicine practitioner,' or it could be another word for '*Tibetan* medicine practitioner.' This is very useful!"

Over lunch that day Gyatso and I discussed the benefits *(pentok)* and obstacles *(gekpa)* that labels like TMP can create. I summarized Stacey Leigh Pigg's (1995, 1997) arguments that it is possible to "find in most traditional societies" people called a Traditional Medicine Practitioner or a traditional birth attendant. Pigg argues that the deployment of such acronyms used in the context of health-development interventions can efface the specificity of place and practice, and may in fact *reinforce* marginal social positions among people like Gyatso, as well as aggravate micropolitics at play within groups of practitioners such as Nepal's *amchi*.

"It will always be difficult for the Nepali government to listen to us," responded Gyatso. "But there are still benefits to using words that are known throughout the world."

Gyatso picked up his pen and wrote the letters T-M-P on his notepad. He then carefully spelled out the English words *Tibetan* and *Tradition*, with my help. Both words extended down, vertically, from the T of TMP. For Gyatso, the acronym was also a foil for the tricky political category "Tibetan" in the Nepali context. With this move, I understood how Gyatso saw the T of Tibetan conveniently couched within the T of Tradition. The entire acronym connected Nepal's *amchi* to a broader frame of reference, albeit articulated in terms that reproduced biomedical hegemony and emerged from development discourse. He had harnessed the rhetoric of health-development programs and institutions such as the WHO to assert the value of *amchi* practice to an otherwise skeptical Nepali state by employing a term that is global in orientation. However, at key moments and in safe spaces, this T of Tradition could be cast off for a more pointed and strategic assertion of authentic Tibetanness, itself a play of lineage and legitimacy that illustrates Pordié's (2008b) assertion that *amchi* rely on forms of "neo-traditionalism" as a way of defending and transforming their practice. Gyatso liked the potential of TMP, even though this acronym simplified divergent social ecologies of Sowa Rigpa for specifically political ends. He was strategically mining linguistic incommensurability, maneuvering within the spaces lost in translation.

Two years after that conference in Kathmandu, I was again beside Gyatso at another international gathering, this time the Second International Congress of Tibetan Medicine held in Washington, D.C., in 2003. As we prepared his presentation on Lo Kunphen and the HAA, for which I would serve as his translator, Gyatso said, "Let's write TMP here, next to *amchi*," as we made an introductory slide about the social status of Sowa Rigpa in Nepal. "Then I can explain that we are both *Tibetan* and *traditional!*" Thoughtful, he continued, "In truth, people like us hold traditional culture." This time he used the Tibetan phrase *rikné nyingba*, which literally means "old systems, traditions, or fields of knowledge." "We make our medicines in ways we learned from our fathers. We don't use much Western medicine. We live in the high mountains. We eat *tsampa* and drink butter tea!" Gyatso chuckled as he spoke. This was all true, even as it was a playfully ironic assertion about how he understands the ways other people see him. Yet in the eyes of people like Gyatso's roommate at this conference, a high-powered doctor from the Men-tsee-khang in Dharamsala, this position was double-edged. I spoke with this doctor about the possibility of recruiting senior Lo Kunphen students for further study at Men-tsee-khang. The doctor hedged.

"We would like to help such students," he began, addressing me in English. "They come from places with a long history of Tibetan medicine. But entrance to our program is competitive. Students need English as well as Tibetan. They need to have passed the School Leaving Certificate. We only have limited positions open for students from the borders," by which he meant people from places like Ladakh and Mustang. In other words, these are the "borders" of cultural or ethnographic Tibet, which bear little relation to the Tibetan government-in-exile's domain of authority. "Most of those seats go to Ladakhis because they are already part of the Indian education system." These comments were not spoken with condescension or bad intent, but they reaffirmed a sense that Nepal's *amchi* are at once valuable *and* peripheral to contemporary Tibetan medicine. People like Gyatso represent a certain kind of authentic knowledge, bound to Himalayan social ecologies. Yet their possibilities for advancement are also profoundly limited by these same characteristics, including their positions as marginalized citizens of Nepal, that little yam stuck between two boulders, as the first king of Nepal, Pritvi Narayan Shah, famously described this landlocked territory between India and China.

GENDER, AUTHORITY, AND EVALUATIVE FRAMES

On a warm day in June 2004 I hail a taxi and head toward the Tibetan Medical College in Lhasa. Silvery willows and poplars glinting green-gold line the streets as the taxi races by newly constructed rows of mixed-use buildings: shops below, apartments above, Tibetan façades overlaid atop cinderblocks. The driver crosses two double lanes of traffic, does a U-turn, and jolts to a stop in front of a pagoda-style gate that frames the entrance to the college.

I've been to the college many times during my two years in Lhasa, but this is a special occasion. My colleague, Mingkyi, is presenting her thesis to a committee of senior doctors. This public oral examination is the penultimate step in earning an advanced degree, known in Tibetan as *rabjampa* but viewed by the Chinese educational authorities as equivalent to a master's degree. Mingkyi and I have been working together for more than a year now on a maternal-child health project, including preparations for the first randomized clinical trial of a Tibetan medicine in Tibet.

I walk through the gates of the college, past the looming marble statue of Yuthog Yonten Gompo, the figure often referred to as the fa-

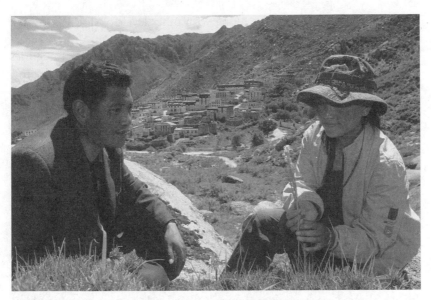

Mingkyi Tshomo (R) and a colleague from the Tibetan Medical College identifying medicinal plants on the hillsides above Lhasa, Tibet Autonomous Region, China, with Sera Monastery in the background, 2004. © Thomas Kelly

ther of Tibetan medicine,[8] and on to the auditorium. Other students, teachers, family members, and friends have begun to file in. Mingkyi's kind, freckled face peers out from the wings of the stage. She greets me, looking anxious in her neatly pressed *chuba*. She is already an accomplished doctor. Born in a nomadic community on the northern edges of the TAR, Mingkyi began studying medicine at thirteen. After completing the equivalent of high school, she sat for the entrance exam to the Tibetan Medical College. First she was admitted to a three-year course of study, the equivalent of a technical college degree. Then she spent another two years earning the equivalent of a bachelor's degree. Throughout her formal education she has also sought out private tutorials with master teachers to whom she has had access in Lhasa and elsewhere.

Mingkyi began teaching at the college several years after completing this five-year course. For the past two years she has simultaneously been a master's-degree student and an instructor. How is this possible? Earning an advanced degree in Tibetan medicine is a relatively new phenomenon, although the college has been graduating practitioners from three- and five-year courses since the mid-1980s.

The designation *rabjampa,* along with other levels of distinction such as *lhaje* and *menrampa,* have been used for centuries in a range of Tibetan social contexts. However, the translation of indigenous categories into Euro-American educational equivalents—masters and doctorates—is new. In 2004 nobody had yet completed a Ph.D. in Tibetan medicine, although this transition was on the cusp of occurring both in Lhasa and Xining, as well as at the Central Institute for Higher Tibetan Studies in Varanasi, India. A new marker of Tibetan medical legitimacy and a new form of lineage have been created through these advanced degrees.

"We will begin soon," Mingkyi says, taking my hand in hers.

"Are you nervous?" I ask.

"No, but I am only worried the examiners will not be open-minded to my methods or results. College leaders sometimes think in old ways."

Some senior practitioners in this institution felt strongly that graduate studies should build on the tradition of writing commentaries on classical Tibetan medical treatises. Some felt *rabjampa* projects should have a clinical research component. Other leaders encouraged students to conduct research that used biomedical analytic categories, technologies, or methods to examine aspects of Tibetan medicine. Students I met in Lhasa in 2002–4 were focusing on textual studies of particular Tibetan medical disease categories, while in Xining in 2010 graduate students leaned more about projects with an applied public health and epidemiological focus.

Each of these models has specific benefits and drawbacks. At times biomedical technologies can service Tibetan ways of doing science; however, the desire to "prove" the merits of Tibetan medicine in biomedical terms or to valorize the ideology of biomedical science over Sowa Rigpa can create conflict or confusion (Adams 2001b; Adams and Li 2008; Adams, Schrempf, and Craig 2010). Mingkyi's project was a critical examination of Tibetan medical theory and practice with respect to women's health and an engagement with biomedical clinical research. She was concerned it would be perceived as controversial.

Beyond this, Mingkyi's fear of being confronted by "people who think in old ways" during her examination reflects the gendered dynamics at the college. Of the fourteen graduating students, only three are women. Aside from Mingkyi, one is the daughter of a prominent physician at the Mentsikhang; the other is from Amdo, the daughter of a famous *menpa,* as Tibetan medical practitioners are known in that region. Mingkyi and other women *amchi* have often shared with me their struggles to balance the demands of marriage and family with being doctors. Other female practitioners I know have not married. Mingkyi is divorced and is raising a son with the help of her mother. Although she and her female contemporaries have not been overtly constrained by their gender, very few senior college or Mentsikhang leaders are women. As in other cultural contexts, Tibetan gender norms do not make it easy to be an outspoken woman or to challenge elder male authority figures.

Eight senior leaders of the college, none women, take their places on the stage; they are the examiners. Each student takes his or her turn at the microphone. Sleepy PowerPoint presentations give way to lively Q and A. There is no overt indication of whether a student will pass, but I sense advanced degrees will be conferred on all. Ultimately it is in the interest of this institution, and the enterprise of state-supported Tibetan medicine in China, to increase its visibility and legitimacy by bestowing translatable credentials and concomitant social and scientific prestige on a new generation of experts.

When it is Mingkyi's turn, a wave of nervous energy passes through me. I want her to do well. She begins by discussing the importance of women's health for the well-being of society, and of health problems at the village level. She summarizes what the *Gyüshi* has to say about women's disorders and complications of labor and delivery. She compares biomedical anatomical drawings of women's reproductive organs with Tibetan medical paintings and texts, describing the womb of an expecting mother as being like a "palace."

"Important Tibetan doctors did not take care to address women's health problems, because they were powerful men," she says. "Too many women still suffer and die in Tibetan areas." While Tibetan medicine has the innate capacity to address a range of obstetric, gynecological, and public health issues, Mingkyi argues that a lack of social and political will has meant this has not been a priority, either in the "old society" prior to the 1950s or, in her opinion, in the present. Several examiners shift uneasily in their chairs. Mingkyi then outlines the research projects with which she has been involved: a child nutrition project, public health research, and the maternal-child health research on which we are collaborating.

"Some people feel that to use the tools of Western medicine is dangerous for Tibetan medicine, that it will pollute our knowledge. Others follow Western medicine blindly, as if intoxicated. But must we follow either path, exactly?" she asks, rhetorically.

"In times past, Tibetan doctors did so many kinds of work. They collected ingredients, taught students, and made small research projects investigating the nature of their own knowledge and experience. This is very different from how we work today." Mingkyi notes how distinct the meanings are behind the term *research* in Tibetan, Chinese, and English.

By this point she has forgotten her slides and simply speaks from the heart. Just as she launches into a detailed description of her thesis research, the examiners cut her off. She has run out of time. Questions begin. I cannot follow each query, but I understand that many focus on the ways medical evidence is construed in Tibetan and biomedical sciences. One examiner says, "Something in your presentation did not seem correct. You talk about Tibetan medicine in relation to 'science.' Is Tibetan medicine not a science? We have thousands of years of history, so what do you mean here?"

Mingkyi takes a deep breath and answers, "We have history, yes. But *rig,* what we call 'science,' is also a particular kind of knowledge. It is different than Western science, *tsen rig.*[9] In our tradition, discoveries have been made based on individual experience and what we might call qualitative methods, rather than methods that can be reproduced in the same way in different environments. Our approach is useful, but its benefits are limited. In the same way, if we only look at numbers or use quantitative methods, this will limit how we see a problem."

Mingkyi faces more questions. Visibly nervous now, she stands her ground, pointing out how Tibetan medical theory illuminates causes and conditions of suffering, but also how its own patterns of "conventional thinking" can limit its utility. As is the case with social studies of science more generally (see Kuhn [1962] 1996; Latour [1979] 1986; Hacking 1990), Mingkyi wants to hold both biomedicine and Tibetan medicine up to scrutiny. She challenges the uncritical use of "tradition" as an excuse for reproducing power relations and stifling what she calls the "boundless" creative potential of Sowa Rigpa. I wonder about the extent to which such "conventional thinking" might also be a veiled expression of frustration with the constraints of institutions in general along with the proverbial "elephant in the room": state control of knowledge in China and the privileging of scientific materialism.

"The world is changing," she goes on. "We need to hold our heritage even as we face modern challenges. In teaching, research, and treating patients we must skillfully combine Tibetan and Western medicine." She uses the phrase *chilug gi men,* "outside medical system." "We can learn from how Western medicine sets specific goals and tests them. However,

Tibetan medicine must not be taken advantage of—not treated like a child." The simile illustrates how heterodox medical practices can be infantilized or co-opted through engagements with "integrative" medicine that essentially enfolds CAM or Traditional Medicine therapies within a biomedical framework (Quah 2003).

Mingkyi passes her examination, but she seems dissatisfied. In the weeks after this experience something seems to change in her. By summer's end she has decided to pursue an advanced social science and public health degree in Europe. This is not an easy decision. It requires securing sponsorship, procuring a passport, being granted permission to leave her teaching post at the Tibetan Medical College, and sending her son off to boarding school. But she is determined. "If I do not leave," she says, "it will limit the ways I can be of benefit in my life, and what I can do when I return to Tibet. This is for me. But it is also for modern Tibetan medicine."

TWENTY-FIRST-CENTURY *AMCHI*

When I think about Tshampa Ngawang, I imagine his graceful hands and his manner of speech. This *amchi* is at once forceful, humorous, and eloquent in Tibetan, Nepali, and even halting English. I have known Tshampa for almost twenty years, since he was my mentor and key interlocutor through an initial foray into long-term fieldwork (Craig 2008a). He comes from an *amchi* patrilineage (Sihlé 1995). His father and Gyatso's father were contemporaries, although the latter outlived the former by two decades. Like Gyatso, Tshampa wears many hats within the social ecology of Mustang. He is a *nakpa*, a painter and woodworker, a hotelier and an educator, as well as an *amchi*. Tshampa has led efforts to improve the standing of Sowa Rigpa in Nepal, chairing the HAA from its founding in 1998 until 2003. It is his photograph that graces the cover of this book.

In August 2008 I return to Mustang for the first time in five years. My daughter, nearly four, is traveling with me. Aida was born within days of Tshampa's first grandchild, also a girl, who now lives with her mother in New York. *This too bespeaks lineage*, I think as I approach the Dancing Yak Lodge in Jomsom, holding Aida's hand. Tshampa and his wife, Karma, greet us warmly. Tea is served. As I look at Tshampa, I think about the ways we've changed over the years. Although he has gone through many phases of vocation in the past two decades, physically he seems to have hardly aged. He once told me he would live to be

125 years old. "Just like Yuthog Yonten Gompo," he said. On this morning in Jomsom it seems a reasonable proposition.

Tshampa and I have a lot to catch up on. While my daughter naps, I follow him into the small clinic beside his lodge. The room is well designed. The doctor's desk faces the door, framed by a wall of handmade medicines in glass and plastic jars. Other shelves are crammed with cotton bags of raw materials. The opposite wall is lined with books: Tibetan medical texts, field notebooks from Tshampa's years of research, reports on health care and rural development, and copies of the student papers, graduate theses, and stories that were inspired by Tshampa, some of my previous work among them. A white cloth is draped over the desk, on top of which rests a silver measuring spoon, studded with coral and embossed with a lotus flower motif. This once belonged to Tshampa's father. Beside this desk is a locked cash box, atop which sits a receipt booklet. Tshampa prescribes on a sliding scale, but unlike some other Nepali *amchi* with whom I work, he routinely charges for his medicines, especially when transactions occur within the clinic walls or patients are not local. A row of pictures, letters, and certificates crowns this space, in uniform golden frames. Each document is a visual evocation of legitimacy: Tshampa beside Rumtek Monastery in Sikkim; Tshampa with Jhampa Thinley, a famous scholar-practitioner in Lhasa; Tshampa before His Holiness the Fourteenth Dalai Lama.

"Do you like my new clinic?" Tshampa asks in Tibetan.

"Yes," I nod. "Do many people visit each day?"

"Oh, *many* people," Tshampa affirms. "Sometimes they wake me up in the early morning. Other times they come late at night. But this is my duty." Humility is not Tshampa's strong point, but he is a compassionate, effective doctor. Sometimes social tensions have impinged on the perceived efficacy of his practice. Similar criticisms have been leveled against Gyatso and Tenzin in their efforts to run Lo Kunphen. Mustang is a place of gossip and rumors, where being overtly "uppity" is not condoned, but everyone is looking to get ahead nonetheless.

"How is Tshéwang doing?" I ask after Tshampa's youngest son. He has recently completed grade 12 in a Tibetan medium boarding school in Kathmandu and now has begun medical training, although not under the tutelage of his father. Instead Tshampa decided to enroll his son at Chagpori Institute in Darjeeling, West Bengal. In its original form Chagpori was a monastic college of Tibetan medicine, founded in Lhasa in 1696 by the Fifth Dalai Lama's regent, Desi Sangye Gyatso. Chinese Red

Guards destroyed the institution in 1959. Under the guidance of the late Buddhist master and renowned *amchi*, Trogawa Rinpoche, Chagpori was reestablished as Chakpori in Darjeeling, India, in the early 1990s. Although its examination structure and many of its teachers hail from the Men-tsee-khang in Dharamsala, Chagpori retains its own institutional sensibility.

"Why did you decide to send Tshéwang to India to learn *amchi* medicine? Why not train him here, with you?" Personal politics between *amchi* families in Mustang means that Tshampa never would have sent his son to Lo Kunphen; there is too much "bitter speech," in the Tibetan phrase, between Tshampa and Gyatso for this to have occurred. Besides, after a decade of schooling in Kathmandu, Tshéwang was essentially an urban Nepali youth. He returned to Mustang each year, but he was acculturated to the city, and his educational aspirations were coupled with the eventual goal of earning a salary.

"Sending Tshéwang to India is in perfect harmony with the main goals of the HAA," Tshampa responds. "This organization aims to continue Nepal's medical lineages, to pass on knowledge." Tshampa folds his long brown fingers in his lap, looks me straight in the eye.

"First we had Yuthog Yonten Gompo. Then we had Desi Sangye Gyatso. From that time on, Sowa Rigpa began to see for itself the goals of its development." Tshampa uses the word *yargyé* for "development," but this Tibetan term also means "to be uplifted or elevated," with respect to spiritual practice. "You need family lineages but also other teachers," he continues. "My grandfather and father were important teachers. But I have had other teachers of *bodhisattva* mind *[jangchub sem]* from whom I have had oral instructions *[lung]* and received empowerments *[wang]* in Tibet, Bhutan, Nepal, India. There is no difference where you get real teachings, with people who share right motivation."

"What about Tshéwang?" I ask. "He is studying with good teachers in India, but he is not here, learning from you."

"Oh, yes he is!" Tshampa responds. "He studies in India, but he comes to me on vacations. Tshéwang is benefiting from two systems of knowledge. And in life, two is always better than one! Two horses, two sons . . . well, maybe not two wives!" Tshampa jokes. "Too much trouble!" Regaining his composure, he explains that they chose Chagpori because of the lineage of teachers with which it is associated.

"To be *twenty-first-century amchi*," Tshampa says this phrase in English, "we need *twenty-first century* goals. We need to do research and support different forms of education. Tshéwang passed class twelve before he went to Chagpori. He has good Tibetan language and also English, Nepali, Hindi. You need languages for communication. You need this for patients. Patients will come from many countries. The world is becoming a small village, oh yes! Tshéwang should speak many languages. I can get by with Nepali, Tibetan, Hindi, and some English. For Tshéwang, this is not sufficient. He needs superb English. It would be good if he could learn other European languages too. Or Japanese. The Japanese love our medicine!" Tshampa's experience with Japanese donors, film crews, and foundations has led him, aptly, to this conclusion.

"I have invested wealth in Tshéwang to send him to Chagpori, but he is doing well. Among all students, he is *top ten.*" Tshampa then turns to my original question. "I have made this decision to protect my lineage [*gyüpa*]. From the eighth century to the twenty-first century, in this way Sowa Rigpa will remain strong." He sees an institutional education as a way of maintaining lineage-based legitimacy.

My fieldwork in China reveals parallel sensibilities, although the social and political pressures at play in these shifts from local lineages to institutions are distinct (see Schrempf 2007; Hofer 2011b, 2011c). A lineage doctor from the shores of Qinghai Lake sends his daughter to train in Xining; she now practices at the Tibetan medical hospital in her county seat. While sitting in on a lecture in the master's-degree program at the Qinghai Medical College, I learn that one student is the son of a lineage doctor from Huangnan Prefecture. The son is being educated in the provincial capital. And yet I notice a profound shift in that classroom in Xining, when compared with how Tshampa, Gyatso, and others of their demeanor have described the education they received. In a word: *textbooks.* Knowledge is codified and presented in new ways. It is ordered differently. People still study the *Gyüshi,* but instead of mnemonic devices and prose poems of medical theory, they rely more on reordered chapters, summaries, and new commentaries.

"Tshéwang will be able to practice many places, not just Mustang." I note how global this vision of Sowa Rigpa's future is, and how this resonates with Mingkyi's thinking and even aspects of Gyatso's and Tenzin's hopes and dreams. I know Tshampa well enough to ask him a difficult question in response.

"This is good for Tshéwang, but what about treating people here in Mustang? Expanding Sowa Rigpa in the world is beneficial for *amchi* development, but who will care for people here, once you die?" I wonder what the repercussions of this trend will be for health care in Mustang, as patterns of health-seeking behavior continue to shift with outmigration as well (Craig 2011b).

"Tshéwang may choose to live in Mustang for at least some part of each year, to help the people," Tshampa answers honestly, "but I cannot force that. When Tshéwang comes home, he helps me in the clinic. I teach him about making medicine. This is a weak part of the school learning. Now these ready-made medicines are too much *modern fashion*," he says, speaking of the Tibetan medical industry in India and China, as well as the few burgeoning factories in Kathmandu.

We are interrupted by a knock at the clinic door. A woman arrives with her four-year-old daughter, who is weakened by diarrhea. Tshampa feels the girl's pulse by touching her ears. "The disease is seasonal, not serious. Do not feed her meat or dairy products until the diarrhea stops," he directs the mother. He prepares three satchels of medicine, for thrice daily administration, and then asks the woman to pay 100 rupees ($1.50) for the prescription. He records this transaction in his ledger.

Next a local woman with a toothache enters. Tshampa examines her and says the toothache has "gone to [her] brain." He switches from the Central Tibetan we have been speaking to the more guttural local dialect, describing this problem in terms of *sin*, a class of disease-causing agents sometimes translated as "bacteria." The woman says she has been to the Jomsom hospital. Tshampa gives her five days' worth of medicines. He does not ask her for money. Once she leaves, he confides, "She is a little bit crazy."

Tshampa and I chat in the lull between patients. Soon in walks a thirty-two-year-old Hindu Nepali man from Pokhara. He has a stomachache. Tshampa takes his pulse and examines his tongue. "You have too much acid," he addresses the patient in Nepali. "It is a water-changing phlegm disorder," he then says to me, in Tibetan. "If you don't have *gyastric*, you're not Nepali!" Tshampa jokes, in Nepali, with this new patient.[10]

Tshampa hands the man several satchels of pills and powders and labels them "morning," "afternoon," and "evening" in Devanagari script.

"This is my first time taking *lama ko aushadi*," says the Nepali man. This phrase means "lama's medicine." The patient's choice of words marks this therapeutic encounter as an ethnic encounter, a slightly exotic healing practice inflected with Buddhism.

"We call ourselves *amchi*," Tshampa explains.

"I believe in *herbal medicines* more than *chemicals medicine*," he says, the latter referring to biomedicine. Tshampa pulls out some newspaper clippings about the HAA and himself, explaining in brief the tradition to which he belongs. "Now that you show me these newspapers, I remember hearing about you from a friend in Pokhara. I will introduce many new patients to you, Tshampa *ji*. We cannot keep your talent hidden in the corner!"

Tshampa grins. The patient asks for a bill.

"The medicine really costs 600 rupees, but you can pay only half since you will send me patients," Tshampa answers. This act links his practice with altruistic ideals and reciprocity: the promise of patient referrals in the future begets a discount now.

While this strategy may be employed in this instance by a twenty-first-century *amchi*, it is, as they say, one of the oldest plays in the book. In the Tibetologist Janet Gyatso's forthcoming work, *The Way of Humans in a Buddhist World: An Intellectual History of Medicine in Early Modern Tibet*, she highlights the concept of *mi chö*, or the "way of humans." The term, she argues, highlights distinctions between Buddhist ethics and the moral compass of a practicing physician, bringing to the fore questions about legitimate behavior and efficacious practice for an *amchi* as opposed to someone whose primary focus is Buddhist philosophy.[11] *La chö*, meaning Buddhist *dharma*, articulates a moral sensibility trained on dispelling illusions of self that define cyclic existence (Skt. *samsara*). *Mi chö*, in contrast, are practical moral principles.

"In medicine," this scholar recounted when reading from her translation at a conference in 2010, "*mi chö* eclipses Buddhism and is the main topic of interest. Buddhism is along for the ride, giving a patina of religious legitimacy to something based on an empiricist, scientific reality, the direct reality of patient suffering, and the possibility of death." Gyatso's work shows how Tibetan physicians are impelled to "learn skillfully, speak compliantly, and control toughly." Chapter 31 of the *Instructional Tantra* of the *Gyüshi* condones the practice of doctors doing what they can to get ahead in the world, but warns, "If you are lazy, or become too confident, there may be a lawsuit." Such words, likely written in the twelfth century, should dispel any Orientalist illusions that, unlike stereotypically greedy or inhumane Western doctors, Tibetan practitioners are somehow beyond ego or material concerns.

This chapter also discusses *namdzö*, a sense of artistry we might equate with the Greek term *techne*, evoking the embodied artistry and skill learned through apprenticeship. These skills are not only technical. As a doctor, one must "choose one's words carefully" as a way of responding to life's unpredictability and the practical impossibility of addressing all human suffering. *Mi chö* advises a type of "doublespeak," in Janet Gyatso's words, by which the physician hedges against too much hope or despair when talking with patients and their families. Although seemingly antithetical to Buddhist ethics, these culturally sanctioned tactics make practical sense. Outcomes of medical interventions are often beyond a physician's control. The stakes are, in a sense, higher than the esoteric if ultimately practical goal of taming the mind, which is the paramount aim of Buddhist practice. *Mi chö,* this way of humans, is a profound commentary on *being* human. I have witnessed *mi chö* in action while watching *amchi* in Nepal and China diagnose with compassionate firmness and prescribe medicines with an air of confidence in their efficacy and a desire for recompense.

Gyatso's translation of the chapter from the *Instructional Tantra* notes, "Be nice. Do what is asked. Gain a reputation. Then you can act tough." This "toughness" includes being able to ask for payment from patients as well as transportation fees: in other words, "getting what you are owed." This text goes on to say, "It is helpful if everyone is a little bit afraid of you." In a culture that can treat excessive ambition as negative, rivalry with other physicians is also taken to be inevitable— necessary to secure a livelihood. This fact is explained "without embarrassment," Janet Gyatso notes. I recognize here behaviors common among *amchi* I've worked with, including Tshampa.

Before Tshampa bids farewell to his Nepali patient, he suggests the man take a look at a larger-than-life-size *thanka* painting that hangs from the second-floor railing of Tshampa's trekking lodge. This work depicts Tshampa seated in lotus position, wearing the robes of a householder priest in the *nyingma* Tibetan Buddhist tradition. Images of Tshampa's father and grandfather rest in the uppermost corners, as do pictures of other teachers. The painting resembles traditional Tibetan art—brocade silk frames the canvas—yet there is something magical-realist about it. This is the work of the Virginia-based artist Jane Vance. Jane first met Tshampa in 2000. The *thanka* was produced in the United States and brought to Mustang in 2007, a journey chronicled in a documentary film, *A Gift for the Village.*[12] As Tshampa and the Nepali man talk about the painting and Tshampa's trips to America, I stare at this magnificent yet alarming work of art, thinking about *mi chö* and the pressures on *amchi,* whether of the twelfth- or twenty-first-century variety, to secure repute, and with it a living, and how this can require efforts to cultivate an image of oneself as well networked and well regarded by patients far and wide.

Yet something else strikes me as I stare at this painting. Women are absent. This pictorial reality is mirrored in Tshampa's choices regarding which of his children will inherit his medical lineage. Tshampa's three daughters are educated, two as laywomen and one as a nun. But none was ever considered for the study of *amchi* medicine. In this way Tshampa seems more socially conservative than Gyatso and Tenzin, the founders of Lo Kunphen, since one of Gyatso's daughters and a niece have studied at Lo Kunphen. Although Gyatso and Tenzin acknowledge that training women has been an adjustment, they feel that young women are more likely to remain in Mustang, to practice locally.

Over the echoing lines of a Skype call with Mingkyi in 2009, while she was studying in the United Kingdom, I asked her about these issues of women, lineage, and the transmission of Sowa Rigpa knowledge. She stressed that family lineage is not only *becoming* less salient but that, in her reading of the *Fourfold Treatise,* patrilineage has *always* been less important than religious lineage and oral instruction from master practitioners, regardless of one's family background or gender.

"Family lineage is 'smaller' than the profound continuum of medical and spiritual teachings," she said. Family-based knowledge might provide a certain form of security, she argued, but this alone should not be the basis of a doctor's legitimacy.

"Family-lineage doctors have problems now. They say they have knowledge from their father or uncle. But they only understand the surface of Tibetan medical teachings. They practice case-by-case. In my experience, this can be very dangerous. The *Fourfold Treatise* is so deep! Many people cannot understand it fully, so they find their own approaches to healing. Sometimes this works, but when diseases are more complicated, they have more trouble solving these problems because there is no systematic theory supporting the individual cases."

This emphasis on patrilineage, Mingkyi went on, "is not about who can practice good medicine. Tibetan women often have not received deeper medical educations or achieved higher positions due to cultural ideology, not innate difference. But men like to think women are weaker."

Mingkyi's social commentary with regard to gender, coupled with her assertion that family-lineage doctors were, at times, not up to snuff, not only contrasts with Tshampa's claims to expertise and his hopes for his son, but also puts a gendered spin on the pragmatic advice given to doctors in historical medical texts such as those Janet Gyatso translates. Historical references to female Tibetan medical practitioners are rare

(Adams 2000; Tsering 2005; Fjeld and Hofer 2012). How would *mi chö* be regarded if practiced by a woman? Mingkyi's thoughts on these matters are compelling because she advocates, in a sense, for standardization in response to gender inequity. Her standards are not derived from government certificates or family histories, however; they are rooted in immersion in Tibetan medical theory and oral instruction from Sowa Rigpa and Buddhist masters. Mingkyi promotes a devotional adherence to Sowa Rigpa fundamentals instead of an approach to practice constrained by patrilineage. She posits that twenty-first-century Tibetan medicine should inspire a "tradition" of change—of new gender norms and, as we have already seen, of innovative research practices, if not a re-visioning of the root sources of authoritative knowledge. This too is a certain kind of liberation.

THE INNER LIFE OF AN ASSOCIATION

On winter solstice 2007 I wrap myself in a shawl and head to the Himalayan Amchi Association office in Boudha, a Tibetan neighborhood on the eastern edge of Kathmandu. Dense fog clings to everything, resisting the flirtations of December sun. The HAA office is located in a shoddy structure. Its pale yellow exterior is water-stained. Iron rebar spirals toward the sky as a monument to a third story that was never completed. I sidestep a poorly designed sewage pipe and climb a flight of concrete stairs with no railing before entering the office: one room painted toothpaste green.

The HAA board meeting has already begun. Seated around a plastic table, in flimsy plastic chairs, are Gyatso Bista, the current HAA chairman and the cofounder of Lo Kunphen, whom you have already met; Menla Phuntsok, a smart Bönpo monk from Dolpo with a perfectly round face and a penchant for big ideas; Lama Namgyal, a *nakpa* from Dolpo with a crooked grin and an unassuming demeanor; Ngodup, a *tulku,* or reincarnate lama, and *amchi* from Dolpo, whose cloak is lined in snow leopard fur and who speaks only rarely; Karma, a diminutive elder *amchi* from Mugu District, west of Dolpo, who rarely comes to Kathmandu and, even on this morning, smells of dung smoke and rain; and Nyima, an articulate *amchi* from Mustang's Muktinath Valley who hails from a Bön family and was trained at a small school of Tibetan medicine in Dhorpatan, Nepal.[13]

Also in attendance is Tsering, a Tibetan travel agent who has supported the HAA over the years, and Tshénor, a young man from Humla who is the HAA's jack-of-all-trades: program officer, grant writer, secretary, translator. Puskar, the Nepali accountant, sits with a ledger on his lap, scratching his head at a pile of receipts. I am not the only foreigner in the room. Yoji Kamata, a Japanese development expert and anthropologist who has worked with *amchi* in Ladakh and Nepal, is also present. A decade my senior, Kamata looks young, save his graying temples. He and I serve as advisors to the organization. Our collaborations have focused on HAA conferences and on assisting board members with lobbying efforts, networking, and fundraising.

Three HAA board members are conspicuously absent. Tenzin Darkye, whom you will meet again in chapter 4, runs a private clinic in Kathmandu. He has promised to show up but is not yet here. Wangchuk is also missing. This senior doctor from Gorkha District has operated a small Tibetan medicine and incense factory in Kathmandu for many years, although he is now semi-retired and makes less medicine. He has connections to a Buddhist center in Italy and is currently in Europe. After handing over the HAA chairmanship to Gyatso in 2003, Tshampa has chosen to focus on projects in Mustang and is not in attendance. Menla Phuntsok and Lama Namgyal have just returned from Taiwan, where strong priest-patron *(chöyon)* connections between Dolpo lamas and Taiwanese Tibetan Buddhist devotees provide them with a source of income. Other board members have recently arrived in Kathmandu from their mountain homes. They travel to the capital in the winter for meetings, pilgrimage, religious teachings, and to purchase raw materials they need to make medicines. As I take a seat, *amchi* are discussing work with CTEVT.

"We have gotten 50,000 rupees from CTEVT to develop *guidelines*," Gyatso reports, an English term in an otherwise Tibetan sentence. "We need *guidelines* so we can make the *durapa* course. We should recruit students not only from Lo Kunphen but also from other Tibetan medium schools. This is my idea, but give me your ideas."

Namgyal responds, "Many students in such schools could study *amchi* medicine if we had a proper *durapa* course, in a place like Pokhara, not in any of our home regions." I note that the future of Sowa Rigpa in Nepal, as envisioned by this generation of lineage doctors, includes a strong desire to educate in classrooms, far away from where these *amchi* practice and how they were taught. At one level this is a practical acknowledgment of the challenges of rural life and the desire to provide opportunities for new generations in line with the shifting socioeconomic realities. However, this choice also speaks to the difficulty of recruiting teachers to rural areas. Ironically, although recent graduates from places like the Dharamsala Men-tsee-khang have been sent to Lo Kunphen to teach, they often leave after one season in the mountains. Rural mountain life is a social ecology to which they, as urban exile Tibetans, are unaccustomed.

My Japanese colleague asks, "The *durapa* curriculum is finished, right?"

"Yes, but now we need to make *guidelines*," Gyatso repeats, switching into Nepali.

"Have you all talked about what these *guidelines* should be?" asks Kamata.

"No! We all just came down from the mountains or back from Taiwan!" Gyatso responds, to the laughs of others. The comment is prescient. The HAA is firmly established yet also a fluid, even seasonal organization.

"How are *guidelines* different from *curriculum* you have designed?" I ask.

"*Guidelines* means what qualifications graduates of *amchi* programs should have. *Curriculum* is what we put in the lesson books," Tshénor clarifies.

"*Curriculum* is a *Gyüshi shortcut*," Gyatso adds. "*Guidelines* is also about who can join the *durapa*. We made rules that only students who graduate from Class Eight could join the *kanjenpa*. For *durapa*, we are thinking they need SLC-pass or to have completed the *kanjenpa*. But there are many questions. Will we give scholarships? Will students have to pay fees? Where will the teachers come from?"

Menla Phuntsok pipes up, ironic. "Because of course *we* are not qualified to teach in schools! We who learned from our fathers and grandfathers."

The group discusses whether a future *durapa* course—three years of intensive Sowa Rigpa study along with modules in the natural and health sciences—should be separate from Lo Kunphen or connected to that institution, since it is the only one in Nepal with any formal state recognition. Most lean toward connecting the *durapa* to Lo Kunphen. This is Gyatso's preference, but he is still wary of the responsibility.

"I've had lots of problems with the *kanjenpa*," Gyatso reflects. "We are getting two kinds of students. Some have Class Eight but bad Tibetan language. Some have good Tibetan but have not completed Class Eight. For example, one boy from Humla earned his SLC in Dolanji, India. He is very good in English and Tibetan, but he has no Nepali.

According to CTEVT, he needs Nepali language to begin the *kanjenpa* course. So Nepali language is stopping this student from learning *amchi* medicine."

"Governments are crazy," Ngodup contributes, arms folded.

"To give another example," Gyatso continues, "we got scholarships from an American NGO to send students *not* from Mustang to Lo Kunphen. We were supposed to find a student from Rasuwa District. This is a place where people want *amchi* medicine but there are no *amchi* in the region. We could not find a student from Rasuwa who had passed Class Eight and who had basic Tibetan language. So we found a girl from Solu." This is a district in eastern Nepal, south of the Everest region. "Her English and Nepali are fine. Her family said she knew some Tibetan, but she has had to start from the beginning—*ka, kha, ga, nga*," Gyatso sounds out the first four consonants of the Tibetan alphabet. "She is nervous, being far away from home and not being able to understand very well." I had met this young girl the previous week. She was homesick, miserable.

"I don't know if she will complete the *kanjenpa* because of the language and culture problems, even though she has a scholarship," Gyatso confides. "The young man from Humla could make a very good *amchi* and be of great help to his people. But now he is bored. He has chosen to leave Lo Kunphen and go to Amchi Gege's school in Dhorpatan."

"So he is still studying to be an *amchi*, just not at Lo Kunphen?" Kamata asks.

Gyatso affirms. "Yes, because he was frustrated by sitting in Nepali class with the little children!"

The school in Dhorpatan is the one from which Nyima graduated. Although his nine years of study were not recognized as medical training by the Nepali government, Nyima speaks highly of his education and reveres his teacher. "I know this young man," Nyima adds. "He has chosen to move from Lo Kunphen to Amchi Gege's school also because of family background. He wants to learn Bön medicine." The divide between Bön and Buddhist medicine is not openly discussed at this time, but it reveals points of tension in the HAA. Nyima and Menla Phuntsok are both Bönpo, while the rest of the group are Buddhist. Questions about how to account for this diversity within *amchi* identity have been silenced internally, usually with the excuse—voiced by the HAA's majority Buddhist members—that introducing Bön *and* Buddhism as frames of reference will only confuse the Nepali officials they are lobbying for support, particularly since the HAA needs to pitch *amchi* medicine as a coherent, standardized system of knowledge.

In the past, Nyima has voiced his skepticism to me about the HAA's pursuit of government recognition. In this meeting he says, "Methods of teaching are more important than government certificates. I learned from Amchi Gege for almost ten years. Besides, who knows what will become of the Nepali government? It is always changing." Nyima thinks the HAA should pursue connections with schools of Tibetan medicine in India. At an individual level, Tshampa has already made this choice by sending his son to Chagpori.

Ngodup passes around a business card for the director of the Tibetan Medicine Council, based in New Delhi. "Why don't we make connections with this organization? Maybe they would even invite an *amchi* from Nepal to serve on the council."

"Tenzin met with members of that council the last time he went to India," Gyatso responds, referring to his brother. "I don't think they would have someone from Nepal in this group, unless he was a Tibetan refugee who lived in Nepal. Everyone wants to be big kings of small kingdoms."

"Gyatso is right," Menla Phuntsok contributes. "We probably would not get a place on the council. But if we were able to have our *curriculum* approved by this council it would offer a little protection for the students we train—some kind of proof of their qualifications from the powerful schools in India. Today *amchi* need to protect themselves. In the past, if someone died under an *amchi*'s care in the village, this was not said to be the fault of the *amchi*. Care is his responsibility. But death is not his fault. Now the responsibility is different."

"This is also why *guidelines* are important," Tshénor says.

"Right now we are like children." Gyatso directs this comment to Kamata and me, in Nepali. "This is the first time we are trying to educate people in this new way. We need help for this reason." While Gyatso's sentiments are true in a sense, this lapse into a self-infantilizing tone from an otherwise strong-willed, creative person bespeaks entrenched power relationships, reflecting something of the "internal colonialism" (see Scott 2010) of Nepal's history, the neocolonial tendencies of development work, and the dynamics of being a *jindag*.

"We have heard examples of how some *kanjenpa* requirements, the ones that are part of the Nepali national curriculum, are holding students back. Learning some Western science and getting a diploma is beneficial for young people, but it takes time to study these other subjects," adds Nyima.

"If there is some Western science in what our students learn, fine," says Menla Phuntsok. "But if we have nothing but Tibetan language and Nepali subjects in the first year of a *durapa* course, then the beginning knowledge of Sowa Rigpa that students gained from the *kanjenpa* will be forgotten. There will be no continuity."

"What is the point of saying you are doing a three-year program in Tibetan medicine if you don't even start studying it until the second year?" Nyima interjects. "For our culture, I don't believe that mixing Western science from the very beginning is the right decision. It is mentally confusing."

"This is what they do in China," says Menla Phuntsok. "But it has created many problems. Tibetan medicine gets swallowed up by Chinese medicine and Western medicine."

"The root problem is language," adds Gyatso. "We can't really translate our way of science into English or Nepali. Government workers don't believe in our knowledge. As for education, nine years of study of *amchi* medicine will make you an *amchi*." He looks at Nyima. "The most important issue is individual capacity and right motivation. But what we study *does* make a difference. Problems arise when we try to make a new system. Sometimes we do not know which path to follow. If we succeed, it will bring great benefit for future *amchi,* for sick people, for Sowa Rigpa in the world."

"We can't say 'if' we will accomplish these tasks. We must say 'when' we will accomplish them!" Namgyal posits, oddly triumphant in a meeting that has been riddled with complexity.

Not to be outdone, Gyatso rises to meet Namgyal's statement. "This is hard work, but we can't be like a mother who doesn't give her baby milk just because she looks happy. We need to work hard, no matter what the obstacles."

"All this sweet talk is like yelling into the fierce wind," exclaims Menla Phuntsok. "We need to consider what the benefits of a government paper really are. After all, we could just have our good students start clinics and do what everyone else in Nepal does—just pay a bribe if someone comes asking for papers!"

"Yes," Nyima adds dryly. "And patients do not care if you have a government certificate. They care about the benefits your medicine can bring."

Although these comments are made in good humor, the underlying questions are serious. As a marginalized group of practitioners who have operated under the radar of the state for many years, the HAA members consider the costs and benefits of practicing "the art of not being governed," as Scott (2010) puts it, with reference to highland peoples of *zomia*, a mountainous region of Southeast Asia that spans at least seven countries (see also Shneiderman 2010). While Nepal's *amchi* are certainly not stateless peoples fleeing state projects of conscription or resource extraction—they are all citizens of Nepal who are trying to determine what, if anything, they might eke out of their government—they operate at the margins of the state, hedging bets in their search for self-determination. Most HAA members agree that the constraints posed by Nepali governmentality are possible to ignore or sidestep in the short term, but that disengagement now will cause problems in the future.

Gyatso reports that three Lo Kunphen students, all natives of Mustang, will take *kanjenpa* examinations soon. Each will apprentice in Mustang, but they will also need other job opportunities. Several students may be able to assist Darkye and Wangchuk. I ask if a graduate might find work at a Tibetan medical institution run in central Kathmandu by Tibetan doctors originally from Nyalam, near the Nepal-Tibet border. "Those Tibetans like to keep to themselves," Namgyal counters. "I'm not sure they would allow our students."

"What about some of the Men-tsee-khang branch clinics?" I ask. There are several in Kathmandu and Pokhara.

"We could ask, but they can be closed in their thinking," Tsering responds.

"They tell us our students are not qualified because they have not spent five years in Dharamsala," Namgyal interjects. Here we see the paradoxes of professionalization and the limited efficacy of an education that is an evolving hybrid of place- and family-based legitimacy, on the one hand, and institutional education, on the other.

At this moment Darkye arrives, motorcycle helmet in hand, apologetic.

"So, you have decided to bless us with your presence!" Menla Phuntsok chides. Darkye sits down, greets Kamata and me. Kamata asks Darkye if he would take on an apprentice in his private clinic. He says yes. As you will see in chapter 4, Darkye is an example of what can be done without a formal medical license, though with appropriate certification to run a pharmacy and with an entrepreneurial spirit.

"If our students can find good apprenticeships," Gyatso picks up, "and open clinics or find good jobs, as Darkye has done, this will help HAA's reputation, and the work we have ahead. Hopefully some students will work in remote areas, areas where they come from. We are saying this is a requirement, but sometimes young people want to live in the city and do not listen . . ." Gyatso's voice trails off for a moment. "It does not really matter if the boy from Humla is trained at Lo Kunphen or by Amchi Gege. If he studies well, he could open a clinic in Simikot," the district headquarters of Humla. "He could do well."

The final item of business is the question of whether to revive the HAA's small clinic. The members opened a clinic several years ago to promote their visibility and attempt to raise some money. The current office has been broken into, and the association's computer has been stolen. The storeroom where they keep copies of their literature and textbooks is prone to mold. They need a better space. The clinic presents a challenge and a possibility.

"Should we reopen our clinic?" queries Gyatso. "When we had one before, it helped us. But it was difficult for one of us to stay and be the doctor. We all have work at home."

Darkye offers, "If we make a new HAA clinic, then we need to devote ourselves to it. We can't just claim a physical space as our own but leave it empty on the inside. That is the way of the government, of *bikas*," he jokes, using the Nepali word for "development" ironically (see Des Chene 2002).

"We would need to fill the space with good work," says Menla Phuntsok, "and a talented *amchi*." All the board members nod in agreement, but when Gyatso asks for possible names of such an *amchi*, the only people they can think of are Tibetan refugees trained in India or Tibetans from China. I ponder the paradox of an HAA clinic staffed by an *amchi* who is not Nepali.

"You would also need to come up with money," Tsering adds.

The accountant Pushkar agrees. "You cannot just point toward foreign sponsors or the government as the solution. You all go off to Taiwan and Hong Kong and America and make money. Why not invest some of this into the HAA?"

In response to this direct criticism, Menla Phuntsok defends his right to use the money he earns from religious services abroad for personal commitments, including monastery restoration projects. Namgyal looks embarrassed at first, but then implicates Gyatso in his response. "I *have* to use money I make in Taiwan to keep my clinic going," he says. "Unlike some other people, I do not have many foreign sponsors." The social strain in the room is palpable. I feel it personally, not only as a researcher and an advisor but also as someone who has raised funds for clinics in Mustang and Dolpo. But this truthful, charged moment passes quietly.

Absorbing the tensions and the ties that link this group of *amchi*, I think about the meanings of lineage and legitimacy. In English the term *lineage* connotes descent from a common ancestor and a sense of belonging. It bespeaks the blessings and burdens of inheritance. Buried within the word is the idea of a *line*, and with this a sense of teleology, a well-defined path toward a specific end. In Tibetan the term *gyü*, translated as "lineage," also means "continuum"—of life, of mental processes, of sacred knowledge, of consciousness. Like the English equivalent, *gyü* can mean a very grounded sense of succession tied to birthplace, family, or clan. Yet *gyü* can also refer to an experiential moment when an initiate learns something that is, or will be, fundamental to his practice. This latter sense is evoked by the Tibetan title of the *Fourfold Treatise*. The term *gyü* contains the capacity for innovation within boundaries, as in a river shifting course. As you have seen, belonging to a lineage of healers can be an asset and a liability. Family lineage can connote primordial, embodied authenticity borne in blood *(trak)* and bone *(rü)* that is not reproducible in the context of institutional learning or, sometimes, even through intimate connections to a root teacher *(tsawé lama)*. Yet one can become imprisoned by lineage—bound to place or social relations (including gender inequity) that limit one's possibilities. In still other settings, lineage becomes the tail wagging the dog: legitimating a practitioner even though he or she lacks aptitude.

Legitimacy can be equally double-sided. The concept of legitimacy is imbedded within the notion of lineage in both English and Tibetan, by virtue of its reference to the circumstances of one's birth and ideas about everyday morality. In English, to be "legitimate" means to be genuine as well as normal, to be justified as well as legal or lawfully born. It means acting according to established rules, principles, or standards. The array of Tibetan terms used to approximate the English word *legitimacy* speak to Tibetan ideas about inherently existing *(rangzhin)* phenomena, reliability, authenticity, and genuineness, which lead to a sense of trust, confidence, and truth. In the case of Tibetan medicine, the perpetuation of lineage and the maintenance of legitimacy require social validation, a sense of pedagogical coherence, and an ability to defend one's intellectual and professional territory. The efficacy—in the Tibetan sense of beneficial and potent practice—of belonging to a medical lineage emerges within specific social ecologies that either grant or deny a practitioner's legitimacy. HAA members struggle to reconcile that which makes them legitimate in their home communities or among fellow practitioners—their connections to specific lineages of patriline and practice—with the more opaque, if still important goals of gaining governmental recognition and support. Likewise they wrestle with questions of allegiance, at times torn between individual endeavors and the compromises collective action requires.

At once politician and pragmatist, Gyatso tries to dissipate the tension, summarizing, "At home in our villages, we remain true to our lineages. This is one meaning of 'duty' [T. *chö*, Skt. *dharma*]. Now that we have some experience and *facilities,* we need to keep thinking with a big heart, not a small heart, and to work together. We also need a computer."

SUMMARY

When Sowa Rigpa practitioners become legible in the eyes of the Nepali or Chinese state through mechanisms such as nationally approved curricula, licensing, and incorporation into education and health care policy, new benefits and concerns arise. Gaining state support for Tibetan medicine, or even a combination of governmental and NGO sponsorship, can help promote culturally oriented education, including Tibetan literacy, in settings that do not always provide such opportunities to young people. We see this in the example of Lo Kunphen and other small institutions of Sowa Rigpa in Nepal (see Millard 2002). Nepali government schools do not teach Tibetan, even in regions where dialects of Tibetan dominate, and despite pushes by Nepali ethnic activists for the support of "mother tongue" education in the wake of political changes in the country since 1990. Likewise Tibetan medical colleges such as those in Lhasa and Xining lead young Tibetans in China toward a socially valued career that allows them to use Tibetan language more than Chinese in professional life. However, this opportunity to develop such expertise is partial, provisional, and shifting in today's PRC. Indeed peaceful protests over language policy in Qinghai Province—a pushback against privileging Chinese—has dominated Tibet-related news since 2010.

As this chapter has shown, gaining state legitimacy and support for Tibetan medicine can require that Sowa Rigpa theory be "integrated" into biomedical frameworks as well as national(ist) language and education policies. Nepali *amchi* struggle to translate Tibetan medical texts into Nepali so that this core curriculum might be comprehensible to the Ministry of Education. Similarly Tibetan medical colleges in China often mirror the framework of state TCM colleges. In both cases, contemporary curricula become Sowa Rigpa hybrids, structured according to both Tibetan and biomedical subjects. While knowledge of subjects such as anatomy and biochemistry are becoming increasingly important, these pathways toward legitimacy and licensure do not always succeed in producing outstanding Sowa Rigpa practitioners, even as the values of modernization, "rational" governance, and an allegiance to the *ideology* of science are emphasized, especially in China. In a previous publication (Craig 2007) I noted a "crisis of confidence" with respect to what young practitioners felt a Tibetan medical education conferred on them, with ethnographic comparisons from Nepal and China. Following Hofer (2011c), I'm now not so sure if *confidence*, necessarily, is the heart of the issue; rather, questionable employment prospects, concerns about access to medicines, an increasing reliance on new medical technologies (from blood pressure cuffs to ultrasounds and IV antibiotics), and meeting patients' desires are central to how young practitioners experience the efficacy of their training and their claims to legitimacy as practitioners.

The perpetuation of Tibetan medicine depends on practitioners' abilities to convey what they know to a new generation. This includes the oral transmission of knowledge; text-based learning, including the mastery of principles of diagnosis, treatment, and pharmacology; and hands-on apprenticeship. Patterns of knowledge transmission have shifted over the course of Sowa Rigpa's history, from institutional settings to private spaces. We can draw distinctions between knowledge learned in institutions and that which is passed down in more personal and secret modes, from master to disciple (see Hsu 1999). However, we should not view these two ends of a spectrum as Weberian "ideal types." In practice they can overlap. Despite differences between Tibetan medical education in Nepal and China, senior practitioners in both settings still test a young doctor's expertise. Increasingly, national governments must validate this knowledge. Yet the possession of a state-issued medical license does not necessarily mean that fellow practitioners or patients will recognize a doctor's praxis as valid. This type of legitimacy still rests, I argue, within culturally meaningful frameworks of authority and specific social ecologies. It is to such contexts—places where the work of healing plays out—that we now turn.

CHAPTER 4

Therapeutic Encounters

Illness is the night-side of life, a more onerous citizenship.
Everyone who is born holds dual citizenship, in the kingdom
of the well and in the kingdom of the sick. Although we all
prefer to use only the good passport, sooner or later each
of us is obliged, at least for a spell, to identify ourselves
as citizens of that other place.

—Susan Sontag, *Illness as Metaphor*

SPACES OF HEALING

Tenzin Darkye's clinic is located across from Swayambhunath, the "monkey temple" on the northern edge of Kathmandu. On a winter day in 2007 we meet at the base of the temple and I follow him across the ring road.

"This way," he says, guiding me by the arm. "My clinic is very *convenience*. Many local people from Mustang come. Others, like Nepalis, Sherpas, Tibetans, are also coming." I note the way my colleague parses ethnicity: "locals" are from Mustang, even though we are in Kathmandu; an array of "others" include lowland Nepalis, other high-mountain groups, and Tibetan refugees.

The sign he's hung above the door reads "Himalayan (Tibetan) Medicine and Clinic." Unlike Lo Kunphen, in which a reference to Tibetanness is conspicuously absent, here it is parenthetical, a loose marker of affinity.

Darkye is in his midthirties. He was born in the village of Dhi, an enclave east of Lo Monthang. After attending government primary school, he went to study with Gyatso and Tenzin's father. When his teacher died in 1996, Darkye continued his apprenticeship with Gyatso and Tenzin. Darkye came to Kathmandu in the early 2000s. He began working for Wangchuk, one of the HAA members, at his small medicine and incense factory. At first Darkye was only allowed to assist the senior

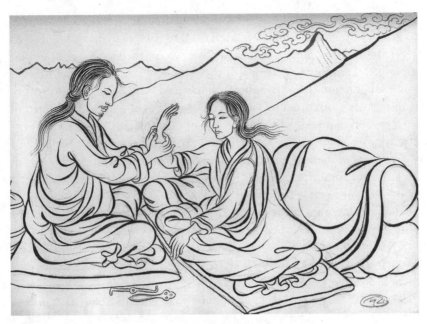

Depiction of an *amchi* from Dolpo, Nepal, reading the pulse of a patient, 2011.
© Tenzin Norbu

amchi, but after two years he helped Wangchuk open a satellite clinic in Kirtipur, the town on the Kathmandu Valley rim where Tribhuvan University is located. There his patients were primarily local villagers and university students, particularly women. Darkye developed a reputation for successfully treating a range of "women's disorders" *(moné),* including menstrual irregularities and infertility. After several years of work with Wangchuk, he struck out on his own. Darkye does not hold a formal medical license—he would qualify as a D-grade *amchi*—but his small clinic is registered as a private-limited pharmacy, currently under the auspices of Wangchuk's practice.

In a short time Darkye's practice has transitioned from a rural, community-based endeavor to an urban business. He goes to an office each day, dons his white coat, and treats patients. In his second-floor office, his blood pressure cuff and stethoscope rest beside the pillow on which he places patients' hands during pulse-taking. His human anatomy chart hangs beside a *thanka* of the Medicine Buddha. A copy of *Where There Is No Doctor* rests alongside a reprint of the *Fourfold Treatise* and several other Tibetan medical texts. Carbon copy pads, on which Darkye makes notes and writes prescriptions, are stacked on his desk.

These external indices of professionalization are connected not only to geography, indicating a shift from rural to urban environs, but also to ideas about development, modernity, and what a medical practice *should* look like. The notion that health care should occur in a clinic has become salient among contemporary *amchi* and their patients. This reality is differently configured in Tibetan areas of China, where governmental intervention in people's lives and state support for Tibetan medicine penetrate more deeply into the countryside than they do in Nepal, and where ideas of medical professionalization, modernization, and forms of "traditional" practice cannot be decoupled from the historical reach of a strong socialist state. Yet in both contexts, private and hybrid spaces of healing proliferate. In Nepal these practices tend not to be connected with government health care, though they are sometimes supported by NGOs. In Chinese settings such clinics are sometimes established by Tibetan medical practitioners who have retired from their posts as government health workers (Hofer 2011c).

Darkye's clinic has been open about a year. On this Saturday morning the place is busy. The clinic comprises four rooms: Darkye's office, a pharmacy, and two treatment rooms, one of which contains five single beds. All but one bed is occupied at the moment with mostly elderly patients, hooked up to IVs.

"What types of injections are you giving them?" I ask Darkye, who has received no formal biomedical training.

"Vitamins, mostly. B complex and C," he answers. "Sometimes glucose or antibiotics. It helps patients to be strong." Although the everyday consumption of intravenous medicines is less common in Nepal than it is in China, the sense that this form of medicine produces a quick and powerful positive effect is pervasive here, as elsewhere (Wyatt 1984; van der Geest and Whyte 1988; Reeler 1990; Schrempf 2010; Hofer 2011a).

The pharmacy is stocked with vitamins, biomedical pharmaceuticals, Chinese herbal formulations, and Tibetan medicines produced by the Men-tsee-khang in Dharamsala, several China-based factories, and local pharmacies. Darkye relies on ready-made Tibetan formulas. He no longer has the time to produce his own medicines, although he spent many a day drying, pulverizing, and mixing plants and fashioning handmade pills during his apprenticeships in Mustang.

The second treatment room contains a desk at which a Nepali doctor sits, writing a prescription. Kuman, Darkye's associate, is from Dhading District. He studied in Lhasa, but in a TCM program, and then later, informally, with a Tibetan doctor. He is fluent in Tibetan and Chinese. "Mostly I serve as the pharmacist," Kuman explains. "I write out and fill prescriptions. But I also give acupuncture treatments and IV drips."

As Kuman and I talk, one of the patients in this room interjects, "This is a very good place to come for medicine. Not so much waiting or unpleasant sounds and smells like at the big Nepali hospitals, and the price is good too! It is like a *supermarket* for medicine where we can get all we need. Tibetan medicine, Western medicine, even Chinese needles to make the pain better. And the doctors *take care*. They practice with compassion *[nyingjé]*. They speak our language. We have trust in Dharkye because we come from Mustang. But look around. There are all sorts of people here."

These comments are perceptive. This boisterous older man from the village of Chuksang in upper Mustang values the diversity of treatments available. A certain degree of "integrative" practice appeals to him, and to other patients with whom I speak at the clinic; issues of formal qualifications or even sophisticated laboratory testing remain secondary, if they are mentioned at all. Equally important are considerations of cost. This clinic's prices for Tibetan medicines are in keeping with other Kathmandu clinics; IV infusions and pharmaceuticals are comparable to what one would pay at a pharmacy but less expensive than at a hospital; and the consultation fee is nominal, at 10 rupees (13 cents) per visit. Also significant is the manner in which medicines are administered. Based on my observations at the clinic, Darkye and Kuman spend, on average, seven to eight minutes with each patient in a setting that can hardly be called "private."[1] Stereotypes about "traditional" practitioners giving patients more time or attention than biomedical doctors often do not match empirical reality.[2] Yet themes of trust and shared language are consistent across my interviews with patients in clinic settings in Nepal and in China. People like to be treated by practitioners with whom they can directly communicate. Given the ethnic makeup of urban hospitals in Tibetan areas of China and in Nepal, this is not always possible. As such, clinics like this one fill a very important niche. Beyond language, the way advice about diet and behavior is given makes a difference. Darkye tells patients not to worry, not to eat too much chili, but also to go on pilgrimage, to recite mantra, and not to engage in immoral behavior. He rarely links the causes and conditions of an illness directly to nefarious spirits *(döndre)*, but he sometimes suggests that a patient should seek religious teachings or have rituals performed as part of the healing process.

Darkye sees a succession of people this morning. He reads the pulse and then takes the blood pressure of a young Nepali woman, a returning patient. Her previous *béken* disorder has resolved, but she is left with a *tripa* imbalance. Darkye asks her how many days of medicine she wants, giving her some agency in the process of medical decision making, and records this information on the carbon copy pad. She adds this sheet to a stack of other records, some from this clinic, others from biomedical and Ayurvedic practitioners.

I ask Darkye about the most common ailments he treats. "Many stomach problems—*gyastric* and ulcers—but also *tsa* disorders, the things you call *nerves* problems, along with arthritis, high blood pressure." The practitioner's answer reveals a practical and epistemological fluidity at work in this space of healing. When I ask Darkye how he understands the relationship between biomedical and Tibetan medical diagnosis and treatment, he says, "Sometimes you can miss problems when only looking from the perspective of one system. If you use tools from both systems, then you can know with more certainty what is wrong, and also how best to treat it." Perhaps, I think, but this elides a certain crucial and perhaps taken-for-granted translation that occurs when a blood pressure cuff reading signifies a *béken* disorder, or an illness of the *tsa* is at once equated to a neurological disease and causally attributed to a disturbance of the *sa,* earth spirits. In other instances, points of conflict can arise over how to read a patient or a set of test results, sometimes creating difficult choices for doctors and patients when it comes to deciding on a prognosis or a therapy (Adams and Li 2008).

Darkye treats between fifteen and twenty-five patients a day; on busy Saturdays he can see as many as forty. The *amchi* seems grateful for his expanding practice and says he is happy in Kathmandu. "I help more patients here than I would in Mustang, especially more *rongba* [lowland Nepalis]. This is good for their health and my livelihood. It also brings benefit for Tibetan medicine. More people who come here end up believing *[yijé]* in Tibetan medicine, having faith *[dépa].* Many come to me when they are frustrated with *gyamen* or if the Nepali doctors tell them their case has no hope."

Given the diversity of medicines and therapeutic practices at play within these walls, Darkye's insistence that this is a Tibetan medical space is significant. So is the sense that this clinic can produce hope and, in some cases, positive outcomes for disorders that have been deemed incurable by biomedicine. Here language is crucial. The question of what to call biomedicine in Tibetan is complex. Terms vary,[3] but *gya-*

men remains the most consistent signifier, in my experience. *Men* refers to a medicine, drug, or therapy. *Gya* is more multivalent. It means "extent, broad, and vast," but when coupled with the qualifiers "white" *(kar)* and "black" *(nak)* it denotes India and China, respectively. It signifies law and order and can also indicate urban or politically significant places. So the thing we might call "conventional biomedicine" means, in Tibetan, a medical system linked to power and authority, to urban centers, and to highly influential neighboring civilizations. *Yijé*, in turn, is a type of mental engagement that assumes belief that is not blind but rather well considered, apprehended through focused attention, meditation. *Dépa* is one of the Virtuous Mental Factors in Buddhism (T. *semchung gépa,* Skt. *kusalacitta*), but it also connotes serenity and trust, confidence and faithful acceptance. When I think about the deeper meanings of Darkye's comments, I come to understand that, far from clinging to miracles or superstitions, many of his patients visit this clinic not only after careful consideration of cost and convenience, but also with a keen experiential grasp of the limits of biomedicine and the ways it is enmeshed in particular relations of power, both social and economic.

It is early morning in a county town in Huangnan Prefecture, Qinghai. This dry landscape with its ochre-colored cliffs and dramatic bends in the Yellow River reminds me of places in the southwestern United States, that is, except for the Tibetan Buddhist monasteries and Muslim minarets. Rinchen, one of my research assistants, has arranged for us to meet a private doctor with a thriving local clinic this morning.

"He is very famous around here, mostly for acupuncture and moxabustion, but he also gives Tibetan medicines," Rinchen explains. "He is strict with patients. He yells at people who drink too much, and will not keep seeing people if they do not follow his advice. He will only see people if they agree to come for at least a week of treatment. Otherwise, he says it is not worth it. Even so, people come from far away to get his medicine."

We walk through the sleepy county town, past the police headquarters to a residential neighborhood of single-family dwellings surrounded by concrete walls. The gate to the doctor's home-clinic is open. There is no sign on the door. One would only know to come here through networks of local knowledge. The courtyard brims with fruit trees and flowers: nectarines, peaches, zinnias, and carnations. The clinic itself takes up three rooms of the house, including a glassed-in sunporch that has been given over to boxes of acupuncture needles, Chinese herbs, and Tibetan medicines.

Several patients are waiting to be seen. Some sit in the main room, while others squat in the courtyard. The doctor acknowledges us, then keeps on working. The room smells of burned hair and bitter herbs. Posters in Chinese and Tibetan depicting acupoints and organ systems hang on the walls beside two framed certificates. One is from the county health bureau. The other indicates that the doctor has received Tibetan medical training at the prefecture hospital. Rinchen comments that people like this doctor are often fearful of being regulated by government health authorities. "The certificates could be real or not," Rinchen says quietly. "This is China, after all. You can make anything here. But it is important for him to have these, not so much for patients—they trust his medicine—but in case anyone ever asks if he has permission to practice. Everyone comes here, even government officials and Party cadres, but you never know what will happen." Beside the certificates are posted images of the Medicine Buddha and several deities. Both the government certificates and the religious iconography are symbols of protection and authentication, in very different ways.

One treatment bed is positioned on the far side of this room. A thin Salar Muslim woman rests there, needles protruding from the region around her kidneys. A Tibetan nomad woman sits very still in a chair facing the doctor's desk. The doctor, dressed in a baseball cap and a slightly dingy white coat, is busy inserting more than a dozen needles into this woman's head, neck, and hands. Once the needles are positioned, the doctor prepares small pinches of moxa, places them on top of the needles, and lights each one. I learn that the Muslim woman on the bed is suffering from kidney and stomach problems. The nomad woman has a headache and neck problems. Another woman lying on a second treatment bed in a side room is suffering from a *tsa* disorder. She has been undergoing treatment several times a week for four weeks, traveling an hour each way by tractor to see this doctor.

Rinchen's sister, who has accompanied us this morning, sits down to get her blood pressure measured. She is feeling fine, but just wants a checkup. The doctor takes down an ancient cuff, which he says is "an authentic item from the time of Mao," as his first order of measurement. He then retrieves a newer blood pressure cuff and takes another measurement, comparing the results. "You have a small heart problem that could become a big problem," he tells the sister. "Don't eat too much

meat. Watch your diet!" Rinchen's sister nods. As we observe this interaction, Rinchen tells me the doctor is divorced and remarried, and that
the doctor's new wife is related to his mother. Rinchen's sister chats with
the doctor. The doctor brags that his four nephews have all passed the
college entrance exams. In these interactions I sense the smallness of this
community, the connections of alliance and descent that help delineate
pathways to treatment and circumscribe social ecologies of healing.

Moxa trickles down the needles in the nomad woman's head and
neck. The doctor removes some of the needles, palpates the area, and asks
her if the pain has decreased. The woman nods gingerly, so as not to disturb the needles that remain in place. Interspersed throughout these interactions are comments about where I'm from, and if I can speak Amdo
dialects. I follow the flow of conversation, but my attempt to insert
Lhasa-dialect Tibetan into the mix only confuses things. "She sounds like
she is speaking some real language, but I can't understand her!" one patient calls out from the side room.

Nearly all of the patients are women. I ask the doctor about this. "In
one year, I see more than five thousand people," he responds. "About
eighty percent are women. Mostly I give them Tibetan medicine and do
acupuncture and moxa. I also treat dislocated bones and sore joints.
Sometimes people come for women's problems. Around here, women do
not get to rest after birth. They work very hard all the time. So when
they come here they can get relief from their pains." The doctor seems
gruff but not disinterested in these gendered patterns of suffering. I note
the parallels with the gender composition in Darkye's clinic and even the
inpatients at Arura's medicinal baths unit.

"Sometimes people come to me from other hospitals. I take their [lab
and x-ray] tests and use them when deciding on treatment." This pattern of using biomedical diagnostics to confirm Tibetan medical diagnoses points to a crucial aspect of innovation and fluidity across social
and technoscientific systems, confounding notions of a medical system's
boundedness.

Through Rinchen I learn that most patients come to see this doctor
for between ten days and a month. When I ask about the economics of
this pattern and the choice of this clinic over public health care options
at the township, county, or prefecture levels, Rinchen explains that people
do not like the way they are treated at the big hospitals, or how they
struggle to communicate in Chinese. For many, hospitals represent a
last resort after seeking care from people like this doctor, making temple

visits and offerings to lamas, and self-medicating. On the town square I counted three private pharmacies, one run by a doctor who stocks Tibetan and Chinese medicines and biomedicines, and another branch pharmacy of a famous Tibetan medicine clinic in a neighboring county. Many of these medicines are not supposed to be sold outside a registered hospital or clinic setting, but this does not stop the commerce.

"At the hospital, even with medical insurance, you still have to pay two to three yuan for a registration fee to see the doctor," Rinchen continues. "But most people, especially women, think 'I can buy salt for a month for that amount of money,' so they do not go. Besides, if they go to the hospital they will always be told to have tests and buy medicines. It is more expensive. This doctor charges seven yuan [$1.25] for each treatment, but this includes all medicines, the moxa, and the acupuncture." This clinic is not only culturally appealing but also an efficient use of resources.

As the doctor treats a patient with sterile, disposable acu-needles, he jokes with me, "My needles come all the way from America!" Yet over the course of the morning I watch him use new needles and reuse others, after they have soaked in a disinfectant liquid, much like a barber would bathe his combs.

The final treatment encounter we observe that morning is with a toddler. He has trouble breathing and is not walking, although he is nearly two. The youngster starts crying as soon as he hears the doctor's voice. His mother plays songs on her cell phone to quiet him. The parents are from Rinchen's village. Both are government workers.

"They have money for the hospital, but they choose to come here," says Rinchen.

The mother explains that she is worried, and that her son has not been helped by visits to the county hospital. "We have given him their medicines and spent a lot of money, but received no good results." I note the idea of "receiving" results, as if one were being handed a divination. The doctor listens to the mother and responds not with words but with action: a quick sleight of hand that leaves the young boy with needles in the soles of his feet. Then he moves on to another patient.

Over the course of this morning I have witnessed no money change hands, no records written down. On paper it seems this space of healing hardly exists. But the practical importance of the clinic seems undeniable. As Rinchen and I prepare to leave, we pass another six people sitting in the courtyard, waiting to be seen.

STORIES OF SUFFERING

I now consider two illness narratives, one from Qinghai and the other from Mustang. Data from these interviews elicit common themes. Both are from older women in their midsixties to midseventies. Each woman uses a combination of Tibetan medicine, biomedicine, and ritual healing to address the causes of illness and choose treatment options. In both cases the cost of medicine remains an issue, as does accessibility to health care resources. These women suffer from illnesses that have, at least in part, distinct biomedical diagnoses: Parkinson's disease in the first case and tuberculosis in the second. They impact each woman's sense of biopsychosocial well-being. In addition, each illness, in how it is understood and experienced, contains what one might call cosmological or spiritual dimensions, tied to place. As such they exemplify the social ecologies concept.

Huangnan Prefecture, Qinghai Province, July 2010

A sixty-seven-year-old woman greets Rinchen and me on the porch of her home, inside a courtyard surrounded by high adobe walls. A cement incense urn stands in the center of the courtyard, surrounded by flowers. A well is located in another corner, a convenience brought about by a government-subsidized village development project. The house is wood-framed, although a small addition has been built of concrete, tile, and glass. This is Rinchen's natal village, although he no longer resides here. His uncle, who lives locally, accompanies us. As we begin the interview the woman's daughter-in-law is also present. The woman sits in a chair propped against the side of the house. She has few teeth, many decayed. A walking stick rests beside her. She shakes constantly. Her right foot taps, incessant and disembodied. Her hands rest on her thighs, half clenched. The woman's clothes are stained, her hair unkempt. We learn she has not been to school and has lived in this village for most of her life.

We begin, in the vein of other illness narrative work (Kleinman 1988; Groleau et al. 2006), by asking her about the illness she suffers from. What is it called? When did the problem start? She supplies halting answers, the tone of her voice unusually high.

"I have had this problem for three years," she begins. "It started with a pain on the left side of my head. Then my left thumb began shaking. It spread to my left side and then my whole body." She cannot feed herself or do household work. Her speech is labored. Sometimes she has trouble breathing. Her walking stick allows her limited mobility, but only if someone helps her up.

The woman has six children. One of her daughters attends school in Xining; two sons and two daughters no longer live in the village. A son and daughter-in-law live here, her primary caretakers. Her husband is an itinerant carpenter and is often away. Her youngest son works construction in another county and sends money home to help pay for health care, "since he does not yet have a wife."

We ask what she has done to address this illness.

"For the shaking, we visited hospitals in Xining two times. The first time we left with five thousand yuan [$695] and came home after eight days because the money was gone. I also visited Xining one other time, in autumn. I had a lot of tests. Then the money was gone." A round-trip between this village and Xining costs about 200 yuan ($26) for travel expenses. "The first time, my three sons accompanied me, but none of them speak Chinese. The visits were unhelpful, except for getting one medicine. The second time I went with my husband and elder son, but again we could not communicate. We asked the name of this problem. Doctors said something we could not understand." The woman adds that at first she also went to the county-level Tibetan medical and conventional hospitals, but in both places they told her to go to Xining.

"I do not know the name of this sickness. . . . Before I went to the hospital in Xining I could not even walk the distance from here to the road." She motions from her place on the porch to their gate, a distance of about thirty feet. "After that, when I came home from Xining with one medicine I could walk a bit more, with the walking stick."

I ask what medicine she was given in Xining. "IV and pills," she answers. Her daughter-in-law produces a brown paper bag that holds several boxes of Roche-manufactured Levodopa + Benserazide Hydrochloride .25g tablets. My suspicion that the woman may be suffering from Parkinson's disease is confirmed. I have this visceral sense that I am watching the progressive degeneration of neurons, the erratic seeping away of this woman's ability to control her movement, the brain starved for dopamine. Even so, I realize that while this designation might be helpful to me, it is a meaningless label to this woman and her family. A sign on a map written in a foreign tongue. A loose shard, not fitted to the mosaic.

While some studies have reported that China has the lowest rates of Parkinson's disease in the world, more recent studies that have taken into account regional and socioeconomic variation have reported prevalence rates much closer to those in the United States and other countries in the global North, suggesting the disease burden here is underestimated (Zhang 2005). Some clinical research has shown that Chinese herbal medicines and acupuncture can have a positive effect on the symptoms of Parkinson's. I wonder what a senior Tibetan doctor like Aku Nyima would prescribe for a patient like this, where he would locate the problem.

"I got these pills last year, after plowing season. The pills cost two hundred thirty yuan [$30] for one bottle. I take one pill a day, after eating. This year, my husband knows a person going to Xining, so we will send money with him to buy this medicine again." The woman seems satisfied with this medication even though she does not know precisely what it is for.

"I also suffer from kidney and cold-related disorders, but the shaking is the biggest problem. It is not a stable condition. Sometimes it is better, other times it gets worse. Walking is difficult. I cannot even scratch my own head." The woman's voice cracks. She begins to cry. I ask Rinchen quietly if we should stop, but before he answers the woman continues. "Now all the money goes to buy my medicines and pay for my daughter's school tuition. Because of this, I waited a long time to see a doctor. It was two years from when I started shaking until we went to Xining. The illness is now strong." Her decision to delay treatment was based on a pragmatic understanding of her family's economic limits and priorities— a decision common around the world—and she thinks these decisions have exacerbated her illness.

"The *menpa* may be right," says the woman, referring to a local Sowa Rigpa practitioner. "He tells me I have a disorder of the *tsa*." This comment signifies a moment of epistemological crossover between Tibetan and biomedical understandings, but also between material and cosmological causes of illness. As mentioned earlier, *tsa* can signify neurological disorders. They are located in the material body, but they also link to nonmaterial forces (Gyatso 2003; Garrett and Adams 2008). Problems of the *tsakar*, or "white channels," are referenced in relation to paralysis, seizures, and other forms of uncontrolled shaking or tremors (Samuel 1999). The term *tsakar* is the name for a specific bodily channel and can also be a euphemism for problems caused by malevolent spirits, especially those of the earth *(sa),* who are dangerous enough that sometimes people avoid speaking their names directly.

"It is also an illness of the heart," the woman goes on, using the term *nyingné*. Literally this means "heart disease," but it is not a cardiovascular problem; it is a particular idiom of distress used in this part of eastern Tibet to describe a range of biopsychosocial disorders that manifest as profound melancholy, sometimes with a violent streak (Bassini 2007). "When someone startles me, I cannot turn around. I am always afraid, especially at night."

"Did anything special happen when this problem began?" I ask.

"I got sick suddenly," she answers. "I had the thumb shaking and a pain in the left side of my head, but there was no accident." However, this discussion of the start of things reminds her that, when she gave birth to her first child, she had a sudden pain on the right side of her head and then her neck. "At that time I did not care about it or pay much attention. I was young. But this may be connected to these problems," she contemplates.

"When the shaking got worse, I took some Tibetan medicines. I visited two lamas and another famous *nakpa*. They said we should do rituals, but we cannot even provide good meals for them, let alone pay for rituals!" The market for ritual practice is enmeshed in a hierarchy of local social and economic capital (Dorje and Stewart 2009). A formal prayer ceremony costs, on average, 1,500 yuan ($210), Rinchen explains. Even the performance of a divination *(mo)* requires in-kind gifts and a small sum of cash. Clan members can perform ritual healing by chanting for an ill person, although such acts may not be considered as efficacious as a lama's performance, and may still be a burden for some families.

"Twenty or thirty men chanted for me. We gave them food. I do not know if this helped. Nothing but the medicines make me feel better. Still, we do these things as our custom." The woman adds that when she went to see the lama he did not tell her what was wrong. "He touched my head and blew on me and said prayers to Tamdrin [Skt. Hayagriva]. This is all he did."

When I ask the woman if there is anything she would like to do to improve her health or that she thinks would help, she says she would like to have more money for chanting and maybe for going to Xining again. Both ritual healing and biomedical treatments hinge on the income her son sends home from construction work and seasonal collection of *yartsa gunbu*. She is not registered for the Cooperative Medical System. I ask why. She says their village headman demanded that medical insurance funds collected from families be put instead into a monastery restoration project. She felt she had no choice but to comply. As such, any treatment she seeks is an out-of-pocket expense.

I ask her how she sleeps. "I need to sleep sitting up," she answers. "Lying on my back gives me a strong fear. But I do not shake in my sleep. It is a peaceful time when I am away from people and feel safe. . . . When I have to awaken, this makes me feel very bad." The specific local word she uses for this "bad" feeling is *anuk,* which Rinchen describes as a "profound" term that implies deep unease, which comes from the sense that someone or something has caused or sent this problem to her. Rinchen clarifies that, in its central Tibetan pronunciation, this term is *nö,* the word for "harm" or "injury." Rinchen goes on to explain that, in this region, "being harmed" is synonymous with being sick.

I sense this woman's discomfort in her own skin and come to rest on this concept of "sent" illness—a sickness brought on by the harm another person or a nefarious spirit wishes on you. Such an understanding of illness causality is not unique to Tibetan culture. Indeed the idea that some localized force or individual (in the form of a person, a cosmological entity, or a specific nefarious spirit) can "send" someone an illness remains a hallmark within anthropological studies of medicine and religion. For example, Paul Farmer (1999) describes "sent" illness in relation to folk epidemiology of both tuberculosis and HIV/AIDS in rural Haiti. He emphasizes that explanatory models that rely on the concept of "sent" illness are not necessarily replaced or discarded even when microbial or political-economic understandings of illness causality also enter the picture; I've found the same to be true in my fieldwork. Such explanations of illness causality can be expressions of interpersonal tension among family members or community rivalries; they can also be linked to environmental imbalances, social inequities, or problems of karmic inheritance, whether voiced by fellow villagers or whispered, as it were, by a disgruntled local god.

Muktinath Valley, Mustang District, Nepal, September 2008

A seventy-five-year-old woman, small-boned and frail, sits on a saddle blanket in the sun. Her graying hair is loosely braided. She wears a traditional Tibetan-style dress *(chuba)* around which is wrapped a hand-woven apron and cummerbund, their once rich indigo and vermillion stripes now faded. The woman's home is not far from the river. Like all other villagers in this part of Mustang, she fetches water from a village tap or, when winter comes, from the mostly frozen river. High clouds linger over Himalayan peaks in the distance. A nephew of the host is also at home and sits in on the interview. The woman has nine immediate family members, including a son and daughter in Kathmandu, both of whom are monastics.

When asked about illnesses from which she has suffered, the woman answers, "I have many health problems. Even though I have been taken to the hospital in the district headquarters, I was still not cured! I was going to die due to vomiting blood. The doctor told me it is TB. At that time I had been sick for more than a month. At first I only had a cough. It was bad before rising, but once I got up it would get better. But it turned to continuous pain. I thought, 'I will not be cured.'"

"What happened after you went to the hospital?"

"I was given an x-ray and then diagnosed. They gave me medicines for two months. I stayed three days in there." Directly observed therapy short-course (DOTS) TB protocols call for at least six months of treatment. I wonder how this woman's experience might be reconciled with Nepal's national TB policies and programs (Harper 2010). "When I felt very sick, my phlegm was yellow or white, and sometimes filled with blood. Since I began taking the medicines this has improved." Unlike the woman from Qinghai, this woman's narrative describes a positive experience with biomedical treatment available in a rural area. Of course, tuberculosis is a curable disease, but Parkinson's is not.

The woman's nephew interjects, "I think this sickness is caused by eating too many chilies and drinking too much alcohol!" He uses the word *chang-rak,* which signifies local barley beer and distilled grain alcohol.

The woman answers, "I drink only a little." Both men and women drink in Mustang. Alcohol can serve as a front-line painkiller. Most local festivals, community gatherings, and political oaths are sealed with spirits. I have witnessed the social and physical effects of alcoholism here. The idea that excessive chilies and alcohol cause a range of illnesses is also quite common, voiced by local *amchi,* government health care workers, and laypeople alike.

"First, all I had was that cough," she continues, avoiding for a moment this question of diet and behavior. "I went to the village health post and took some of their medicines—injections—but these did not help." When asked what sorts of injections she took, the woman cannot be more specific, aside from saying "medicines you get by needles, with water going into your body." Based on visits to local health posts, this could have been either a glucose-saline solution or an intravenous antibiotic.

"I got weaker and weaker after taking the health post injections. Then I vomited blood, almost two big bowls. I coughed. Then the blood came. I vomited blood like this continuously for ten or eleven days, so the health post doctor took me to Jomsom," she continues, using the term *doctor* to refer to the local community health assistant. "In Jomsom, my illness was diagnosed. I was given medications and told to return home. I thought about going to Kathmandu because my daughter is there, but that hospital doctor told me to take the medicines and go home. I also thought that Kathmandu is too warm and this will not help my illness. Maybe if I am better next winter, I will go to Kathmandu."

Family and medical dynamics continue to reveal themselves. "When I was very sick, I could not work," she elaborates. "During that time the doctors were kind. My son-in-law and my son the monk were here. But my daughter and son-in-law have their own child to care for and, yes, there are economic problems in our household. It is always like this, in this poor place. People travel out to foreign countries to earn money. If you are really sick, if you don't have money for a plane ticket to Kathmandu, you die. This happens so often. For me, at least the medicines from Jomsom are free." The woman's comments counter other narratives I've gathered from Mustang, which posit that good biomedical care can be found only *outside* Mustang, or even outside Nepal (Craig 2011b). This woman did not feel the medicines available at the health post helped her, but she trusted the government health worker enough to let him facilitate her referral to Jomsom, where she was given both free and, by her account, effective treatment.

"No, it is not the chilies or the alcohol that caused this problem," the woman continues. "I have TB." I note the different ways this woman talks about her diagnosis. First she says the doctor in Jomsom furnished her with the diagnosis. Then she insists that diet and behavior have not caused this problem, even though she does not offer an alternate explanation for disease transmission. I am not surprised to learn that the woman is familiar with TB as a concept. It is estimated that as much as half of Nepal's population of more than 29 million are infected with *tuberculosis bacillus* and that about 40,000 new cases of active TB occur every year.[4] While Nepal was one of the first countries in Asia to adopt the DOTS protocol for treating TB, and while there have been some remarkable successes (including cure rates of 90 percent and an estimated

75 percent of active TB cases detected), the implementation of successful treatment strategies has sometimes foundered due to the remote environments in which so many Nepalis live, the effects of a ten-year civil war, patterns of wage labor migration that often make it difficult for people to follow a single course of treatment, and other cultural and policy barriers (Harper 2010). As in other settings, multidrug-resistant TB and extremely drug-resistant strains further exacerbate these problems (Farmer 2004).

"When I ate those TB medicines, I felt *tséring,* like my life would be longer. The doctor told me to eat well and take this medication—all of it. Here is some of the medication." She pulls out a dusty package containing rifampicin and isoniazid, tuberculosis medications. "But now after some time, when I eat the medication I feel lazy. It has been a month now. I am having nine pills, always. When I started taking the medicines the blood stopped, but I was not able to walk because I felt dizzy. I think this is due to the powerful nature of these medicines. When I sleep for a long time, it is much better." This woman is not alone in reporting difficulties with tuberculosis drugs, both in terms of side effects, pill burden, and problems of adherence.

"The health post doctor brings her medicines," the nephew interjects, "and tells her not to drink alcohol or eat spicy foods, fatty things—like that." It is as if this dietary advice vindicates his sense of how she has contracted this disease.

"TB is a common illness in our village," the woman continues. "Last year someone else I know also got this illness. She went to Kathmandu for treatment and, oh, how much she spent! This is an easy illness to cure, but taking all the medicines is boring."

The nephew adds, "Earlier, my father also got the TB illness." I find this admission compelling and wonder if the nephew would also attribute his father's TB to diet and alcohol use.

"Now I am getting better with the doctor's medication," the woman summarizes. "How did I get such a bad illness?" she asks rhetorically, adding a final layer to the story of her suffering.

"My elder son, the monk, did a divination. He said I had taken food from a bad person and that there was a problem with a *shindre.*" The term *shindre* refers to a particular type of nefarious or malevolent spirit that has the capacity to remain attached to a person or particular activity after a person's death (Tucci 1980: 187). Sometimes this attachment is associated with a commitment that remains unfulfilled or an unresolved vendetta (Millard 2006: 11). "I remember meeting one person when I went for a checkup," the woman continues. "We had a cup of tea. After that moment I think I was followed by a *shindre*. My monk son did rituals to stop the *shindre* from following me. . . . Actually, there were two men who passed away at that time. I went to their family to apologize for celebrating the Yartung festival when they were mourning. I think the *shindre* from those dead men followed me continuously during Yartung. I also became sick for this reason." So this woman's understanding of tuberculosis—an illness common in this area, and treatable—is also conceived as a misalignment of local spiritual forces, being in the wrong place at the wrong time, and an inadvertent lack of respect for the dead during an annual celebration. The avenues for making sense of this sickness and returning to a state of health are equally diverse: from self-control over one's diet and behavior to a sense of folk epidemiology, from the prescience of divination to the strength of pharmaceuticals.

MAPPING ILLNESS

Back in Darkye's clinic in Kathmandu, I meet a man from Mustang who, in praise of the clinic, compares it to a "supermarket." As we talk, I learn more about his illness experiences.

"I have suffered from *khogma natsa,* a throat problem," he reveals. "I could not talk. When I did, it hurt. Yes, I have been to Om Nursing Home and other hospitals. The doctors could not explain my illness. They told me the cause is my being talkative. So they told me to stop talking. This cost a lot of money." The man laughs and throws up his hands. "After that I went to a lama to find out which type of medicine I should use, Tibetan medicines or *gyamen*. I was told Tibetan medicine is better. After that, I did treatment in Pokhara, but it didn't work. Later I heard from some relatives living in New York about a good *amchi* from the Muktinath Valley. I got medicines from him, but I still could not speak. Then I heard about this clinic. So I came and took medication for almost two years. From the beginning I have been helped by Darkye's medicines. Even though I live in Pokhara, I come here for treatment. The medication really works. Still, I am taking them. I bring my wife and my grandchildren here—the whole family, many generations!

"I will give you another example of the benefits from this clinic," the man continues. "I have a Tibetan friend. He is suffering from cancer in his intestines. Through a lama, he was told Tibetan medication is better. After taking some Tibetan medicines from the Dharamsala

Men-tsee-khang for a year, the illness didn't end. I told him to come here for treatment. Now it has been ten days of treatment *only,* but he did all the checkups and he is improving. They say the cancer is shrinking. He can eat. He feels well."

This man's narrative reflects the fact that health-seeking behavior cannot be reduced to a set of predetermined possibilities based on exposure to health education or socioeconomic metrics, or to a teleology of care that begins with diagnosis and ends with treatment at one health facility. Social ecologies of illness are more complex. Seeking care is like making a map—a set of experiences that can be charted, that occur in many different locales, and that involve instinct, direction, guidance, tools. Reading such maps requires weighing evidence generated from diverse systems of thought. This man first sought out biomedical treatment for something he identified as a throat problem. By Mustang standards, he is not poor. He visited several biomedical institutions in Kathmandu. Yet the biomedical practitioners could not provide a name for his illness, nor could they alleviate his pain. Their response to this man, at least as he recounts it, was flippant, a judgment of character. He simply needed to talk less.

This failed experience led the patient to a crossroads, for which he sought guidance from a lama about the course of treatment he should pursue in his quest to get well. Should he follow the pathway of Tibetan medicine or biomedicine? I find this distinction notable, given the array of medicines used in the clinic. In his consultation the lama not only gives practical advice. He also points toward frameworks for understanding *illness causality.* When told to pursue Tibetan medicine, this man from a village in Mustang turned to his relatives *living in New York* for advice about which local Mustangi *amchi* he should see. Mapping illness is at once conceptual and geographic, encompassing translocal (Zhan 2009) realities through which the distances between New York and Nepal become small.

When one *amchi* failed to deliver effective medicines, the man was referred to Darkye. Here he found relief. Indeed the faith he now has in Darkye is such that he continues to bear the expense of traveling to Kathmandu from his home in Pokhara to seek treatment. The absence of any discussion of specific medications or the costs of those medications is notable in this narrative, as is the bleeding of a first-person story into another person's experience. Maps of illness can be shared cartographies, pilgrimages to specific places in the nation of the sick. The mention of cancer is also notable. While this term has many possible interpretations

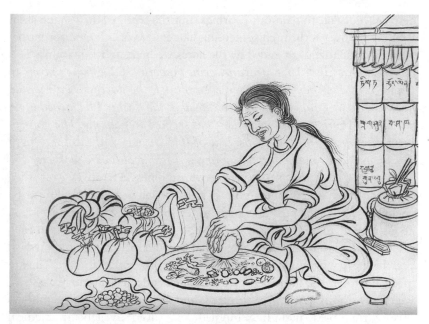

Depiction of an *amchi* from Dolpo, Nepal, grinding *materia medica* and preparing medicines for local patients. The compartments pictured in the upper right corner of the drawing are labeled with the names of medicines, 2011. © Tenzin Norbu

in Tibetan medicine (Czaja 2010), it is recounted here as an illness that can be addressed by practitioners such as Darkye, but that is also "seen" by biomedicine. Biomedical technology remains authoritative in this narrative, even as a way of confirming the effectiveness of Darkye's treatments.

As you can see, mapping illness is not only about naming a disease and following its progression; it is an iterative process, rooted in particular bodies and locations, tied to geography and economic challenges of travel. Maps of illness defy standardization even when standards exist, in the form of specific treatment protocols, a predictable range of family expectations, religious precepts, or state health care systems. The ground truth of a specific map trumps truisms: *Tibetan medicine is good for chronic disorders or common problems; biomedicines are good for trauma and serious diseases, but they have harsh side effects; doing rituals is always beneficial.* Different types of authoritative knowledge are encountered along the way, from a lab test to a lama's divination. At such pivotal moments one must decide which way to turn, what to believe in. We might be tempted to view maps of illness as still images that help us to orient, to gain our bearings. But the truth is, they shape-shift. Routine pathways through something like cancer or a *lung* disorder become particularized, amended by the notes we make in the margins: *This practitioner is kind. That medicine seems powerful. I did many prayers to Green Tara and then I felt better, even though the doctors said I would not recover. We could not communicate with the doctor. I happened upon a group of tourists with medicines that seemed to help me. The government reimbursed me for 50 percent of this lab test, but not that one. I don't trust drugs made in this country, or local health care workers.*

In both China and Nepal people whose illness narratives I recorded often spoke of practitioners who live in particular places, followed by comments about the positions such healers occupied within or outside of an institution, making explicit the social-ecological groundedness of each healer. Many interviewees distinguished Tibetan *medicines* from medical practitioners whose medical practices were grounded in core Tibetan medical principles, informed by a Buddhist-inflected morality. A Sowa Rigpa sensibility (Adams, Schrempf, and Craig 2010) can encompass diverse therapies, including biomedicines used by Tibetan medical practitioners. Such a sensibility elides dichotomies—tradition versus modernity, Western versus Asian medicines—and does not allow for biomedicine to be imagined either as a (foreign) white knight entering into this kingdom of the sick or as anathema to Tibetan ways of healing. Most interviewees did not rely exclusively on Tibetan medicines or pharmaceuticals; nor did they only seek out Sowa Rigpa practitioners, ritual healers, or biomedical health workers.

That said, some did say that Tibetan medicine is limited because it is perceived to work slowly. Other people who did not have money to pay for biomedicine used Tibetan therapies as a first resort. Some opined that people choose not to take Tibetan medicine because it is not "modern." For other individuals, negative experiences with either Tibetan medicine or biomedicines deterred them from using such medicine thereafter. Such instances were rare. More common was the sense that Tibetan medicine demanded a commitment to therapy, while biomedicines were generally viewed as "easy" or "convenient" to take. This provides an interesting counterpoint to the assertion one encounters in some global health literature that the formulations of traditional medicines are somehow more culturally acceptable or likely to promote adherence.[5] Rather while the financial costs of purchasing Tibetan medicine are usually less than biomedicine, taking these therapies requires discipline. Tibetan medicines are often prescribed for several weeks, if not months; should be taken at particular times of the day; and may include dietary strictures.

Many interviewees were also ambivalent about pharmaceuticals, biomedical practitioners, and *gyamen* institutions. Some echoed the sentiment expressed by a nomad woman in Qinghai who said, "Tibetan medicine is cheap and easy to get. Biomedicines are more expensive, but more powerful and cure diseases more quickly." Others cited mistrust of biomedical drugs or, more often, the intentions of people working in biomedical facilities. In both Mustang and Qinghai several interviewees referred to fears about having their kidneys or other, unspecified organs removed without their consent if they visited biomedical hospitals and to a lack of confidence in the motivations of doctors, nurses, and health workers.[6] In some cases this mistrust followed urban/rural lines, with urban practitioners being viewed as more skilled but also greedier. Many viewed urban hospitals as institutions where patient care was less important than profit. Some noted that while they felt biomedicines were powerful and effective, problems of expired medicines, limited stocks at rural clinics, and difficulty deciphering indications and dosage due to illiteracy and the poor training of health workers made them wary about taking such medicines. In other instances interviewees spoke about the complementarity of Tibetan therapies and biomedicines. Practitioners who treated tuberculosis or hepatitis B listed a number of Tibetan medicines that could be used to counterbalance the weakening effects of biomedical drugs, especially those taken for a long time and that impact liver and kidney function—a biological reality validated by both Tibetan medicine and biomedicine. In both national contexts people often used divination to decide how to pursue treatment, to mitigate treatment failures, or to clear away physical and cosmological obstacles that might hinder successful treatment (Schrempf 2010).

When interviewees were asked about the most common illnesses that affected their community, answers varied by place, livelihood strategy, and season. In agricultural and agropastoral communities in Mustang and Qinghai, disorders of the lower part of the body were common, including joint and musculoskeletal problems connected with the physical demands of farming; in nomadic communities, diseases related to the cold environment and connected to the upper part of the body were more common. People associated liver disorders with the consumption of alcohol in these locales and to specific infectious diseases, most commonly hepatitis.[7] Interviewees complicated questions about which illnesses were most common in a given "community": some felt uncomfortable speaking of others' suffering; others took pains to explain local socio-economic and political divisions that complicated notions of community and patterns of illness therein (Craig, Chase, and Lama 2010).

In interviews with people in Mustang and Qinghai, as well as many other moments of observation in Nepal and Tibetan areas of China since the mid-1990s, I've often witnessed people wait until they are seriously debilitated by a health problem before seeking care. In some instances people cite a lack of knowledge or confusion about the symptoms of specific diseases as reasons for treatment delays, but most link such delays to economic hardship, often associated with the costs of travel to seek care. In other instances people link delayed care-seeking to a lack of access to basic laboratory facilities. While speaking about tuberculosis prevalence in Mustang, a schoolteacher said that people usually do not go for treatment until a disease like TB, or at least its symptoms, become pronounced. "Otherwise, people are coughing. Maybe they have TB, maybe not. We don't have the ability to know. So the *amchi* treat for respiratory problems and cough. Either way, patients will not know what they have or will only get Western medicine once the problem is very serious."

The balance between structural inequality and individual agency also emerged as a theme in my interviews. At times a pattern of delayed care was connected to notions that people were "lazy," "indolent," or "backward." Interviewees sometimes spoke of themselves, their neighbors, or their family in these terms. At other times health care workers would make such disparaging comments about their would-be patients. Such judgments about the character or capacity of individuals in a way that potentially limits their access to care, respect, or simply social acknowledgment illustrates Pierre Bourdieu has called symbolic violence: the tacit or even unconscious modes of cultural and social domination that occur in everyday habits and mannerisms (Bourdieu and Wacquant 1992). They also indicate an aspect of the internalized impacts of colonialism or the sorts of neocolonial processes to which Tibetans in China have been subject (Yeh 2007). These dynamics indicate relations of power and state control over individual bodies that can permeate experiences of medicine (Foucault 1973; Nandy and Visvanathan 1990).

Yet there are more localized barriers to seeking care, including access to *amchi*. These barriers are often bound up with social divisions—

hierarchies of class, ethnicity, and religion that can shape relations with a healer or health care provider in a particular place. For example, a young man from Mustang noted that while commoners *(misé)* would visit *amchi* bearing in-kind gifts in exchange for treatment, the upper classes or nobility *(kudrak)* treated seeing the *amchi* as "a right, not a privilege." These people "do not treat *amchi* with the same respect they would show to a doctor in Kathmandu, or even an *amchi* from the city." In Qinghai and the TAR many interlocutors noted differential access to a range of health care practitioners—*amchi*, lamas, biomedical doctors—based on Communist Party membership or political appointments. Ironically Party membership can afford you the best and quickest access to ritual specialists, even if these acts of divination or ritual healing are performed clandestinely, given their overt association with religion.[8]

Compelling differences emerged between interviews from Nepal and China, reflective of overarching social and political distinctions between these places. In Nepal interviews often ended with a rhetorical move requesting that I get involved in providing health care or to encourage other foreigners to provide aid. Interview transcriptions contain refrains such as *It would be good for you to bring doctors here! Sometimes there are camps where foreigners bring medicines. Can you do that? We need eye medicines and especially medicine for leg pains. Next time, bring those!* In China explicit requests for assistance almost never occurred. Given the political sensitivities in Tibetan areas of China, which have only become more intense since overt political unrest resurfaced in 2008, I was cautious and chose to delegate a good deal of formal data collection to my research assistant. Interviewees in Nepal were much more quick to criticize the government and to expound on the ways Nepal was "weak" and "undeveloped" when it came to providing good health care for its citizens. Some interviewees from Mustang even noted that villagers had taken it upon themselves to collect money for biomedicines they felt should be available at their local health posts but were not. In China, however, a sense that it was fundamentally a *family* responsibility to avail treatment pervaded the interviews, even though citizens of China have much more recourse to state-provided health services than their contemporaries in high mountain Nepal.

Foreign medicines were viewed as repositories of social meaning and indices of social change. The efficacy of such medicines were linked to the distances they traveled to reach a patient, affective connections to the person who sent them, and a sense that the most powerful treatments come from the most rare or exotic sources. A paradox emerges: *the most efficacious treatment is local* versus *the most efficacious treatment is foreign.* This is not necessarily a new theme or unique to Tibetan contexts.[9] Yet the circumstances by which a nomad in Qinghai comes to possess high-end multivitamins made in California, and the fact that Ben-Gay® bought in drugstores in Brooklyn and Queens has become a drug of choice for Mustangis suffering from joint ailments, are novel. These changes are linked to patterns of labor migration in the global economy and the political-economic forces driving some Tibetans into exile, and to the prestige and social capital such commodities symbolize.

Consider this example: a woman in Qinghai suffered from "heart illness" *(nyingné)* after the death of one of her sons. She tried Tibetan medicines, had rituals sponsored for her at three major monasteries, and spent a small fortune on biomedical treatments in Xining, funds sent by another son living in New York. The only thing she felt helped, however, was a gift of shark liver oil capsules sent by her son. Another Tibetan man, a neighbor of the son's in Astoria, recommended this supplement because it had helped his mother, who was also suffering from *nyingné* back in her village in Sichuan Province. The fact that this woman even had this special medicine from America produced jealousy among her neighbors and conjured, through the possibilities of gossip *(mi kha),* other sorts of risks to her health and well-being. Yet these were risks she was willing to take. More disconcerting to her was the thought of what would happen when the bottle was empty.

DHARMA, KARMA, AND DISEASE

Rinchen and I sit by the side of the road in a county town in Malho Tibetan Autonomous Prefecture (Ch. Huangnan), Qinghai. It is hot. The stench from a nearby garbage bin stings my nostrils. We arrived here about an hour ago, hoping to interview a local religious specialist about his role as someone to whom people turn when ill. As we walked up to the locked door of this large compound, three women, each of whom was waiting with offering scarves, bricks of tea, and loaves of bread, greeted us. Children accompanied two of the women. One child had a wound on his foot and was being carried. The other appeared healthy. After several loud knocks, the metal door cracked open, revealing the face of a middle-aged Tibetan woman, handsome and well-groomed.

"The lama is meditating," she said. "He will not see anyone now. If you want to see him you can give me your gifts and come back later. He may see you in the afternoon." The gatekeeper's tone was firm. The mother who brought her son with the foot injury explained that she traveled for more than an hour to see the lama and that she must return to her village soon.

"Please, can the lama see us now?" she asked.

The gatekeeper repeated, "The lama is meditating. Come back this afternoon." The door shut. The mother, visibly upset, tucked her offerings into her purse, hitched up the now crying toddler on her hip, and walked off. The other women mumbled to each other about the brisk demeanor of the lama's attendant and said they would return later.

Now, sitting on the curb, Rinchen holds forth in a moment of frankness. "The lama is powerful. He does most *mo* for people around here, but he is a 'government-employee lama.' If they put lamas in such positions of power, it is easier to control people," he grumbles. "People think they have to do a *mo* or get blessings or make rituals. This delays their treatment. Then, if the *mo* doesn't work, the lamas blame this failure on the patients, saying they lack faith. But they get rich in the process. Think about it! Every day this lama probably has thirty visitors, maybe more. So if everyone brings ten yuan plus some other gifts, he is making three hundred yuan a day, easily! But people will keep coming—exactly *because* they have faith."

Rinchen's microeconomic and political commentary is astute. Many scholars have noted how the politics of Tibet's status within China impacts embodied well-being (Adams 1998; Janes 1999b; Prost 2008). I consider the irony that there are "government-employee lamas" and think about the power dynamics in such a relationship. Imagine being told by an authority figure that you lack true commitment to the process of healing, even as you make serious sacrifices to be healed. Conversely, sometimes lamas are used to confirm a *patient's* conviction that she wants to pursue a particular course of treatment but does not feel she has the right to make this decision for herself. At other moments lamas recognize the economic constraints of a family and advocate for inexpensive and culturally sanctioned therapeutic options: visiting a hot spring, going on pilgrimage, taking "precious pills" *(rinchen rilbu)*. A lama's divination can read into a patient's fears or deflect a patient from seeking a particular path of treatment—a surgery, say—because he knows the patient's family would incur financial hardship if they were to pursue such a path (Schrempf 2010). A *mo* is not simply a predictive device; it can be a tool for communication, a culturally sanctioned means of justifying difficult choices, a way of expressing opinions about the relative efficacy of one course of treatment over another.

A woman who has been turned away from the lama's door joins us. She asks Rinchen where I am from and what we are doing here. He explains that I am interested to learn why people come to this lama if they are sick, and how the lama helps. The woman offers her story.

"I have come to have the lama do a *mo* because I have a problem with my tongue. The doctors at the hospital say I have to do a surgery. But I do not want to be cut."

"Do you think this lama can help you?" Rinchen asks.

"Oh, yes! He is very powerful. Yesterday I was here for another problem, a toothache. The lama did a *mo* for that. He told me I had upset a *lu* and this caused the toothache," she continues. The *lu* (Skt. *naga*) are part of a hierarchical retinue of deities in Tibetan tradition that remain within the realm of samsaric existence, as opposed to deities who transcend this realm and serve as divine protectors. *Lu* and other such "earthly" deities are often associated with places in the natural world such as mountain passes, rivers, caves, trees, and rocks. While the *lha* reside in the sky (associated with the color white), the *tsen* (associated with red) and *nyen* (associated with yellow) live in the intermediate realm on earth, and the *lu* (associated with blue) reside under the earth and are associated with water (Millard 2006: 10).

"It is because I offended the *lu* that I have a toothache. This is what the lama said. He told me to do chants with my rosary and that he would also recite prayers. So I did that. Last night the toothache went away!"

"Do you think the money you spent on gifts was worthwhile?" prompts Rinchen.

"Yes. Also, after the lama told me about the *lu*, I remembered brushing against a tree near our local spring. Right here," she motions to her cheek, "right where the toothache was. So it must have been at that moment that I disturbed the *lu*."

Rinchen's comments and the experiences of this woman help me think concretely about the relationship between medicine and religion, on the one hand, and between individual behavior, the social construction of nature, and concepts of illness causality, on the other. Consider this woman brushing her cheek against a branch and inadvertently disturbing the *lu,* or the interviewee from Mustang offending a *shindre* while participating in a community festival.[10] These and other examples illustrate interactions between the "three bodies"—individual, social, and the body politic—about which Margaret Lock and Nancy Scheper-Hughes (1987) write, as well as what Elisabeth Hsu (1999) calls the "body ecologic" and Geoffrey Samuel (2001) distinguishes as the "mind-body-world" orientation in Tibetan cultural contexts. Lock and Scheper-Hughes offer a counternarrative to the Cartesian legacy that would cleave body from mind. Hsu's analysis challenges distinctions between nature and culture when it comes to medicine. Her work helps to ground an understanding of human health not only in the person within her community or social setting and the larger political-economic context in which she lives, but also within distinct ecologies, inclusive of nonhuman forces that animate a landscape. In the Tibetan context this includes the cosmophysical forces of the five elements *(jungwa nga)* that animate life, and deities who inhabit, influence, and bind together internal and external worlds.

What does the lama's divination and the assertion that this woman's toothache is the result of offending a *lu* have to do with Tibetan medical theory? In short, a lot. Various classifications of disease etiology in Sowa Rigpa distinguish between illnesses that can be treated by standard, materialist therapies and those that require ritual intervention; primary *(gyu)* and contributory *(kyen)* causes and conditions of illness are also articulated (Millard 2006; Samuel 2007; Vargas 2011). Ritual specialization, erudite medical knowledge, textual sources, and lay knowledge often intermingle.

Many Tibetan medical practitioners with whom I have worked refer routinely to the twelfth chapter of the *Explanatory Tantra,* which lists three main etiological categories: illnesses that are caused by disturbances in the *nyépa,* illnesses that arise from negative karma accumulated in past lives, and combinations of these two. This core text is also referenced by practitioners to explain that diseases can occur from internal (or what Tibetans would call "self-arising," *rangzhin)* and or external *(chi kyen)* factors, which include material disturbances from such things as poison and weapons as well as actions of harmful spirits (Millard 2006: 16).

While some categories of spirits hold constant across many Tibetan environments, others are *literally grounded* in specific places. This woman got a toothache because she offended a *lu* that resides in a tree beside a local spring, on which she depends for water. This consensus between the lama and the laywoman regarding the cause of her toothache was reached without consulting a Tibetan physician. Disease etiologies are the domain of specialized Sowa Rigpa knowledge, but they can bleed into lay understandings of the causes and conditions of suffering. Illnesses that arise from karmic action bridge, in a sense, ideas of internal and external factors; they are also conceived of as problems that require both materialist and spiritual therapies. At times an *amchi* might be able to provide both such courses of treatment; more often, Tibetan medical practitioners refer patients to ritual specialists. In Nepal these referrals often are made overtly and involve collaboration between different local healers. In places like Lhasa and Xining these recommendations to seek or sponsor ritual are often made quietly—a testament to the overt secularization of clinical Tibetan medicine in China (Janes 1995, 2001; Adams 2001b, 2002a).

Types of illness that biomedicine might categorize as "psychological" often are described as a combination of exogenous, spirit-caused forces, karma, and biophysical imbalance.[11] At times these disorders can also be linked to imbalances in relation to the *la,* or vital life essence, or the *sok lung,* "life force wind" (Jacobson 2002; Gerke 2012). Consider the following example, excerpted from an illness narrative interview with a forty-one-year-old man in northern Mustang District.

"I can't sleep," he begins. "This is my problem. Before I had a headache. I say 'before,' but it has been five years! The headache came to me because my heart-mind was not happy. I was like this, and then also there was a blood pressure problem. I was thinking a lot, and this created poor health. During the illness, I was in bed for a month. I felt more comfortable when the room was dark, when the door and windows were locked. Light disturbed me. I felt nervous. I called lamas to perform rituals, but I can't remember. I was *nyomba*—crazy—at this time. My *la* was disturbed. I am getting much better."

At this point in the interview Amchi Gyatso, who is with me, adds, "Due to rituals and therapies such as golden needle acupuncture *[ser khab]* he is much better." The patient mentions that Gyatso's brother Tenzin took charge of his care. In the patient's view and the assessment of local *amchi,* an efficacious treatment for this illness required ritual intervention and materialist medicine. My mind races with thoughts of migraines, the nebulous yet pervasive set of meanings I have been conditioned to associate with terms such as "anxiety" and "depression," and the exorcism and soul-calling ceremonies I have witnessed during my years of fieldwork in this region. I then ask the interviewee if this illness had a name. He responds, "I don't know what it is called. . . . I think it is a problem of the *tsa*." Again we see the notion that disturbances in the channels can lead to biopsychosocial imbalance, perhaps somewhat similar to the ways *nervios* is described in Latin American contexts (Low 1981; Scheper-Hughes 2007). The patient understands a general correlation between the *tsa* and the disturbed state of his heart-mind *(sem)*.

Interestingly Gyatso and I have not actually come to this house to talk with this person, but with a cousin of his. This cousin is seated on a platform bed in the corner of the room, his back deformed and hunched, his legs shriveled. I wonder about extrapulmonary tuberculosis, polio, palsy—biomedical points of reference that inform my observations of this person—and all I do not know about the causes and conditions of his disease. The man's voice is much higher pitched than an average adult male. His face seems disproportionately large for his body. I learn that he must be carried around, piggyback style, or "walks" on his back, propelling himself forward with his arms. Despite his disability, this man cards and spins wool and helps as he can with other agricultural tasks.

This man describes his problem as "self-arising" *(rangzhin)*. Different from the term *natural* as an English speaker might use it, this term connotes a certain innateness linked to karma and can be used to describe what a Christian might call a "miracle" affixed to particular places in a landscape: the formation of a holy person's footprint *(shabjé)* in a rock or the image of a deity or ritual implement *revealed* by an adept of the *dharma* but *not created by* him, and whose contours have been smoothed by centuries of human touch, polished, in delicate acts of homage, by fingertips and foreheads. So to say that an illness is "self-arising" references a sense of causality beyond human control.

"Until I was twenty, I could walk. There was no problem. Then one year when there was lot of snow I got worse. I tried the various methods—doing rituals and going to the *amchi*. I went to Kathmandu once, but I did not go to the hospital at that time because I had no money. Instead, I did a lot of circumambulations *[kora]* at Boudha," says the man, referring to the pilgrimage site in Kathmandu. "This caused me to get a cold disorder." I imagine this man moving around the girth of the Boudha *stupa*, knuckles rubbed raw on slate flagstones, surrounded by a sea of footsteps belonging to the pilgrims beside him.

"I have a lot of pain, but I can't be free of it. I am thinking about the problems from my previous life. There is no other explanation for why this would happen. It is also a *lu* and *sap dak* problem because of the work that I have done in the earth, in my younger years," the man continues, referencing not only karmic inheritance but also his possible disturbance of serpent and earth spirits. I am not sure if this "work in the earth" refers to specific tasks beyond routine agricultural labor and ani-mal husbandry. Either way, the mention of obstacles carried over from his previous life, along with a sense that his actions in this life, in this par-ticular social ecology, have contributed to his illness is significant.

"I have spent twenty-seven years like this. Without the help of the *amchi,* I would have been dead a long time ago." I appreciate the man's acknowledgment of the importance of *amchi* in his care. However, I am quite conscious that I am sitting beside Gyatso. His presence, like mine for different reasons, shapes what is shared.

"When I'm working," the man continues, "I feel good. After I finish, my body is in pain."

When Gyatso and I emerge from the house, this Tibetan doctor and tantric householder priest turns to me and says, "This house has many *barché,* obstacles. Even though they do rituals and take our medicines it has only helped *fifty percent.*" He says this last phrase in English. "Yes, they have economic problems, but many people here are poor. Maybe there is some *bu* that causes some problems also. Or *tension—* you know the man with the headaches, his wife died. But it is not just money obstacles, like not going to hospitals in Kathmandu, that makes these problems." While *bu* is a culturally specific term that can mean ei-ther "insect," "bug," or "microorganism," depending on context, *tension* is a Nepali-ized idiom of distress, imported from English. My friend looks pensive. I notice he has combined, in a sense, two narratives of suf-fering into one master story couched within the framework of family. Gyatso speaks about the balance between internal and external causes of suffering in biological, spiritual, and socioeconomic terms. His thoughts echo refrains about the ways purely material intervention for illnesses whose etiological basis is in the karmic or cosmological realm will not be efficacious.

Interpersonal friction and social change, whether proximate or global in orientation, present us with additional layers of explanation when it comes to the relationship between karma, *dharma,* and disease—and the ways medicine exists betwixt and between the ideological poles of science and religion. Much has been written about the ways modernity's ills be-come embodied in Asian contexts (Cohen 1998; Langford 2002; Hsu 2009). Consider the following examples. A Mustang man links his eye problems to disturbances of the *lu* that resides near his home and to a more general critique of improper care for village water sources; this, in turn, is connected to patterns of out-migration and disregard for, or inability to steward, local resources. A woman from Lhasa opines that bad relations with her daughter-in-law and the anger that brews in the household as a result of economic pressure have caused her *sok lung* disorder. A nomad from Yushu tells me that government-sponsored resettlement programs are leading to higher rates of joint problems and heart disorders not only because of the decreased sense of control and agency one has in life, but also because of the physical location of these settlements, which are planned without regard for local earth and water spirits and because the materials used to build homes are inherently "cold" in nature.

Likewise Tibetan medical practitioners sometimes remark that increasing trends toward mentally demanding yet sedentary lifestyles often lack a contemplative practice or a set of moral bearings. Likewise, incessant focus on economic gain gives rise to higher rates of mental affliction, physical problems caused by diet and behavior, and a disregard for the balance between the human and natural worlds. Such social and political commentary, expressed in the language of Tibetan medial theory, is directed not only toward cosmopolitan settings in the global North—wherein such critique is apt—but also toward rapidly transforming urban and periurban places in Asia. Here discourses on climate change and habitat destruction come into dialogue with indigenous knowledge about forces that animate the landscape as well as ideas about public health and community well-being (Gyaltsen et al. 2007; Cuomu 2011).[12]

The belief that immoral behavior can give rise to illness also surfaced in narratives that mentioned people who have robbed religious sites for material gain, for example. Infectious disease and epidemics such as sudden acute respiratory syndrome (SARS) were embedded in moral discourses. In the case of SARS, Tibetan religious symbols, practices, and medicines used to protect all manner of people from contagion and essentially *political* commentary about the differences between Tibetans and Han Chinese; expressions of Tibetan nationalism were couched in language about the moral underpinnings of infectious disease (Craig and Adams 2008). People linked SARS to Buddhist prophesies about this age of degeneration (Skt. *Kaliyug*). These examples add to our understanding of how laws of cause and effect and *dharma,* in the broadest sense of moral duty, relate to patterns of sickness and people's ideas about disease transmission as well as experiences of illness and prospects for efficacious treatment.

SUMMARY

This chapter has not been strictly about Tibetan medicine. Rather it has related stories of human suffering and wellness, including intersections with Tibetan medicine in diverse social ecologies. I devoted more attention to the perspectives of laypeople than practitioners, although you were privy to intimate engagements between doctors and patients. As such, this chapter has addressed some of the most persistent questions in medical anthropology: How might we understand the therapeutic process? Why do people respond to illness in particular ways? How do people allocate scarce resources to procure medicines or seek treatment? How do "religious" and "scientific" frameworks exist as a continuum of healing strategies? How do moral explanations for the causes of illness square with understandings of disease that are based in the material world? How might we understand the interconnected, dynamic relationship between the environment of the body, the "natural" environments in which people live, and the forces that animate such environments, with respect to the causes and conditions of health and illness?

The capacity of the government in culturally Tibetan areas of Nepal differs from that of the Chinese government when it comes to providing health care to their citizens. This difference manifests at many levels. Sufficient medicines and a year-round presence of competent government health workers remain the exception in most of Nepal's remote, high-altitude regions; *amchi* are not integrated into the state health care system. In contrast, the Chinese model of rural cooperative medicine, in combination with road building and other infrastructural developments across the Tibetan Plateau, has afforded many rural Tibetans access to basic medical services and, in many cases, to state-supported Tibetan medicine (Janes 1999a; Hofer 2008), albeit imperfectly. Even as the most remote parts of China shift toward more market-based health care and insurance schemes, away from socialized medicine, the Chinese state's political will and ability to provide health care to its citizens is far greater than it is in high mountain Nepal.

Despite these differences, small clinics that integrate Tibetan medical praxis with a repertoire of biomedicines are common in townships, counties, and prefectural centers in the Chinese context, as well as in rural and urban Nepal. Such spaces are neither supported nor necessarily sanctioned by governments or NGOs, but they remain crucial sites of health care delivery for many people. Contrary to the methodological boundaries, epistemological blind spots, and ideological debates that characterizes much clinical *research*, as you will see in chapter 7, within the space of clinical *practice* you've seen in this chapter a great deal of fluidity between the practices of Sowa Rigpa, biomedicine, ritual therapeutics, astrology, and divination. Medical pluralism is alive and well across the Tibetan-speaking world. Yet as we will see in the next chapter, other forces of socioeconomic and cultural change are transforming Sowa Rigpa on the ground, with respect to who makes Tibetan medicines, how they are made, what they cost and, ultimately, who consumes them.

CHAPTER 5

Good Manufacturing Practices

I am scorched
to realize once again
how many small, available things
are in this world
that aren't
pieces of gold
or power—that nobody owns

—Mary Oliver, *Thirst: Poems*

(AD)VENTURE CAPITAL

Steam wafts from the cup of jasmine tea around which my friend Pema wraps his hands on this cool autumn morning in Lhasa in November 2002.[1] Beyond the tea house, commuters scuttle along Jiang Su Lu, a north-south corridor on which the Inpatient Division of the Mentsikhang is located.

A few weeks ago a strapping Irishman, strawberry blond and somewhat brazen, appeared on the expatriate scene in Lhasa. He said he was looking for potential investment opportunities. Tibetan medicine was one avenue for the venture capital at his disposal. The Irishman picked up on Pema's English abilities and that his wife was a doctor at Mentsikhang. He approached my friend about arranging a meeting with Dr. Dorje, a senior leader at this premier state institution of Tibetan medicine. Pema agreed, but asked me to accompany him. "I don't trust this guy," Pema said. "But if he is interested in Mentsikhang, it is my duty to help."

A taxi pulls up beside the teahouse, outside the Mentsikhang gates. The Irishman steps out. "Hello," he says, tipping his baseball cap with bravado. "Shall we get started?" Pema and I lead the Irishman toward Dr. Dorje's office. This leader is stately, his hair slicked back to reveal a caramel complexion marked by few lines. As he shakes my hand, I imagine what his grip might feel like as he takes a pulse: light, smooth, subtle. He has spent the past decade as an administrator, but he has been practicing Tibetan medicine for more than three decades.

Dr. Dorje has been briefed about the Irishman's interests. After formalities and introductions he says, "In the history of Tibetan medicine, there was never really a need to *sell* our medicine. There was especially no idea about selling medicine to foreigners. These days there is a big opportunity for the world to benefit. Before, nobody knew about our medicine. Now it is gaining a reputation in China and throughout the world."

The Irishman answers, "I'm sure you're right about market potential. But I wonder about export regulations, clinical testing, things like that. In Mongolia and Russia I hear things are a bit easier.

"I want to help preserve Tibetan culture," the Irishman continues. "Investing in Tibetan medicine might be a good way to do this. But you'll need to improve production methods and do more marketing if Tibetan medicine is going to keep up with TCM and other alternative medicines— you know, aromatherapy, acupuncture, things the New Agers go for. As standards improve, we can address regulatory issues for export to the U.S. and Europe, even other underdeveloped countries, like parts of Africa, where Chinese medicine is already popular.[2] My associates and I could help add value to your products and increase the quality of the medicines produced in your factory. Of course, you would need to follow strict regulatory protocol—Good Manufacturing Practices, GMP, and all of that."

Pema tries to translate this flood of jargon. He whispers to me, "How do you say *quality outputs* in Tibetan? What is *added value?*"

Dr. Dorje interjects. A flash of recognition has passed across his face. "*GMP,*" he says in halting English. "*Yes, very important.*"

The Irishman goes on to say Mentsikhang would need to improve its fiscal planning and marketing capacity if he and his associates were to invest in the factory. Of course, he has yet to see any financial records for the institution, let alone the factory to which he is now laying a certain entrepreneurial claim, as if he were the local and Dr. Dorje the visitor. Pema squirms and translates selectively. I find the exchange both shocking and fascinating, in part because the language of venture capital is different from the vocabulary of development, with which I am more familiar. Yet both discourses tend to assume that a certain trajectory of modernization is inevitable and that Tibet is in need of "saving" (Adams 2005b).

"There are difficulties," continues Dr. Dorje. "But Tibetan medicine is being developed. You will see when you visit our factory." Pema translates. Dr. Dorje arranges for a driver to take us to the Tibetan Traditional Medicine Pharmaceutical Factory of the TAR. From my place in the back seat I glimpse the golden roofs of Sera Monastery rising above the edge of Lhasa's urban sprawl. Concrete buildings with low ceilings, in which one can buy anything from shellacked pressboard desks to pirated Mariah Carey CDs and a freshly slaughtered pig, are nestled up against shops selling produce imported from Sichuan Province. Poplar saplings line the road. The trees, like the Chinese migrants who make their living under their dappled shade, have been transplanted here but have begun to put down roots in this place.[3]

"How long has the factory been in this location?" I ask as we pull up to the gates.

"About seven years," the driver replies. "But many of the buildings are new. Some are still under construction. You'll see, once you go inside."

A senior-level manager meets us at the entrance to the new GMP-certified building. The imposing three-story structure is bedecked with banners: Tibetan and Chinese characters painted in crisp white tempera across what can only be described as communist red cotton. The banners announce the recent ground-breaking ceremony for a sales and marketing complex.

"Welcome to our factory." The manager extends his hand in greeting toward the Irishman.

"Impressive," says the Irishman, speaking to nobody in particular.

"Since Mentsikhang was founded in 1916, we have been working continuously to produce the best medicines," the manager begins. I note how he smoothes over history, creating a narrative of continuity where there has been much contestation and upheaval and at least three distinct phases of drug manufacturing norms. "Now we are combining modern technology and scientific methods with traditional practices. We have many important drug registration numbers.[4] The nectar [dutsi] of Traditional Tibetan Medicine is becoming a national heritage trademark in China. Today the factory is worth more than one hundred fifty million yuan [$18.7 million]. We employ more than two hundred people." The manager speaks as if reading from the factory brochure. He ushers us inside.

As we pass through heavy glass doors into the factory foyer, the Irishman leans in toward me. "This is prime real estate. I'd guess they had to use this land as collateral to secure bank loans for construction.

I'm skeptical they could be selling enough medicine to afford this expansion. Either that, or they must have some pretty big investors already." I soon learn that the TAR and Chinese central governments have indeed made provisions for low-interest loans and other state subsidies to help spur the growth of this industry. Although the sources of industry figures are often opaque and certainly imperfect, it is reported that by 2008 the TAR government had invested an estimated 200 million yuan ($27 million) in this process of bringing Tibetan medicine to market (AsiaInfo Services 2008). This support includes government loans and subsidies, incentive and training programs, and other forms of support for Tibetan medical factories, particularly those that are partially or fully state-owned.[5]

"We must dress in the special clothes," directs the manager. I pass through a set of metal doors. A Tibetan woman instructs me to sit on a low steel bench that divides the room.

"Put these slippers on over your shoes," the woman explains. I slip the flimsy plastic sheaths over my soles.

"Gown, hat, face mask." The woman hands me a paper surgical gown and a hairnet. "For keeping the factory clean," the worker explains. "Otherwise the medicines won't be good." The worker wears the same protective gear. Underneath she is dressed in a baggy beige uniform that lends her an androgynous look. I tuck my hair into the plastic cap and position a mask across my nose and mouth. The worker leads me down a long corridor, where the rest of the group is waiting.

The Irishman turns to me and confides, "I don't know what you were expecting, but I was picturing huts and people squatting in the dirt."

"Really?" I stammer. My mind races and I feel oddly defensive, even as the scale of this enterprise makes me dizzy. Ethnocentrism comes in all shapes and sizes. We look out through double-pane windows onto the factory's courtyard. The manager explains the building was designed in Lhasa, but that final approval was granted only after consultation with Beijing experts. In one room, half a dozen workers operate an elaborate machine that counts, sorts, and weighs *rilbu*, Tibetan-style pills. In the next room workers use another machine to shrink-wrap groups of three *rilbu* in foil packets. Others are sealed in blister packets. We are not allowed to see the actual sites of medical production, the areas where raw materials are sorted, ground, and mixed.

"We produce about forty medicines according to GMP standards. But we plan to make more than fifty by 2004. The other two hundred medicines we make are just for use at Mentsikhang hospitals and clinics.

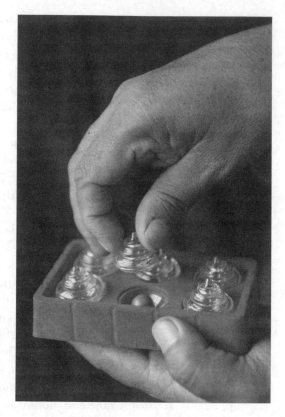

Traditional Tibetan-style pills, or *rilbu,* prepared at the newly GMP-certified Shongpalhachu Factory, Lhasa Prefecture, Tibet Autonomous Region, China, 2004. © Thomas Kelly

They are made in the old building, out behind this one. But in the next few years we will replace that building and make all medicines according to GMP."

"Good," says the Irishman. "This is encouraging."

The manager says they have plans for a wing devoted to producing *rinchen rilbu,* the "precious pills" that are the most pharmacologically complex formulas in the Tibetan medical repertoire (Aschoff and Tashigang 2001). As Saxer (2010a: 73–75) describes in detail, these remedies are at once considered the most potent and the most sought-after commodities in the growing commercial market, symbolizing the "high art of Tibetan pharmacy."[6] The manager explains that by 2004 these pills must be made in accordance with GMP and follow the 2001 Chinese Drug Administration Law, which was drafted soon after China's entrance into the World Trade Organization. Referencing the challenges of production, the manager notes the difficulties, as he sees them, in complying with these regulations and practicing forms of detoxification such as in the creation of mercury-sulfide ash *(tsothal)*, a key ingredient in many precious pills that contains mercury in a purified form and is akin to *rasayana* practices in Ayurveda and Indian alchemical traditions (Samuel 2010).

"Within our medical system we have methods to remove poisons. But it is difficult to convince people who do not know our medicine that ingredients like mercury are safe, so we are making some medicines differently now," the manager notes.

Indeed as I would learn over the coming years, this question of *tsothal* points to a paradox of the industry in China. *Tsothal* is officially recognized as part of Tibetan cultural and scientific heritage; Mentsikhang was even granted a state-issued patent for this processing method in the early 1990s, and *tsothal* was listed as part of China's Intangible Cultural Heritage (a national designation inspired by UNESCO) in 2006 (Saxer 2010a: 76). Official state regulations and compendia on specific precious pills sometimes exclude the mention of *tsothal* altogether—a reflection of the fact that such formulas are generally considered both secret and proprietary knowledge. However, by any non-Tibetan estimation, *tsothal* runs the risk of conflicting with the monitoring and evaluation of traditional medicines for mercury and other heavy metal–based contamination, and was even explicitly targeted as problematic in this regard by Swiss drug authorities, even as countervailing claims have emerged from clinical studies carried out at the Men-tsee-khang in India (Saxer 2010a: 73).

"Have there been any tests to see if changes to production environments affect the quality *[putsé]* or potency *[nüpa]* of the medicines?" I ask.[7]

"We consult with many traditional doctors," he answers obliquely. I am reminded that he himself is not trained in medical production but has a background in administration. "It is difficult to know about changes in potency without expensive studies. For now, we are investing in GMP certification, because, without this, we cannot sell."

The manager is correct to emphasize the increasing pressures to comply with Chinese State Food and Drug Administration (SFDA) mandates on the production of Tibetan medicines. The pace of change is dramatic, the financial capital required to comply with new state laws is massive, and the possibilities for confusion about new regulations is significant.

"Some people I've spoken with say the benefit and potency of *rinchen rilbu* and other Tibetan medicines are decreasing these days," I comment.[8] "Do you think this is true?"

"Such people do not know about science," answers the manager, his tone sharp, polished. "We have to follow the path of modernization. We must use the traditional wisdom combined with modern technologies and knowledge. This is the way forward."

Caught in the middle of this translation, Pema adds, in English, "Many Tibetan people may not know Western science, but they do say that some of these new medicines look fancy but are not as powerful as before." Pema's commentary contrasts with the neat dichotomy this factory administrator draws between "traditional" wisdom and "scientific" knowledge. Why is it that wisdom must be located in experiences that are perceived as non-Cartesian, unscientific, or even (heaven forbid) religious, while knowledge is a catchall for what is ascertainable to a modern, capable of digesting wisdom, processing the past? As Latour (1993) has taught us, this "great divide" emerges from the specifics of Enlightenment ideology and the crafting of modernity as a concept. I wonder how the manager envisions this integration between traditional wisdom and scientific knowledge. Is it enough that formulas produced under highly altered circumstances bear traces of a Tibetan (and Buddhist) *aesthetic* of healing? That they come in packages stamped with images of Himalayan peaks and the Potala Palace?

When I ask the manager where the factory gets its raw materials and if they ever have problems with supply, he answers, "We are thinking about the future. But our Tibet is big. There is a lot of land. We can still get what we need." I encounter such a sentiment many times in my research, this notion that the vastness of the Tibetan Plateau will somehow "naturally" counterbalance the problem of resource depletion in the face of commodification. Yet other practitioner-producers from Nepal, India, and China with whom I've interacted cite the rising costs of raw materials and the difficulty in finding adequate quantities of some ingredients.

"I recognize the huge global potential for Tibetan medicines," the Irishman says, addressing the administrator/tour guide. "Building the Tibetan medicine industry is a good way to help Tibet. The most important thing for us, if we were to invest, is that your factory meets GMP certification, that raw materials pass regulatory standards, and that we can be competititive in business. If this means changing the ways some medicines are made, that is your business. The rest of it—ancient healing treatments for modern problems—people eat that up."

Pema summarizes, "He agrees GMP is needed."

The manager nods. "We will meet GMP certification by the deadline in 2004." He leads us back to the dressing rooms where we began our tour. After shedding our sterile paraphernalia, Pema, the Irishman, and I bid the manager farewell. "Come back another day and I will show you the sales building," he promises. "We can talk more about markets." The Irishman nods and pumps the manager's hand.

I have a feeling that, despite his enthusiastic displays, the Irishman will not be back. Later that day Pema concurs. Although my friend kept cool during the tour, he allows himself agitation now. "He has a lot of pride," says Pema, "like a thief [kuma]. I want to tell Dr. Dorje not to bother with him, but I cannot do that. Mentsikhang needs support. But people like that manager do not really care for Tibetan medicine. I think about the duty of being a doctor, like my wife. There is no comparison. This is not medicine. It is business."

Pema's assessment is apt. By 2004, when all commercial factories had to be GMP-compliant or risk state-enforced closure, the Tibetan medicine industry was well established. Estimates of the overall value of the China-based Tibetan medical industry are difficult to discern; annual reports of profits may be unreliable. However, it is safe to say the industry is now worth tens, if not hundreds of millions of dollars, and is growing rapidly.[9] The largest number I have found cited is $146 million in annual output as of 2003, thirty times more than in 1996 (Huang 2006). This number does not fully account for the range of assets and access to capital at the industry's disposal, including low-interest government loans, prime real estate, and some foreign direct investment. Though still small when compared with the commercial TCM and Ayurveda industries, the desire to consume Tibetan medicines continues to grow in China and beyond. The commercial sale of Tibetan medicines has been touted as an "economic cure" for Tibet's perceived "backward" economy—which remains heavily dependent on central government subsidies—and as the "economic backbone" in the development of a historically marginalized and politically contested region (Dickie 2004).[10]

The question of foreign direct investment in the Tibetan medical industry may have loomed large in this meeting with the Irishman, but the political sensitivity in which Tibet is enmeshed has actually continued to *hinder* rather than foster such expansionist visions of (ad)venture capital in the Land of Snows, marking Tibet as what Agamben calls a state of exception (Agamben 2005). Adams (2002b: 666) notes the presence of global pharma representatives at an international conference on Tibetan medicine in Lhasa in 2000, and Saxer (2010a: 38) describes foreign investment put toward the creation of Shongpalha-chu Factory in the mid-1990s. But at about the time of this meeting I describe in Lhasa, the TAR government announced that foreign supporters were being withdrawn from the Tibetan medicine council, and in 2005 the SFDA announced a ban on foreign direct investment in companies that produce medicines based on secret or proprietary formulas, including some precious pills (Saxer 2010a: 49).

As the Irishman's market sensibilities reveal, the implementation of GMP regulations for the production of Tibetan formulas in China has occurred within the context of increasing attention to traditional medicines worldwide and, as such, increasing global governance of this industry. Over the past decade the WHO has invested significant energy and resources in the development of policies on Traditional Medicine and CAM, as have national institutes of health, particularly in the United States, the United Kingdom, and the European Union. The WHO's Traditional Medicine Strategy (2002–5) includes as part of its mandate that member states develop domestic legislation and regulatory models for the production and quality assurance of traditional formulas. This strategy outlines a variety of challenges to developing international standards for the production and evaluation of traditional therapies. Chief among these are (1) issues of *policy,* including the integration of TM and CAM into national health care systems; (2) issues of *safety, efficacy,* and *quality,* including the need for evaluation, guidance, and support for regulations; (3) issues of *access,* particularly ensuring the availability and affordability of TM and CAM; and (4) *rational use,* which means the promotion of therapeutically sound use of TM and CAM by providers and consumers (Zhang 2005). Significantly, environmental impacts remain unaccounted for in the strategy.

The WHO strategy recognizes the connections between the safety, efficacy, and quality of herbal medicines and the source materials. Yet they also note these are notoriously difficult to discern, particularly in compound formulas as opposed to single botanical remedies. In sum, the WHO strategy states that the quality of source materials is determined by what it calls "intrinsic" factors, which are essentially defined in terms of genetics, and "extrinsic" factors, including environmental conditions, cultivation and harvesting, field collection, and post-harvest transport and storage (World Health Organization 2005a). Significantly such extrinsic factors do not include a sociocultural component or a way of acknowledging different scientific epistemologies about what makes a source material safe or of high quality. This point illustrates the "forms of compression and representation of actions" (Lampland and Star 2009: 4) that occur when people make standards. Arbitrary boundaries are drawn around particular ways of classifying things that, in turn, validate some knowledge and render other knowledge invisible, unknowable, even dangerous.

Building on the WHO's TM strategy, the Beijing Declaration, adopted by the WHO Congress on Traditional Medicine in China's capital on November 8, 2008, explicitly connects the as yet unmet goals (articulated at Alma Ata in 1978) of providing global primary health care and the aim of meeting Millennium Development Goals by 2015 to the use of traditional medicines. Citing the 2003 World Health Assembly resolution on TM, the document advocated that such medicines should be "respected, preserved, and promoted," even as it recognized that the term *traditional medicine* itself was broad and variable. Despite, or perhaps because of this variability, the Declaration further articulated that while member states may have different legislation, regulatory responsibilities, and delivery models for TM, the development of such policies, standards, and regulations was crucial to ensure the "appropriate, safe, and effective use of traditional medicine" worldwide (World Health Organization 2008).

The Declaration posited that the standards by which TM should be measured emerge from international biomedical "best practices." In a speech she gave at the Beijing Congress, Dr. Margaret Chan, director-general of the WHO, summarized, "Some systems of traditional medicine have histories dating back thousands of years. Over a comparatively short period of time, modern medicine has developed powerful methodologies for proving the efficacy, ensuring quality, standardizing good manufacturing practices, testing for safety, and conducting postmarketing surveillance for adverse effects. Many, but not all, traditional medicines have an inadequate evidence base when measured through these standards" (World Health Organization 2008: 2). One is left wondering which medical systems or practices are presumed to have adequate evidence bases, how this is determined, and if this policy statement is not simply a rehashing of another set of dichotomies between "big" and "little" or "scholarly" and "folk" traditions (Bates 1995).

Chan acknowledges that "modern medicine" presumes a global relevance by virtue of practices she takes to be biological and scientific universals. According to these standards, Traditional Medicine just doesn't measure up. The sense of inevitability and noblesse oblige in her speech reveals the ways TMs should "behave," a "taming" of deviant, heterodox medical practices. It is assumed that safety, efficacy, and quality standards for TMs should be driven by conventional biomedicine. Such policies presume that TMs will become more scientific and therefore more effective (and, I would add, more marketable) in the process. However, quality and safety are context-dependent; they emerge from the admission of particular types of evidence, whether generated in the laboratory or in the clinic.

These WHO positions illustrate a classic double standard, in which traditional medicines must adhere to accepted norms that biomedical therapies, techniques, and practices themselves do not always meet (Waldram 2000). In her speech, Dr. Chan briefly mentioned the underlying social and economic costs of complying with WHO directives and related, state-mandated changes to TM production. The working assumption is that standardizing traditional medicines is not only "good" to do, but that it will also address health inequality. This is an untested, even paradoxical proposition. Indeed, in contemplating the assumptions of people like the Irishman whom Pema and I met, these changes in how TMs are made and evaluated reflects larger issues, namely the alienation of labor and fragmentation of production in (late) capitalist societies. The WHO sensibility that traditional medicines should be "respected and preserved" and also "promoted" shows how global policies impact local cultural forms and what "integrative" medicine really means, but this is rarely addressed (Lock 1990; Adams 2002b).[11] Yet as we will see, China's introduction of the GMP and the new Drug Administration Law cannot simply be viewed as a one-sided inculcation of "Western" or international standards. Rather such changes are integrally bound up in ideologies of science and modernity as they are uniquely expressed in China.

HOLY WATER AND POLLUTING FLOWERS

My watch says 8:30 A.M., though cool early morning light has just overtaken Lhasa's night sky. Thousands of miles from Beijing, we are still on Beijing time. It is late spring 2004 and I'm standing outside, waiting for Mingkyi to pick me up. She arrives, out of breath, cheeks apple red, hands tucked into her jacket, and registers a look of concern.

"Why are you not wearing a hat?" she scolds, by way of saying good morning. The driver we've hired for the day leans back against his SUV, blowing on his hands, smoking a cigarette. We hop into the car and head toward the Shongpalhachu Tibetan Medicine Factory.[12] Located not far from Lhasa, the factory is named for a sacred spring that flows nearby.

"These days it is difficult to find really good quality medicine, made by people of ability [yönten], with proper blessings and the right way to prepare ingredients," says Mingkyi. Although she is a skilled Tibetan doctor, she lives an urban life and rarely makes her own medicines. "Nowadays there is a lama from eastern Tibet who lives in the small temple just up there," she points, "near to the spring. He is very accomplished. It brings benefit to the factory." This comment not only points to Shongpalhachu's history as a place marked by the Guru Rinpoche, the famous eighth-century figure credited with the introduction of Buddhism in Tibet, but also illustrates the notion that efficacy is produced within specific social ecologies. In English, the place is called Holy Water Tibetan Medicine Factory. This references the story of Guru Rinpoche ramming his walking stick into the ground and creating a spring on this spot, and that Yuthog Yonten Gompo (the Elder) was born in the region. To Mingkyi and others, including the senior doctor who founded the factory, it is commonsensical that the specificities of this place and the spiritual power associated with it could *directly* impact medicines produced here. A sense of sacred geography and medical lineage remains central to Shongpalhachu's history and its brand, even as the valley a dozen miles outside Lhasa is filling up with other industries, from greenhouses and cement factories to freight yards.

The factory sits at the foot of a tawny mountain ridge. Ripening barley fields and whitewashed adobe homes line the dirt road leading to the gate. Shongpalhachu is what, in business parlance, one would call a public-private partnership, in this case connected to the Nagchu Mentsikhang and some private investment. It illustrates a larger trend, evidenced throughout the 1990s and early 2000s, of for-profit pharmaceutical factories emerging from state-run hospitals of Tibetan medicine. Shongpalhachu does not benefit from the large state contracts of the Mentsikhang, but it has a good reputation.

It is not yet 10 A.M. when we arrive, but several boom boxes are already blasting Chinese and Tibetan pop tunes and Budweiser cans have been stacked in a pyramid in the courtyard. I wonder if I have forgotten a Tibetan holiday, until I ask the first factory worker I meet what is going on.

"We're having a GMP party!" she says. The factory has just passed GMP compliance. They will be issued their certificate before the June deadline, so the directors decided to throw a bash. After months of halted production and nervous energy, they can now begin producing medicines in the new GMP-standard building.

I last visited Shongpalhachu about four months earlier. This morning I am astounded at the pace and scale of change. A three-story stucco structure with Tibetan-style awnings has replaced the older, smaller buildings devoted to drying and cleaning materials. The garden and herb cultivation plots that used to be at the center of the compound now sit on adjacent land, outside the factory's walls.

The production manager, shows us around the new production facilities, but he tells us we cannot enter the GMP building: "There are not the right people on duty who can give us the right clothes to put on." The manager traces his fingers across an architectural plan of the factory, a map of the manufactured terrain in which a new kind of medical and social efficacy is being constructed. The sales department is not yet finished, but looms large. This exchange illustrates what Saxer (2010a: 177) has called "rituals of GMP" and indicates how central aesthetic forms are to this exercise in rendering Tibetan medicine legible within the context of contemporary China. This concern with uniform aesthetics even extends to the design of factories, many of which were envisioned by the same architects.

Mingkyi and I learn that Shongpalhachu employs about fifty people. Their operation includes departments for raw materials, facility operations and personnel management, standardization, and quality control. I ask what the quality control department does. "Those people are experts," Palsang answers. "They do laboratory checks for dirt, molds, and other impurities. This work is more connected to good supply practice, not GMP, but they are related. Other people who know Tibetan medicine are still testing the medicine ingredients in traditional ways of knowing if something has good potency and quality."

"What happens if there is a disagreement about the quality of a raw material or a medicine?" I ask.

"We are a small factory, so people can still talk to each other and come to agreement. But now that we have GMP, we have to listen to what the quality experts say." I am reminded of Mitchell's (2002) argument about how technological and political barriers—jurisdictions—are created by the idea of being an "expert" and how this can reinforce forms of inequality and hierarchies of authoritative knowledge.

One part of the main production building had been fitted with a greenhouse-style roof. "What is that?" I ask.

"A special room for drying some ingredients," Palsang answers. "It allows us sunlight, like the old ways of drying medicines, but none of the dirt from outside." At the time I was unable to see the inside of this room, so I could not confirm whether this space was used for drying preprocessed plants or finished *rilbu*, although it was likely the latter.

Tibetan medical theory advises that medicinal ingredients should be dried under varying climatic conditions (shade, direct sun, etc.) depending on their nature *(ngobo)*. In many GMP-certified factories, large indoor electrical dryers or even industrial-size microwaves are visible. This factory's innovation meets GMP climate control requirements *and* complies with Tibetan medical theory.[13] Shongpalhachu also uses large mortars and pestles fashioned into mechanized grinders. Palsang explains that, while these grinders are not directly required by the GMP—indeed the presence of mechanized grinders predates these regulations by about two decades—they are being remodeled or replaced, in some instances, as part of the building and retrofitting of factories. At Shongpalhachu they have chosen to fit some grinders with marble mechanized mortars and pestles so that ingredients are not ground with metal, which according to Tibetan pharmacology texts may alter *nüpa*. Here and in other factories, stainless steel grinders are also in play, although the question of whether stainless steel alters *nüpa* remains open to debate (see Saxer 2010a).

"We also have a special filter for our water," says Palsang. "Now we don't have to boil water before we use it to clean the ingredients. The water tastes different, but now we can keep using the water from the holy spring. The filter machine cost one hundred thousand yuan [$12,500], but we thought it was worth the expense, since this factory is known for its pure, medicinal water."

The manager then leads us toward a shrine room. "Shongpalhachu also does *mendrup*," Mingkyi says, referring to the medicine-consecration ceremonies that have historically been part of the medicine-production process, and of which you will learn more in chapter 7. These ceremonies were not conducted during the Cultural Revolution, but they were revitalized in the early 1980s and are now allowed, even at state institutions like the Mentsikhang factory. To many Sowa Rigpa practitioners and Tibetan consumers, these ceremonies are a crucial component of what makes a medicine efficacious.

This morning at Shongpalhachu helps me to articulate the spaces of incommensurability (Kuhn [1962] 1996) as well as spaces of innovation

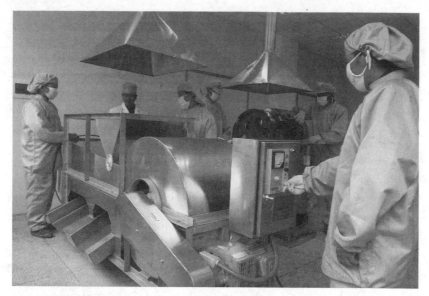

Inside the Tibetan Medicine Pharmaceutical Factory, Lhasa, Tibet Autonomous Region, China. © Thomas Kelly

that surface through an examination of GMP, *even if they are not, in themselves, a product or a requirement of GMP implementation.* Tibetan producers are adopting new practices of production that are accountable first and foremost to national Chinese governance regimes, themselves connected to international conceptions of what makes for "good" medicine, and also to the market. These changes surface in how factories are designed and constructed, how labor is recruited, and how ingredients are sourced, prepared, and compounded.

The advent of GMP certification precipitated the construction of new factories such as this one, and extensive retrofitting, at a breakneck pace in the early 2000s. These GMP facilities are much more expensive to build and operate than non-GMP sites. They consume more energy and rely on high-tech equipment that requires additional expertise to maintain and repair. In the years leading up to 2004, I observed that Tibetan medicine companies were engaged in a type of competition to see who could build the biggest, most expensive facilities, even as they were also under significant time pressures to make these changes. Some factories used government loans for this purpose; at times this has led to factory debt.[14] The new drug manufacturing regulations did not, in themselves, force the closure of sites producing non-GMP medicines, so long as medicines produced at such facilities were destined for use only in Tibetan medicine hospitals and clinics. Nor did they directly mandate price increases. But these have been two powerful indirect effects of what we can call the GMP era.[15] In many cases investments in technology and infrastructure have been extreme. In addition, some personnel must have different qualifications from those who staffed factories during pre-GMP times.

As we stand outside the GMP-certified factory, which cost $1.3 million to build, the manager explains, "With GMP many things have become more expensive: electricity, labor, things like that. This changes what we have to charge for medicines. Using our old system, we could pay someone five hundred yuan [$60] a month, and that was considered a decent wage for a medicine-making assistant. Now GMP means we pay at least three times that, sometimes more, in addition to paying for the trainings. Still, it is difficult for us to find good people. We want to hire from Tibetan medical colleges. People didn't have to know GMP before. Now they do. Getting this experience takes away from their studies of Tibetan medicine. So the overall quality of people studying Tibetan medicine is declining. It is hard to find fifty percent of students who can explain the three *nyepa* and five elements well."

As I begin to understand, GMP is at once a thing in itself—Good Manufacturing Practices as a national mandate—and also a shortcut for referring to a whole range of changes in the manufacture of Tibetan medicines since the advent of the socialist market economy in the early 1990s and that have accelerated rapidly since 2001. While many of the specific articles within the Chinese GMP may seem eminently sensible—stressing the need for dust collection equipment and ventilation systems, or that persons responsible for manufacturing need to have professional knowledge of the medical system in question (e.g., TCM)—they are intimately bound up in a larger framework of the PRC's drug regulations and in the project of rendering Tibetan medicine legible, and in that sense tamed, within the context of Chinese drug regulations and the juggernaut of capitalism with Chinese characteristics. Indeed as Martin Saxer (2010a) shows in his ethnographic and textual comparison of Chinese GMP and relevant passages from traditional Tibetan pharmacological texts, the presumed incommensurability often does not bear out in practice. Yet the anxiety and the impacts of major material investments required at the beginning of the GMP era should not be underestimated.

The production manager continues, "In the West, maybe people think new technology actually makes things cheaper and more efficient. But here, this is not the case. When we made medicines in the old way, we didn't have to worry about buying fancy machines to clean the air and water. We could pay local villagers without much education to work with us, grinding and sifting medicines, helping to make pills. It was good for them and good for us. Now GMP tells us we need experts to make all medicines standard and safe according to what they say. This costs more. We need to bring in people from the outside."

Meeting the demands of new pharmaceutical governance regimes impacts the value, meaning, and structure not only of Tibetan medicine production, but also of Tibetan medical education. The next generations of graduates from Tibetan medical colleges in China are being tracked in new ways. While some will serve Tibetan patients in rural and urban facilities, others will become quality assurance officers, marketers, clinical researchers, and pharmacists. GMP compliance has come to signify changes in labor relations. Before increasing mechanization and now the GMP era, those assisting with medicine production had a strong sensory relationship with the plants, minerals, and animal products. Making medicines required physical strength and drew from local populations. In the highly mechanized era of GMP-certified factories, employees are physically separated from *materia medica* through ritualized acts of donning disposable scrubs, masks, and plastic gloves. While this keeps things "clean"—and is even lauded as a positive change by many in the industry as standards to which other small-scale producers should aspire—it also changes the embodied nature of producing Tibetan medicine. This is not to say that factories are inimical places, but rather that spaces and times for social interaction have become distinct from those devoted to labor. In Marxian terms, this shift corresponds with a transition from conceiving of Tibetan medicines primarily for their *use value,* their direct utility, to seeing them as items that embody specific *exchange values,* linked with market prices and emblematic of processes of standardization and commodification.

The GMP era has ushered in a new set of discourses about what constitutes a "good" environment for making medicines. In the pre-GMP days, Shongpalhachu's courtyard was bursting with flowers. Plots of cultivated medicinal plants poked up from behind the buildings. These have been replaced with clinical, closely shorn sod. "What happened to the flower garden?" I ask the manager.

"We can't accept flowers in the factory area," answers Palsang. "According to GMP, flowers cause pollution."

One professor at the Tibetan Medical College described these changes as follows: "It is not a problem to make money. The problem is how we make the medicines now, what the ingredients are like, how they are collected. Before, we prepared medicines by first harvesting the ingredients well—taking care with the time we collect, the tastes of the medicines, how much we take when, the nature of our minds when we collected. Then we mixed the ingredients together and ground them. If you read the texts, there are even different descriptions of how your body should feel—where you should be in pain—after making medicines. Now they tell us each ingredient has to be clean. But what do they mean by 'clean'? It is different from how we have been taught to make medicines. Now they even make new kinds of *rilbu* that aren't really *rilbu*. They call these medicines *capsule*. They are strange, but people say they're cleaner. They look like Western medicine. We make a lot of them."

These comments illustrate the changed social ecology of medicine production. Even if they don't necessarily mandate production circumstances incommensurate with traditional methods, GMP regulations have, I argue, inspired a fetishization of cleanliness in the sense of hygiene and recast what is considered a potential contaminant. These regulations do not directly address sourcing issues, but GMP compliance, in combination with Chinese Drug Administration laws and Good Supply Practices, has transformed the spaces of medicine making. While it might be appropriate to guard against biohazards and contaminants when dealing with chemical compounds, the argument is more difficult to make with flowers, especially when some are the self-same plants used to make Tibetan medicines.

A pharmacist who worked at the Mentsikhang factory explained this dynamic further: "The Seven Limb Procedure [*yenlak dün*] in the *Fourfold Treatise* says we should use herbs that are harvested by people with good hearts [*sem sangpo*]." He went on to stress the importance of *not* using materials that were defiled (*drip*) in a spiritual sense, and that were also clean (*tsang ma*) in a material sense. "But according to GMP, we could collect plants even from a place at war, like Iraq or Afghanistan, and use these ingredients in medicines, so long as the bags of ingredients were not mixed with grass or stones or dirt. To us, this would be very bad, if people collecting were also engaged in killing and fighting. This would have a karmic effect on the quality and benefits of medicines. GMP does not think of such things. GMP is about making sure everything is clean according to their ideas."

Clearly there is an ethical tenor to these debates over "good" practices, a sensibility that integrates a moral epistemology, tied to Buddhism, that undergirds aspects of Tibetan medical theory. Becoming GMP-certified has corresponded to an increasing concern with avoiding material contamination and promoting new sensibilities with regard to "clean" and "dirty" environments. Some have come to equate sterile factories with a higher order of cleanliness, stemming from a modern, technoscientific aesthetic. This can supersede concerns regarding the loss of medical efficacy linked to poor ethical conduct of those harvesting raw materials or producing medicines, or the sacrificed relationship between medicine production and the social ecologies in which it has historically been embedded.

This theme of cleanliness and contamination can produce cultural incommensurability, if not direct pharmacological conflict. For example, both GMP regulations and Tibetan medical texts speak to the question of shelf life. While the fifth limb of the *Seven Limb Procedure* states that herbs should be processed into medicine within one year of collection, except in cases of decoction, the GMP's article 43 lists a maximum three-year shelf life for all materials "unless otherwise defined" (Kuwahara and Li 2007: 105 in Saxer 2010a: 67). In practice, both the traditional regulations and the GMP stipulations may be altered. Yet to my interlocutors in the early days of the GMP era, they were concerned that compliance with these regulations would render materials unusable well before a physician-pharmacist, or even a factory pharmacist, could determine that they had lost potency. To some people I interviewed, this was a benefit of GMP: it would help ensure Tibetan medicines were made with *materia medica* that had not been sitting on a dusty shelf for years. To others, this underscored the differences between GMP regulations and Tibetan medical knowledge.

Sourcing issues also reflect the paradoxes of an industry that is scaling up as some sources are becoming rare or endangered. This issue predates the GMP but may be exacerbated by it, since related Good Agricultural Practices regulations speak only obliquely to environmental impact with respect to what qualifies as "good" sourcing. Instead emphasis has been placed on adhering to new legislation that requires all *materia medica* enter China through an authorized port by an authorized importer, which requires an expensive license; ingredients are then screened in drug testing offices, also an expensive process. In such milieu, no distinction is made between importing *arura,* one of Tibetan pharmacology's key species, and antibiotics (Saxer 2011). This has changed the social ecologies and economics of cross-border trade in *materia medica* between Nepal, India, and China, thereby compromising a major source of income from the medicinal plant trade for many people and, in some instances, inciting smuggling. These changes have also resulted in a higher value being placed on "audit culture" (Strathern 2000) than on the maintenance of reliable and renewable sourcing relationships.

But this also begs the question *Were Tibetan materia medica being collected and harvested, bought and sold, only in places undefiled and by people of pure intention before GMP?* The answer is clearly no. Likewise GMP has not stopped people from overharvesting plants with high market value, trafficking in endangered species, using highly prized ingredients such as saffron *(kache gurgum)* from embattled Kashmir or Afghanistan, or dealing in fake medicines (Dawa 2011). And even though laws against harvesting endangered species do exist on paper in both China and Nepal, they are not always enforced; furthermore the permitting process to collect limited quantities of rare or threatened ingredients is cumbersome and subject to the forces of corruption and the power that larger producers can wield over local authorities, thereby further marginalizing small-scale and independent producer-practitioners. Yet this does not mean that the pharmacist quoted earlier was insincere. Rather his concerns point to competing ethics regarding the standards by which "good" practice should be evaluated.

For many of my interlocutors in China, the term *GMP* came to stand for much more than constructing new factories and adopting novel processing techniques. GMP often became a subject/animated in people's discussions. One well-respected Tibetan pharmacologist in Lhasa put it this way: "GMP is a very new situation for an old system of knowledge. Sometimes we are afraid that by making Tibetan medicine to GMP standards, it is like making clothes that look good on the outside, but that do not fit, or that are the wrong color. It is hard to compare the old knowledge of Tibetan medicine with these new rules. We have a long history and have used our medicines for thousands of years, but we need to find a way to translate this to the outside." One of Saxer's (2010a: 95) interlocutors expresses a similar sentiment when he says, "GMP for Tibetan medicine is like putting a goat's head on a sheep's body," a metaphor Saxer complicates and analyzes in his ethnography. It would be too simple to cast GMP and traditional Tibetan methods of production in stark opposition, or to assume that these regulations are at the heart of conflicts of best practices on the ground. However, such sentiments concerning medicine that looks good on the outside but whose quality and efficacy is difficult to verify point to a range of ethical, cultural, and practical tensions.

During the first years of the GMP, people I interviewed in Lhasa spoke about these dynamics in terms of rights *(thob wang)*, power *(tséwang)*, and authority *(wang cha)* to make their medicines. Many producers articulated in their own words what social theorists such as Michel Foucault would call the "biopolitics" of pharmaceutical governance. They resented that Tibetan medicine was being made to follow, as some interviewees put it, "the laws of your country" *(kye rang gyi lung ba'i trim)* or "Western science" *(nub chog gyi tsen rig)*. When discussing GMP, interviewees would often refer to the WHO or the U.S. FDA in English or Tibetan (*dzamling tröten tsadzuk* and *ari mendzé dangzé rikdo damchu*, respectively), as the source of irrelevant and even harmful strictures placed on the production of formulas whose safety and quality should be determined by other means. It is crucial to note, however, that this was the case even though they knew GMP implementation in China was the purview of the *Chinese* SFDA and related bureaus, not the WHO or the U.S. FDA.

A monk-physician from Qinghai once said to me, "This thing they call GMP is like the Cultural Revolution. They are both about blindly following rules, with no sense, no respect for culture. But GMP is worse because it is not just in China. It is across the whole world." I often wondered whether some of this ire was easier for my Tibetan interlocutors to direct at international agencies rather than the Chinese state.

In China, GMP and associated standards draw on U.S. FDA policy as well as WHO guidelines, but they are fundamentally the domain of the SFDA. Chinese GMP regulations were first created for biomedical pharmaceuticals in 1998 and have gone through several revisions in the past decade (Xie 2007). The regulation of traditional and herbal formulations in China began in earnest with the 2001 Drug Administration Law, which has seen many subsequent revisions and amendments. These regulations emerged from a long history of collaboration and contestation between indigenous and biomedical practices in China. Official doctrine on traditional medicine has shifted many times since the collapse of the Chinese imperial order in 1911 and the creation of the People's Republic in 1949, and then in the Maoist and post-Mao era (Unschuld 1985; Farquhar 1995; Taylor 2005; Scheid 2007). As Mao rose to power after 1949, he initially shunned traditional forms of medicine, calling their efficacy into question and equating traditional practitioners with quacks and charlatans; his position shifted in the mid-1950s, as he realized that traditional medicine in China could contribute to a new nationalist agenda of building a strong, healthy, and modern Chinese nation. It was from this perspective that the (in)famous Barefoot Doctors emerged, along with the creation of what we call today Traditional Chinese Medicine (Taylor 2005; Hsu 2008a).

Since 1958, China has embraced, in various forms, the interpenetration of biomedicine and traditional medicines. However, this Three Roads (Ch. *san daolu*) policy, wherein biomedicine and traditional medicines were used concurrently and points of integration were encouraged, has often reinforced the dominance of biomedicine as practiced in urban China and by the Han majority culture (White 2001; Fan and Holliday 2006). Indeed a strong ideological commitment to science in the People's Republic of China has also driven a state health care system that, while often lauded for its "integrative" ethos, is still one in which biomedicine remains hegemonic and in which even mainstream TCM occupies a shifting position (Farquhar 1994; Hsu 2001, 2008a; Scheid 2007). Nonbiomedical epistemology and practice are often marginalized even within institutions that are nominally devoted to traditional medicine (Fan and Holliday 2007). In an article that includes case studies of Tibetan, Uighur, and Mongolian medicines in China, Fan and Holliday (2007) argue that an "ideology of science," which assumes that all traditional forms of medicine should be produced, evaluated, and reformed according to biomedical standards, rests on unstable empirical ground. Yet the ideology of science, particularly in the context of Chinese socialism, remains strong (Chen 2005).

There is another layer to all of this. Chinese GMP regulations of Tibetan medicine are based, first, on conventional methods for producing biomedical pharmaceuticals and, second, on GMP regulations of TCM formulas. This is true despite significant differences in *materia medica,* pharmacology, and medical theory. The SFDA's decision to model Tibetan regulations on TCM could be taken for granted. Why not model state-supported Traditional Tibetan Medicine on TCM? However, this Beijing-level policy reflects larger political projects in which Tibetanness *must* fit within an overarching model of Chineseness. Institutional TCM and Chinese biomedicine hold powerful sway in shaping today's "minority nationality medicine" policies (Fan and Holliday 2007). But

Tibetan ambivalence about the GMP era extends from the realm of biomedicine and technoscience to social and political concerns about the place of Tibet and Tibetans in contemporary China, and the state's regulation of ethnic minorities (Litzinger 1998; Harrell 2001; Hillman 2003).

GMP implementation exemplifies Foucauldian ideas about states and the citizen-subjects they manage. You have already seen the ways governmentality—the art and techniques by which citizen-subjects are governed—plays out with respect to state legitimation of Sowa Rigpa practitioners in Nepal and China. With respect to GMP, not only is governmentality at play but also what Foucault calls "technologies of the self": forms of knowledge and strategies that "permit individuals to effect by their own means or with the help of others a certain number of operations on their own bodies and souls, thoughts, conduct, and way of being" (1988: 18). The ways Tibetans involved in the industry *experience* these transformations and *respond* to them reveal how regimes of governance regulate people's behaviors through the application of political power, which becomes embodied in human experience, including making medicines.

Not only is the *techne,* the art and science, behind medicine production changing, but so too is the *episteme,* in a Foucauldian sense of this term. In his work on the knowledge-power nexus, Foucault defines *episteme* as "the 'apparatus' which makes possible the separation, not of the true from the false, but of what may from what may not be characterized as scientific" (1980: 197). The GMP era emerges from national governing bodies and is supported by pervasive ideologies of science and modernity that take root within a minority region of China in specific forms. The enactment of GMP compliance requires the creation of and adherence to new domains of authoritative knowledge, even if both "traditional" methods of production and GMP standards are in a sense abstract principles that are often altered through practice. While they may not always or necessarily be incommensurate—indeed, as we will see below, they can even create new possibilities for action—they have also led to new practical and ethical dilemmas.

TRANSLATION, TRUST, AND TRADITIONS TRANSFORMED

In July 2010 my research assistant, Drolma, meets me in the courtyard of the Qinghai Tibetan Medical Hospital. "Demo," she calls, in Amdo greeting. *"Dr. Thoga is expecting now we will arrive,"* she continues, in confident if imperfect English. I follow Drolma into the hospital production facility, where Dr. Thoga greets us. He is in charge of the hospital's medicine production unit. Wearing a pressed white coat embossed with the Arura insignia, the director pours us small paper cups of steaming jasmine tea.

As with other aspects of this institution, as you saw in chapter 2, Arura's leaders have navigated Chinese regulations and medicine production policies with insight and acumen. In the years since GMP was implemented in 2004, several institutions, including the Mentsikhang factory in Lhasa, have begun lobbying to *re-create* non-GMP facilities. Where there was once a certain fetishization of GMP facilities, along with the rapid and high-stakes demand that factories become compliant, there is now more understanding of what GMP does and does not mandate, more disillusion about what certification buys, and perhaps more space to assert standards of cultural heritage over technoscience, at least with respect to medicines made for clinical use in China's Tibetan hospitals (Saxer 2010a). From the outset, Arura fashioned its approach to manufacturing in pioneering ways, maintaining this on-site production facility for hospital medicines even as it created a new GMP-certified pharmaceutical factory. In addition to meeting state requirements for commercial manufacture, Arura doctors still produce *tsothal* on site. Regular *mendrup* ceremonies are also conducted. Arura's leaders thought proactively about how best to meet GMP and SFDA regulations, and at the same time carve out a brand and a niche for themselves within the "moral economy of Tibetanness" in China (Saxer 2010a).

Drolma and I settle into leather recliners near Dr. Thoga's desk, beside a small room brimming with medical texts and herbal samples. All Tibetan medicines being prescribed at this hospital are made in this unit— more than 260 different formulas. This unit is also a site of research and experimentation. Dr. Thoga explains that they are working on new variations of old recipes and new forms of medicine and other health products created explicitly for local clinical use. He shows us an array of products under development in this non-GMP facility: a Tibetan herbal toothpaste and mouth spray, a medicated bandage for joint problems (in some ways similar to the top earner of the rival company, Cheezheng), and a medicinal wine reputed to be good for strengthening bones. The medicated bandage and mouth spray are this doctor's inventions, based on preparations he learned under the tutelage of a senior *menpa* with whom he studied during his vacations from medical school. Here a sensibility that values oral practice, lineage-based knowledge, and pharmacological variation comes to rest *within* a context in which scaling up and standardizing production also remain the goal. What have been points of incommensurability in other domains, or at different points in the recent history of Tibetan medical production, seem to be reconciled here through innovation.

"We want to make Tibetan medicines easier to use, to improve the public health and hygiene," Dr. Thoga says. "The toothpaste has been a challenge. It is difficult to find the perfect combination of modern forms with traditional principles and old recipes." I think back to my time at the Lhasa factory and the way the factory manager espoused abstract ideas about "traditional wisdom" and "scientific knowledge." Here, in this simple tube of prototype toothpaste, is a concrete example of such efforts.

"We try to use only one modern material," Dr. Thoga continues, fingering the medicated bandage. "With this one, we use a new method to make the bandage stick to the body. It is less messy than the traditional ways, convenient. You keep these patches on for twenty-four to forty-eight hours on the knee. We also give the patient herbal medicines to eat." The consumers of these medicines are those seeking treatment at this hospital or, presumably, their family members. Dr. Thoga tells me that the government sets price increases for noncommercial formulas at a maximum rate of 5 percent over five years. For this reason the fact that medicines produced here are *not* GMP-certified may help to *encourage* patients to seek care from a Tibetan physician instead of just purchasing medicines over the counter. "We want to make the best relationship with doctor and patient," the director goes on. "Here we are different from the GMP factory. Here we don't study MBA. We just want to do good for our patients."

Yet it is precisely the for-profit entrepreneurial spirit and market-driven success of Arura's commercial products that allows this branch of Arura to focus on clinical care and practical adaptations. As we have seen, other producers have carved out spaces in which GMP ceases to be relevant, is directly challenged, or is selectively ignored. Some pragmatists within the industry have even told me it was often easier to falsify standard operating procedure registers than to deal directly with issues of incommensurability that have arisen in recent years, in the wake of GMP and related regulations. In contrast, Arura's overt agenda of compliance coupled with innovation seems to meld compliance with an ethics of care and a spirit of medical and social practice.

Knowing that Arura has explicitly decoupled the labor of commercial, GMP-certified production from hospital pharmacy production, I want to learn more about what distinguishes the two sites. I ask Dr. Thoga about sourcing. As mentioned in chapter 2, Arura has one central sourcing program, from which raw materials are sent either to the GMP factory or to this hospital production unit.

"Most hot, lowland ingredients from Nepal and India come through middlemen, sometimes through connections with other factories," Dr. Thoga answers. "We like to send people from Arura to markets and pick the best themselves. But this is not always possible. Plants, seeds, and roots should be harvested at different seasons, but in the marketplace we cannot always tell when something was harvested. But for the benefit of the patients, we want to find the best quality."

"What about ingredients that come from high-altitude areas, from Tibet?" I ask.

"For this we use middlemen but also people who work here, since they are from all over [Tibetan areas]. Whey they go home, they make relations with local people to collect ingredients that grow there. Our doctors explain what to collect and give training to these people in how to harvest. For example, if you use the flower in medicine, you don't pick the entire plant. But when business people do this collecting, they don't always follow such rules." These issues have been echoed by my colleagues in Nepal, as well as in studies showing that commercial production has influenced harvesting patterns (Ghimire, McKey, and Aumeeruddy-Thomas 2005a, 2005b).

"Before we started doing this training, people did not know. Sometimes they would pick the entire plant, even when this was not necessary. This is still a problem, but it has improved," the doctor continues. At Arura the mandate for producing quality medicines includes a set of social-ecological relationships, even though these ingredients are used to produce medicines for *both* commercial and clinical clientele.

"How do people know if a medicine is of high quality?" I ask. "Who makes these decisions?"

"We work differently than other factories, at least from what I know. We have eighty people in our quality department. We use machines to test for dirt and mold, but first we use traditional methods based on taste, smell, et cetera. This is most important.

"Three times a year, someone from the government does special test-ing," Dr. Thoga continues. "Mostly they figure out whether or not the ingredient is the species it is supposed to be and also if it has other things mixed in with it. This is investigated according to medicine production laws. We do not have control over this. But we make decisions about potency and taste.

"The main difference between here and our GMP factory is not about sourcing, but about standards of hygienic conditions for the place where medicines are made, and packaging. We are only GPP—Good Pharmacy Practice. This is enough for us here." At Arura, GMP still embodies the aesthetic practices of scientific production in that it functions as the gateway to commercial sale, but being compliant with this range of drug administration regulations has not translated into complete transforma-tions of production methods or a disavowal of tradition in the name of science. When it comes to sourcing, Arura has not completely escaped issues of incommensurability. Traditional standards of potency and quality are still linked to practices of matching Tibetan plant names with their botanical equivalents, according to Chinese-language protocols is-sued by the central government and used by provincial-level drug admin-istration bureaus. Furthermore Arura's reliance on middlemen to source ingredients, some of which comes from Nepal and India, implicate them in border regimes and new forms of quality testing (Saxer 2011). How-ever, another order of quality testing remains oriented around Tibetan medical theory. State-sanctioned or not, these patterns of determining the quality of raw materials does influence production in the GMP factory because the sources are one and the same.

I note differences in how Dr. Thoga speaks about these issues now, in Qinghai in 2010, compared with similar conversations I had with other Lhasa-based producers during the early GMP era and in the more po-litically sensitive environment of the TAR. In that milieu, a sense of strife pervaded these conversations. Many people thought the way forward was to create a Tibetan-language GMP, since one of the oft-cited com-plaints about GMP regulations was that they are written in Mandarin and that Tibetan factories are inspected primarily by Chinese specialists who know little about Tibetan medicine. Much, they argued, is lost in the translation.

One factory executive with whom I spoke in Lhasa in 2003 put it this way: "GMP regulations are not easy to understand in Tibetan. They are written in Chinese, with a more modern way of thinking. But without being an expert Tibetan doctor, it is difficult to know how to make GMP better for Tibetan medicine, more true to Tibetan knowledge." In the years since GMP compliance became compulsory, translations of GMP regulations into Tibetan have been produced, with some success (Tso 2011). This process required the creation of Tibetan neologisms that can at times create confusion. Consider the challenges of precisely translating concepts like "particle contaminant ratios" into Tibetan and "postdigestive tastes" into Chinese. But translation issues also signify deeper and more complicated points of ambivalence with respect to the regulation of Tibetan ways of knowing by biomedically conditioned Chinese arbiters.

One of the benefits of ethnography is that it can reveal how culture is contingent and can harbor many points of view. In this vein, some people doubted the quality of GMP-certified medicines in what has clearly become a money-making industry because they viewed it as a departure from the ethical purpose of producing Tibetan medicines. Others derided their fellow countrymen for doubting the quality, safety, and efficacy of "modern" Tibetan medicine, as epitomized by GMP, and chastised those who would value "superstitious" and "backward" production practices of the "old society," a veiled reference to Tibet prior to "liberation," over those promulgated in the GMP era. A Tibetan GMP specialist from Lhasa put it this way: "The people of the old society [chitsok nyingba] and today's situation are not the same. Now we must follow GMP, and there are some problems. . . . Before, there was a lot of cultural knowledge [rigné], but not so much experience with economic forces when considering medicine—what makes it high quality, how to sell it. Today the main concern is the economy, not only with healing."

She went on to compare Tibetan medicine to different brands of soda. To some Tibetan pharma producers, GMP compliance filled them with hope. The factory manager from my visit to Mentsikhang in 2002 said, "GMP is the key to the door of the outside world." From this perspective GMP was an emblem of, or an entrance into, modernity: a process that would allow Tibetans to gain wealth and fame as well as benefit humanity.

Of course, this begs the question *Is scaling up the right thing to do? If so, right for whom, and with what long-term implications?* The elephant in the room is depletion of ingredients wild-crafted from high-altitude environments that, in many ways, make this medicine uniquely *Tibetan*. Over the course of my research I've noted ingredients whose prices have more than trebled between 2002 and 2010, and that are becoming increasingly difficult to find in large enough quantities to meet both clinical and commercial production demands. During a frank discussion about the future of Tibetan medicine with a senior factory administrator, he said, "We don't think of the environment. It is not like small countries like Bhutan. In China—as in America—we just use things up and then, after we use them up, we worry about what to do."

THE BUDDHA AND COMMODITY FETISHISM

From the sidewalks of Lhasa to the avenues of other major Chinese cities, one can find displays advertising a range of commercially produced Tibetan pharmaceuticals. On a major shopping boulevard in downtown Lhasa, Mylar and brass constructions dwarf plaster-cast purple and pink mushrooms and day-glo plastic palm trees in this Oxford Circus–meets–Las Vegas aesthetic. The road is lined with shops selling Tibetan medical products. Standard marketing aesthetics in such retail establishments can include a green cross (signifying "natural" and "traditional" medicines), Buddhist imagery such as the deer and the *dharma* wheel (T. *chö kyi khorlo*, Skt. *dharma cakra*), and evocations of the "pure" mountains, lakes, and rolling grasslands that are the quintessence, if also the stereotype, of Tibetan wildlands. Consumers at these establishments are primarily Chinese tourists, in the case of Lhasa, and upper-middle-class Han Chinese in other cities.

It is rare to find a Tibetan of any social class purchasing items in such stores, although I have known some Tibetans to use products purchased through pharmacies run by state institutions of Tibetan medicine and offered at somewhat lower prices. Much of what is on offer in these places are heavily packaged, ready to bring back to a boss or someone with whom one hopes to garner *guanxi*, connections, and sold alongside miniature yak statues and faux Khampa warrior swords. The advertising bespeaks a benevolent, happy minority people; the small print hinges more directly on tropes of science, listing active ingredients and referencing specific biomedical disease categories or biological conditions that the product is said to treat. Prices are steep for these fetishized commodities.

A smiling "traditional" Tibetan nomad girl, arms outstretched in a field of high mountain rapeseed, sells medicated plasters recommended for joint problems. The Chinese-owned Cheezheng Group makes this product, the best-selling Tibetan over-the-counter formula in China and a paragon of what may be possible with "new" formulas dependent less on complex pharmacology and more on aesthetic transformations. With headquarters in Gansu Province and a factory located in the lush south-eastern Kongpo region of the TAR, in a region known for its bounty and diversity of medicinal plants, Cheezheng is the largest Tibetan medical company. The company's medicated plaster is one of the very few Tibetan medicinal products with a large export market, attributable to collaborations with Walmart (Yi 2003). In summer 2011, Cheezheng was gearing up for an initial public offering of its stock. The company's CEO, a Chinese woman and a devout Tibetan Buddhist, has also been instrumental in the creation of a Tibetan spa experience, geared toward Chinese consumers. What is on sale in this and related advertisements is not only relief from joint pain but also the consumption of Tibet and Tibetans, in all their pure, wholesome simplicity, with all their traditional wisdom—reformulated, of course, into modern and convenient forms.

Arura is another big player in this industry. Yet while Arura is certainly a successful business enterprise in a competitive marketplace, several characteristics set it apart from other commercial Tibetan medicine producers. These differences are what make Arura an interesting institution to work with, if also one that highlights the paradoxes of philanthropic capitalism. Some of Arura's market competitors include companies in which Chinese shareholders own majority stock; Arura remains (at least for now) majority Tibetan-owned. As you read in chapter 2, Arura's business model includes an explicit commitment to channel commercial profits back into the Qinghai Tibetan Medical Hospital, as well as to educating the next generation of Tibetan medical practitioners through support for faculty, student scholarships at the medical college as well as apprenticeships, and, down the road, salaries and careers at its clinical or commercial sites, including the cultural museum and the research institute. But none of this would be possible without the commercial sale of Tibetan formulas. The Arura Group's pharmaceutical factory sits in a science and technology park reminiscent of Silicon Valley on the periurban edges of Xining. This is one of three such factories in the vicinity. This particular site houses not only the GMP-certified commercial production facility but also marketing and administrative offices, a large warehouse from which tons of commercial products are readied for market, and an impressive showroom.

If you were to walk into the showroom at the Arura pharmaceutical factory, one of the first things you would encounter is a map of China, illuminated with small lights, under a banner that says "Arura Tibetan medicine chain stores." Although Arura does not sell its medicines abroad at present, expansion to new non-Chinese markets in the coming years is a possibility; about two hundred retail stores were slated for opening in China's eastern seaboard and cities in the north in 2011 alone. Its pharmaceutical factory produces more than seventy-five commercial Tibetan products that hold national patents, twelve of which are classified as national heritage drugs, classifications that bear not only on regimes of production but also on debates over intellectual property.[16] A young Han woman dressed in a Tibetan *chuba* made from pink brocade greets me at the door. Her English is as limited as my Mandarin, but she is adept at recounting prices in my native tongue.

Moving farther into this retail outlet, I find a *stupa*-like shrine to the spiritually minded consumer, reminiscent of the ways Tibetan sand mandala are displayed in monasteries, with an array of Medicine Buddha statues positioned at the top. Along the far wall of the store sits a large statue, not of the Buddha but of Yuthog Yonten Gonpo, the mythohistorical father of Tibetan medicine. His hand gestures mimic the teaching hand gesture (Skt. *mudra*) of the Buddha. Backlit shelves advertising Arura's most expensive commodities flank this figure. Such products include two vials of *yartsa gunbu (Ophiocordyceps sinensis),* the (in)famous caterpillar fungus that is sometimes called Tibetan Viagra and that is also purported to have a range of beneficial effects, from helping to address liver and kidney disorders to increasing clarity of thinking and, as recent clinical studies have shown, helping to address autoimmune disorders, including multiple sclerosis. These two vials of *yartsa gunbu* cost about $950. The best quality *yartsa gunbu* can price to $40,000 per kilogram wholesale (Winkler 2011).

On this visit to the factory outlet, I collect brochures for a range of products, which a research assistant later translates from Chinese. These products include a saffron capsule, a seabuckthorn capsule, Arura-brand *yartsa gunbu,* "Adapt to the Holy Land Capsule," and a yak (actually *dri,* as female yak are called) butter and milk capsule. Each brochure references the stresses, expectations, and desires of modern consumer-driven lives and the inherent benefits of "natural" products, particularly when refashioned through the tools of modern science and technology. Nomadic lifestyles and Buddhism are also referenced: yaks, salt lakes, snow mountains, religious texts, prayer wheels. Some include images of the ideal consumers: Western-dressed, light-skinned, urban Chinese adults. Most include sections devoted to describing in lay biochemical and biomedical terms the ingredients and their healing properties: "high concentration of essential fatty acids," "anti-cancer properties," and so forth.

Both saffron and seabuckthorn capsules are marketed as "feminine" products. Discussions with the marketing department at Arura and other Tibetan pharma factories indicate that the majority of Chinese consumers of Tibetan medicine are women between thirty and fifty years of age. I note parallels here with Arura's medicinal baths department but also with patients in small private clinics in Nepal and other parts of China. The saffron capsules should be used to address blood imbalances, including anemia, caused by the stresses of being a modern woman, and related dermatological problems. The brochure says, "According to Tibetan medical theory, heart controls blood vessels which manifest externally in the face or skin. The treatment process of Tibetan medicine proceeds from the inside out, and is gradually accepted. Pursuing natural beauty formula and healthy and moist skin is now the essential part of modern aesthetic value." Saffron nourishes and improves the quality of blood. The text references the origins of saffron as both an edible and a medicinal plant and its trade throughout Eurasia. The brochure notes that Tibetan saffron used to be paid to "the central dynasty" as tribute—a hint of revisionist history that would have Tibet as a principality of China even in the premodern era.

The saffron and seabuckthorn brochures feature minibiographies of consumers such as Cheng Yiyan, a thirty-two-year-old woman "who is hardworking and one of the key talents in her company," and Kiangmei, a forty-six-year-old vice president of a foreign investment company. These testimonials illustrate the range of stressors impacting such individuals, concluding, without irony, "Due to stress, women, especially those in the working class, can hardly balance hormones in their bodies." When combined with lifestyle and dietary changes, these products claim to be beneficial for a range of problems, from acne to insomnia.

These stories are rich in analytical material—not the least of which is the pathologization of the successful Chinese woman—but it is noteworthy that key ingredients in several of these formulas derive from cultivatable plants or animal products, two of which are more endemic to the southern hills of the Hindu-Kush Himalaya than they are to the Tibetan Plateau. There is some scalable, social entrepreneurial hope here—if not without risk. These products are based more on single key ingredients than on the complex pharmacology required of "precious pills," for example. This has implications both in terms of sustainable ingredient sourcing and with respect to mitigating troublesome issues of knowledge and intellectual property rights that have embroiled several Tibetan medical producers in legal battles (Saxer 2010a). Furthermore

some farmers might make a decent living growing, harvesting, and selling such raw materials to factories like Arura. But this does not really
address market-based dependencies and the transformation of Tibetan
and Himalayan social ecologies that occur through commodification.

One page of the *Adapt to the Holy Land Capsule* brochure harnesses
potent Tibetan images and forms to valorize the Motherland and the
place of Tibetans within it. A poem titled "The Holy Land, the Qinghai-
Tibet Plateau" is framed by images of carved *mani,* Tibetan prayer stones.
The verse begins as follows:

> The unsurpassed spirit of a *minzu* [minority nationality]
> Heart is the Bodhi tree
> Distant, serene, and holy
> Prayer stones are piled by the path
> Rivers flow from the foot of snow mountains
> The fragrant smell of tea wafts through the air
> Flute music from the herders are distant but clear.

The poem goes on to imply that prosperity has come to the plateau
and, by extension, the Tibetan people, since Chinese "liberation."

The opposing page describes the geographical features of the Tibetan
Plateau, emphasizing its clean, pure environment, which is at once beneficial and potentially harmful to nonnatives, be they Chinese or, as depicted on the brochure, Euro-American backpackers. The brochure goes
on to define altitude sickness in terms of biometric signs and symptoms.
Prior to a section that describes the contents of the capsule and its efficacy with reference to a clinical trial, the brochure notes, "The best way
to avoid or alleviate high altitude sickness is to have a good mentality.
Many illnesses are caused by mentality. It is recommended that tourists
follow advice: don't run or do physical work, don't eat heavy meals,
don't drink alcohol or smoke, eat vegetarian food. Don't take many
showers. Don't resort to the use of oxygen supplies so easily. You can also
take *Adapt to the Holy Land Capsule* and some other pills to alleviate
the symptoms like headache." While the ingredients in the capsule are
primarily derived from Tibetan *materia medica,* they have been formulated "based on the latest scientific findings concerning altitude sickness."
The brochure at once heralds Tibetan nature and views it as a potential
source of pathology—in this case, acute mountain sickness and related
complications. The suggestion to use a product comes, rather sweetly, after a set of behavioral injunctions that echo the advice one might actually

receive from a Tibetan medical practitioner. Yet claims of efficacy are validated by science, and by the *ideology* of science. The product creates a Tibet that is culturally intact, spiritually infused, politically docile, and scientifically potent.

In *The Devil and Commodity Fetishism,* Michael Taussig (1983), a physician turned anthropologist, provides a Marxist exploration of the sociocultural significance of devil imagery and stories about the devil told among plantation workers and miners in Colombia and Bolivia. In a nutshell, the devil becomes an image that helps mediate between "precapitalist" and "capitalist" modes of production and diverse experiences of the human condition. In this book, Taussig also argues that anthropology should be concerned with critiquing global capitalism and the ways it becomes intertwined with notions of Western culture. He suggests that we should shift the unit of analysis away from the gaze on indigenous Others toward a more critical analysis of global capital and our places within it. He also points out that, in highland Colombia and Bolivia, indigenous expressions of the devil provide a means of recognizing the magical and, in this sense, productive *logic* of capitalism, even as his interlocutors *experience* capitalism as a system that gives rise to increased poverty, disease, and death in their communities.

Taussig's arguments are a lens through which we can view how images of and references to Buddhism and other symbols associated with Tibetanness are used to market high-end Tibetan medicines for urban, elite Chinese consumers and what the impacts of this choice may be. It is significant that Taussig's book, published in 1980, was aimed at critiques of Euro-American forms of capitalism and that today I am drawing your attention to Chinese forms of capitalism. In these brochures, images of Tibetan landscape, environment, and culture are presented alongside idealized images of Westernized lifestyles, biomedical disease categories, and a desire to harness the healing power of "pure" Tibetan nature. Here the logic of commodity fetishism in South America, as represented by a devil, is transformed into a Buddha, glowing with the aura of capitalism with Chinese characteristics.

While the logic of capitalism might be similar in highland South America and China's Tibet, the affective impact of referencing devils versus Buddhas is not. Taussig's devil is aggressive, at times bloodthirsty and malevolent. The Buddha is a model of benevolence. Such imagery is a proxy, in the Chinese context, for a successful minority nationality that has found a politically "appropriate" and economically valuable outlet for its cultural, environmental, and scientific uniqueness in a China whose present-day commitment to socialism is as ideological as it is superficial. Underpinning both the devil imagery and Buddhist benevolence is an appropriation of land and labor, nature and culture, which contributes to patterns of socioeconomic inequality, political exclusion, and market-based assaults on geographically marginalized highland populations, including their abilities to address health care needs. In Taussig's work, as with my own ethnography, I am at once fascinated and disturbed by the ways integration into regional and global markets produces a range of adverse effects on indigenous social ecologies, places like the Nepal Himalaya and the rural expanses of the Tibetan Plateau, where about 80 percent of all ethnic Tibetans live. In choosing to commercialize Tibetan medicine in ways that exploit a fetishized desire on the part of Chinese or foreign consumers for the peaceful and pristine, the environmentally bountiful and the spiritually enlightened, the mystical and the scientifically proven—and to do so in ways that rely on high-tech production methods and expensive packaging—one could argue that the viability of *other* Tibetan ways of stewarding landscapes and healing people are directly challenged.

This may be the case even at Arura, which, arguably, puts profit to work in meaningful ways. For as the fair and lovely Han woman with Prada on her shoulders and Blahnik on her toes purchases a $40 bottle of seabuckthorn supplements or a $400 vial of *yartsa gunbu* for her husband, somewhere else in this great country a rural Tibetan, perhaps suffering from tuberculosis or a blood-bile disorder, is hooked up to an antibiotic IV drip at an underresourced township clinic because the drip offers the most expedient salve for suffering—and an infusion of modernity. Never mind the biohazards behind the clinic, near a local water source, or the faint outlines of the borax mine down the valley. Maybe this individual travels to a Tibetan doctor who, despite increasing costs of raw materials and the specters of state extortion (for he produces without a proper license) continues to make medicine by hand. These powders wrapped in newsprint are known for their potency because of the person who made them, the materials that compose them, and the prayers that infuse them with a different kind of efficacy. Yet both realities—the commercial products and the handmade therapies—depend on allusions to Buddhism and Tibetan environments, albeit in distinct vernaculars and with reference to divergent moral economies. And herein lies the rub. As unnerving as it is to admit, the Buddha, in his benevolence and repose, is more insidious—or at least more capable of being misrecognized—than the devil.

SUMMARY

This chapter has analyzed the impacts of pharmaceutical governance on the production of Tibetan medicines in contemporary China. I presented evidence of the ways Tibetan knowledge systems and the value of medicines themselves are being transformed through engagements with science, technology, and the market. You have seen from the factory floor, so to speak, how global regulatory bodies influence the creation of national governance regimes, which in turn shape local social practices, and how local practices are refigured and reworked in light of these new systems of authoritative knowledge. We can thus advance our understanding of globalized ideas about science and Traditional Medicine as well as the implications of international and national standards on the ground in a place like Tibet.

In the most politically benign sense, GMP regulations were first created to protect consumers of pharmaceuticals from adverse effects and to enable medical practitioners to prescribe drugs with confidence. However, this rationale emerged from specific cultural systems, which in turn reinforced particular ideas about science and medicine. These ideas assume a certain relationship between patients, health care providers, and makers of pharmaceuticals, one that is defined by the separation of those who *produce* medicines from those who *prescribe* medicines and manage illness. We might take this distinction for granted, at least as conventional biomedicine has been practiced in the wake of Upton Sinclair's *The Jungle* and the Safe Food and Drug Act of 1906. We might even view this separation between medicine production and prescription as a cornerstone of bioethics (Fox and Swazy 2008).

Such assessments might be relevant in an American biomedical context. This does not mean, however, that such regulations can be summarily imported into another medical and scientific system and still be meaningful. In China, GMP implementation has required Tibetan medical enterprises to adopt methods of production that were first created for the manufacture of biochemical pharmaceuticals, as outlined in Chinese-language protocols, and then further derived from regulations developed for the production of standardized TCM. It is seriously debatable, however, whether compliance with these regulations actually produces more efficacious or safe Tibetan medicines. Note the current modifications to GMP production facilities in places like Lhasa and Qinghai.

This exploration of commercialized production in China leads me back to rural practitioner-producers of nonstandardized medicine in places like high mountain Nepal and Ladakh or private Tibetan producers in China. These individuals exist on the literal and figurative margins of the booming commercial Tibetan medicine industry and a similar market for commercial Ayurvedic formulas in India. As we will see in the next chapter, some of these individuals are actively engaged in conservation-development activities and implicated in the recontextualization of nature that this work engenders. These local Himalayan healers hail from regions where medicinal plants and other *materia medica* fundamental to the production of Tibetan formulas exist in situ, where access to biomedical health care remains limited, and where regional plant trade has existed for centuries as both an avenue for health care and a livelihood strategy.[17] Such individuals and communities are implicated in different regimes of value evident in the commercial production and sale of high-end Tibetan pharma. It is to these local doctors, and the *materia medica* on which they depend, I now turn.

CHAPTER 6

Cultivating the Wilds

There is no such thing as an inanimate object.
—Pablo Neruda, *Intimacies*

KNOWING PLANTS

Wangdu tilts his hat against the glare of morning sun.[1] This senior *menpa,* as eastern Tibetans often refer to Sowa Rigpa practitioners, is of slight stature and few words. He is sixty-one. After living through the Cultural Revolution as well as the *longue durée* of the Reform Era, Wangdu has retired from his position as a government health worker in Yunnan Province's Dechen (Ch. Diqin) Tibetan Autonomous Prefecture. He still sees patients at his home and continues to mentor people like Gawa, a thirty-year-old doctor with whom I am also traveling, and Samphel, a *menpa* and social entrepreneur in his early forties.[2] Samphel runs a clinic in Kunming, Yunnan's provincial capital. The younger husband in a polyandrous marriage, Samphel spends most of the year in Kunming, though his hometown is not far from Mt. Khawakarpo, near a bend in the Yangtze River. Gawa is not yet married. He spends as much time as possible in Dechen's county seat, though his official post is in a township clinic an hour's drive away from this relative hub of civilization. Wangdu studied Tibetan medicine locally, inheriting lineage-based knowledge from people who have passed away or gone into exile. Samphel studied with Wangdu and other senior doctors in the region. He also spent years as an itinerant herb salesman and attended a brief course at the Lhasa Mentsikhang in 1988–89. Ten years later, Gawa also went to Lhasa, one of several local students selected for an educational extension program at the Tibetan Medical College.

It is July 2007. This is my first trip to Yunnan, a part of the world Tibetans call Kham. This region has captured the attention of Euro-American botanists and explorers since the era of Joseph Rock. Once a site of major logging operations, the region was renamed Shangri La by the Chinese government in the early 2000s and now features a number of protected areas (Hillman 2003). After spending time visiting Tibetan medical institutions in Gyalthang, I've arranged to travel with Wangdu and his students.[3] We plan to see Samphel's home village, near the Baima Snow Mountain Nature Preserve. I want to learn about the local Dechen Menpa Association, akin to Nepal's HAA. Samphel helped to create this organization, with support from a local Tibetan development broker working for a conservation international nongovernmental organization with offices in Gyalthang. Although the circumstances under which the Dechen Menpa Association must operate in China differ from the political milieu in which the HAA functions in Nepal, members of both institutions share key goals: to improve the quality of and support for local Sowa Rigpa education and clinical practice and to engage with conservation-development organizations with respect to the documentation and use of the region's medicinal plants.

As we load the car that will take us to Dechen County, I notice how each doctor is dressed. Wangdu wears a chocolate fedora and a rumpled navy blue blazer. He could just as easily be wearing a Mao suit. Samphel sports an urban-retro look: long braid, corduroys, and a nouveau traditional Tibetan-style silk shirt that I imagine appeals to the Chinese clientele at his Kunming clinic. Gawa's thick hair has been cropped short. He wears acid-washed blue jeans and a black T-shirt that depicts the faded face of Bono, U2's front man. This superficial sketch speaks to the generational divides that separate these men, yet belies the bonds between them.

Before we head out, Wangdu recruits Gawa to help him purchase medicines from the local government-supported Tibetan medical hospital and a private pharmacy. Wangdu's Lhasa dialect is eloquent, but his Chinese remains rudimentary. By contrast, Gawa and Samphel can hardly speak a sentence without code-switching between local Tibetan and Mandarin. Sometimes this reality produces embarrassment; this morning, as Gawa and Samphel haggle with medicine salesmen, it proves an asset. Wangdu prefers to make his own formulas. He knows how to substitute locally available plants in key formulas, and he feels most confident in medicines he's made himself. However, sanctions against collection within the territory of nature preserves as well as resource depletion and the impacts of growing industry demands have made the cost of making his own medicines prohibitive. He makes a few varieties and buys the rest, within the means of his pension. "I spend about six thousand yuan [$860] on medicines and plants each year," he explains.

We head out, past the ghosts of logging enterprises, the regional botanical garden, horse racing grounds, a defunct ski slope. Fertile hills are dotted with wooden homes built in the signature local style: carved columns, second-story verandas, and pagoda-style roofs, tips curved toward the sky.

The doctors and I chat as we drive. "People say herbs are best on this side of the Himalayas, but minerals are best in India," Samphel opines.

"Yes, we have plants with the greatest potency here," Wangdu adds.

"But it doesn't seem to matter," Samphel interjects, "because Yunnan is the most neglected of all the Tibetan areas regarding Tibetan medicine."

"Why?" I ask.

"The government does not pay attention to us doctors. People only care about plants." *Amchi* from Nepal have voiced similar sentiments. They work hard to remind conservation organizations, which hire them as ethnobotanical experts, that they are also health care practitioners and teachers (Craig and Bista 2005; Besch and Guerin in press).

"This is a place of bountiful medicine," Wangdu says. "But it is also a place of people who suffer. We need plants, but we also need medicines." He tells a story about a famous disciple of Yuthog Yonten Gompo who once came collecting in this region. "The doctor's purse was so filled with medicines that some of the seeds spilled out—just there!" Wangdu motions to a verdant mountain slope on the other side of the road. "Those spilled seeds made the mountain special, overflowing with *ngo*," he says, referring to medicinal herbs and shrubs. This story spins a web of connection between a person with expansive Sowa Rigpa knowledge and the biodiversity of place—another way of envisioning social ecology. A botanist's narrative might attribute species diversity in this area, which is called *ménri*, literally "medicine mountain," to soil quality, precipitation patterns, natural selection, genetic drift, and random seed dispersal by humans and other animals. The local doctor's version credits the synergies of human agency and natural abundance in a different way.

"Stop the car," Wangdu directs the driver. He has spotted a stand of *ruta (Saussurea lappa)*. This plant is used in many Tibetan formulas. I watch Wangdu harvest selectively. "This *ruta* is different from the one in Dechen," Samphel says. "Better for stomach and blood disorders," Wangdu mumbles, stooped to face the ground. "The Chinese say there are four kinds of *ruta*, but we Tibetans say there are two kinds," the elder doctor goes on. Indeed the problem of classification between medical and social systems, as well as languages, is a perennial one, crossing Tibetan, Sanskrit, Chinese, Latin, and English. Classification has long been a seminal area of inquiry for anthropology, ethnobotany, and ethnobiology (Durkheim and Mauss [1903] 1963; Berlin, Breedlove, and Raven 1973; Berlin 1992; Bowker and Star 1999) and with respect to Tibetan medicine in particular (Ghimire, Lama, and Tripathi 2001; Kletter and Kriechbaum 2001; Lama, Ghimire, and Thomas 2001; Cardi 2005; Grard and Pordié 2005; Lama and Thomas 2005; Boesi and Cardi 2006; Salick et al. 2006; Law and Salick 2007; Glover 2010; Dawa 2011; Dorje 2011). Incommensurate classifications give rise to much confusion when it comes to determining everything from sustainable harvesting levels to substitutions for ingredients that are either not available locally or are prohibitively expensive. The seemingly simple act of identifying *ruta* on the side of the road is enmeshed in ongoing cross-cultural and cross-disciplinary debates about classification and regional variation of Tibetan and Himalayan plants. These debates bear on conservationist agendas, even though such subtleties can remain unaccounted for in protected area management plans or on transnational endangered species lists.

Wangdu mentions he worked with an American botanist, helping to identify species and explain their uses. "I enjoyed this work," he says, "because the foreign scientists really cared about what I know. But there were also problems. Anything we collected had to be named according to their systems, or they would not collect them!" This bias is amusing to Wangdu, who operates under different taxonomic assumptions. To him, a plant might have a number of names, some emerging from classical Tibetan texts, others reflecting local idiom. A plant's utility matters more than the name it is given in another scientific system, and this practice of identification itself represents distinct ways of knowing the world.

For example, a botanist might identify the plant(s) Tibetan doctors call *lang na* as belonging to the genus *Pedicularis (Scrophulariacea)*, possessing "two-lipped" flowers and "dark green cauline leaves arranged in groups of four at each node, pinnatified to pinnatisect, with abundant simple and glandular trichomes" (Kletter and Kriechbaum 2001: 85–87). To a *menpa* like Wangdu, *lang na* would likely be distinguished by specific characteristics of its flowers, all of which have beaks reminiscent of an elephant's trunk. Whereas a chemical analysis would reveal that one species of pedicularis contains triterpenoids that may have anticancer properties, a Tibetan doctor might tell you that the nature of *lang na* is warming, the taste is sweet and astringent, the secondary qualities are smooth and flexible, and the flowers are used in medicines that treat disorders of the *chu ser,* which biomedicine might recognize as synovial fluid.

Furthermore, while both the botanist and the Tibetan doctor recognize different varieties of plant under a general category and as an organizing principal *(pedicularis* or *lang na),* and while both create nested hierarchies of knowledge about these plants, they rest on different assumptions and ways of *knowing* plants. This is not to say that these systems are fundamentally incompatible, but rather in each there is the possibility of blind spots according to the other, and that normative assumptions about what makes for scientific knowledge might render the nuances of Tibetan praxis invisible at times. It occurs to me as we drive that this is another way of thinking about Marx's concepts of use value and exchange value. Here exchange value is not solely economic, but is also tied to the exchange of scientific knowledge across regions, languages, and cultures.

The drive toward Dechen goes slowly. We examine many species alongside the road, including poor-quality *solo marpo,* a type of rhodiola that has become commodified of late. Several Chinese companies produce sweetened medicinal shots of rhodiola extract and a Red Bull–esque energy drink with this plant, for it helps guard against altitude sickness. Arura's *Adapt to the Holy Land* capsule contains rhodiola. Gawa scrambles up the side of an embankment, eager to point out this specimen to his teacher. When he brings it down, Wangdu shakes his head. "This is *solo marpo,* yes, but it is the one with a small life *[tsé chung]* and not much potency. The better quality ones are always found higher up the mountain," he instructs.

We stop at a bluff from which we can see the snow mountain at the heart of the preserve, a place known in Chinese as Baima-Meili Xue Shan, but that Wangdu calls Dorje Drak or "Thunderbolt Scepter Cliff" in Tibetan. Wangdu points out a delicate white tuber. "This root medicine is used for headaches," he says, "but it is becoming rare. People are digging it up and not thinking of the future."

I wonder how the overharvesting problem of which Wangdu speaks squares with official bans on the collection of many nontimber forest products from the preserve. Do people abide by these regulations? I ask.

Samphel answers, "The nature preserves are mostly for tourism. Only a few people are really interested in protecting the medicine of this place. Collection for profit still goes on. Money can solve problems of permits. And people still collect from the edges of the park." I have heard similar stories from colleagues in Nepal, regarding the buffer zones of its national parks and protected areas (see Ghimire et al. 2005b).

"Medicinal plants are precious jewels [norbu]," Samphel continues, "but most people do not understand this landscape. They talk about protection [sung kyob], what foreigners call *conservation*"—he says this word in English—"but most people here are more interested in supporting their families and making money. *Conservation* and *development*, these ideas have potency and strength, but they do not have sufficient methods to accomplish their goals."

The comment resonates. So is the nuance behind the term *sung kyob*. Many people have taken up the language of conservation, including those in the Himalayas and Tibet. Yet as powerful as this transnational concept may be, it does not fully capture how meaning is given to biologically rich landscapes or how the pragmatic work of conscientious resource use is undertaken. The Tibetan term *sung kyob* means "to protect, safeguard or defend"; *sung* is the same term used for protective amulets worn to keep nefarious spirits at bay, beings you read about in chapter 4, who can inflict illness and misfortune. A linguistic analysis of the term *sung kyob* indicates that the Tibetan concept often translated as "conservation" is more about the maintenance of relationships between different classes of sentient beings and an ethics of resource use linked, at times, to Buddhist ideals. Even if we agree that this term alludes to *ideals,* it is still worth noting that *sung kyob* and *conservation* are rooted in distinct concepts of nature. These differences are borne out in practice, in what *menpa* think and how they act.

At our next stop we see *honglen*. (As another example of the issues of classification, this one Tibetan plant is listed under at least five different Latin names in the Tibetan medicinal plant books to which I have access: *Lagotis glauca, Lagotis kunawurensis, Lagotis yunnanensis, Lagotis Picrorhiza, Picrorhiza Kurroa.*) Although historically common, this plant is routinely cited by Sowa Rigpa practitioners I've worked with in Nepal as one that is becoming increasingly rare; successful cultivation trials of this plant have begun in Mustang. Here in Yunnan, practitioners have not tried to cultivate this medicine, which has cooling properties and whose roots are used to cleanse impurities from the blood.

"We want to make rules about how to harvest plants," says Gawa. "This is our area, our medicine. So it should be our responsibility to tell people how to use plants."

"This is my number one goal with the Menpa Association," Samphel says. "Now people pick with no care." Notions of sustainability translate in a range of ways in the Tibetan language; there is no single equivalent word. As my interlocutors on this trip illustrate, discussions of what we might label "unsustainable" behavior produce phrases such as "not using plants in the right way" and "harvesting with no thought of the future." Wangdu explains how TCM and Tibetan medical "factory people" give samples of plants to local people who then go to the mountains to collect. This leads to depletion.

"We don't have the power to stop this," Samphel adds. "Not even big NGOs have this power in China. The Nature Conservancy tried. The Mountain Institute tried. Only the government has this power. But they also benefit from making a business out of Tibetan medicine." In China, for better or for worse, NGOs rarely function as independent agents with significant ability to pressure or override state policies, as they do in other parts of the world.[4]

Wangdu exclaims, "Local collectors, even some *menpa* who do not have much training, take all they can and do not leave anything to grow the next year." These comments echo narratives I have heard on both sides of the Himalayas: villagers collect and sell to middlemen, who then broker deals with factories; they have no idea what the ingredients are for, and they do not know where these ingredients end up; often when these villagers themselves need medicines, they end up buying back ready-made Tibetan and Ayurvedic formulas from Indian and Chinese companies.[5]

"How to protect—this is not easy either," Wangdu adds. "Foreigners and Chinese people think with numbers, what they can calculate on the computer or what someone else in some other place tells them is good to collect. But this does not always match what is here, on *this* earth." The doctor glances toward the ground, muddied by rain. "They draw lines on maps and say 'Here is a place to protect.' It would be more beneficial to let the people who live in those places have some power to make the rules. But we would need the government to give us this power. We cannot do this on our own."

Wangdu and his students offer place-based critiques of conservation as an abstract set of scientific practices. They also suggest that natural resource governance might *require* the strong arm of a state willing to cap industry growth for the sake of conservation—but conservation defined in local terms. This makes me think of Bhutan. Sowa Rigpa is incorporated at every level of health care in this Himalayan country (McKay and Wangchuk 2005; McKay 2007). Bhutan's government is robust, the population is small, and the country has a strong ideological commitment to environmentalism. All of these factors support the enforcement of collection guidelines that have been determined, at least in part, by the country's *amchi,* with consideration for local income generation through medicinal plant cultivation and collection. Yet even in Bhutan, in communities where the National Institute of Traditional Medicine not only trains people in proper harvesting techniques but also pays them to collect the nearly sixteen tons of plants they need to supply Bhutanese citizens with medicines each year, lay collectors are turning away from this source of revenue. Some argue this is primarily because *yartsa gunbu* collection is more lucrative and ultimately easier; secondarily, permits for medicinal plant collection can be difficult to obtain.[6]

On this drive toward Dechen, I am reminded of the ways plants embody biocultural life. We examine small blue-black flowers whose leaves address bile disorders and are good for sore throats. Wangdu notes, "If you eat it, then you will have wise speech." Up on a high pass we encounter a red Himalayan poppy. Samphel blushes and talks about how he learned to associate this flower with female genitalia. The men have a good laugh. The female anthropologist feels awkward. I learn that *chang tser (Morina nepalensis)* can make you very emotional if you use it in brewing beer, and that *gangla metog (Saussurea medusa / laniceps),* the "snow deity flower," also called the snow lotus, will make you violent if you eat it when you are sad, or make you think you can fly if you are drunk.

Such colorful conversations continue the next day, as we hike up the valley from Samphel's home village, a temperate place of peach trees, wheat fields, and rows of corn that give way to steep mixed-growth forest and craggy rock faces. Samphel has been walking these paths with Wangdu since he was an adolescent. The work of plant collection and medicine preparation in the elder doctor's company helped him deal with the heartache of his father's untimely death, he confides. As we walk, Wangdu provides a running commentary on the tastes *(ro),* potencies *(nüpa),* post-digestive tastes *(surjé),* and beneficial qualities *(phenyön)* of the plants we encounter. Gawa sings folk songs. When we pause to look back down toward the Yangtze, we catch glimpses of

Khawakarpo's glacial skirts. The sacred mountain itself is shrouded in mist and clouds.

Samphel explains that he has helped to form seven user groups in his village and surrounding areas, encompassing about nine hundred people in this buffer zone of the Baima preserve. In some senses this is a nascent example of the type of local governance about which Samphel and Wangdu spoke on our drive. The fact that such groups exist seems to be a positive step toward a vision of what conservation and development could mean. Yet I also consider local politics. Perhaps these user groups provide a way of dealing with what could otherwise be fierce competition over natural resources in a place where divisive, even violent acts routinely occur around *yartsa gunbu* season and the harvest of matsutake mushrooms, another locally available wild food with major global market value (Yeh 2000; Winkler 2011).[7]

Gawa adds, "Protecting plants is important, but conservation just to say you are doing conservation won't work. Instead NGOs and the government should encourage community groups to control how much is collected, but also to grow, process, and sell plants." These doctors hope to sell wild-crafted surplus to regional medicine producers in Dechen and Gyalthang, but to retain a stake in the trade.

"One goal of our association is to buy solar dryers and grinding machines so we can process more plants here in the village. That way people can sell them in the markets, cut out middlemen, keep more money," says Samphel. These comments make me think about how both *menpa* and villagers are often caught between a proverbial rock and a hard place: between the strictures of conservation measures and the desire to educate on proper collection methods, on the one hand, and the source-force of industry and a real thirst for cash, on the other.

"Our work to make our own NGO is not so we can have a government job, but because we want to be more self-sufficient and guard against losing knowledge, plant wealth, and other resources," Samphel continues. The idea that one would *not* be in the business of conservation-development work for personal financial security is significant; so is the slippage between NGOs and government work units as categories of being and experience. Both are viewed as pathways to financial security that comes from belonging to a bureaucracy, whether governmental or nongovernmental. As we say in Nepali, such jobs secure a life of "plowing with a pen."

"I know plants, but many people even ten years younger than me do not know them," says Gawa. He notes that Wangdu and other doctors like him have many responsibilities, not only because of the imperative to pass on what they know, but also because of the region's rich biodiversity. In Tibetan areas of China, as in Nepal, such efforts to pass on knowledge also embody a linguistic urgency, since state educational policies and social pressure discourage young people from becoming highly literate in Tibetan. Mandarin, Nepali, and English are viewed as languages of advancement.

"I am a good, but not a great doctor," Samphel reflects. He is perched on a large boulder by the side of a stream, where we have shared a picnic lunch of boiled eggs, peaches, and unleavened bread. "Even so, I try to inspire the younger generation." He is worried that Tibetan medical knowledge, such as that embodied by Wangdu, is disappearing.

We continue up the mountain, stopping at a monastery to have tea. As we sit in the kitchen, I listen passively, catching only fragments of the quickly spoken local dialect. Samphel and the monk-caretaker discuss the new house someone is building, and how a mutual acquaintance's son has not done well on the college entrance exam. The monk asks why I've come to visit. Samphel answers that I am interested in Tibetan medicine. The monk scoffs, "Tibetan medicine is just becoming big business now. For Chinese. For Tibetans. There is little place anymore for good old doctors like this one," he gestures toward Wangdu.

We leave the monastery and head down the mountain, toward the village. Wangdu turns and points to a rock face. "Doesn't that look like a People's Liberation Army soldier? He even has a hat like Mao used to wear! We call him a forest treasure guard." Wangdu chuckles and then reminds us, serious again, that many deities dwell in this forest. He gestures to a ridge high above us.

"You see that small cave? There used to be silver and gold up there. People used to go and dig, dig and dig, trying to reach the wealth at the heart of the mountain. Some people were successful, but this made the local god unhappy. He did not want his wealth and power to be taken by these villagers. So he went to seek the advice of the mountain god near Samye Monastery, in Central Tibet. The local god said, 'They have almost reached my heart. What should I do?' The Samye god responded, 'Can't you even shake a bit?' So the local god did, and many people died in the earthquake that followed." With this story I am reminded of how, in the words of Keith Basso (1996), "wisdom sits in places." Yet I also hear Wangdu's tale as a parable at once *for* and *against* the claiming of territory for the sake of material gain or conservation in the abstract. His words bespeak a living, agentive land, vulnerable and resilient.

PRODUCING SACRED LANDSCAPES

"You've arrived." Gyatso smiles from the side of the road. On this cool winter day in 2007 we are on our way to a meeting at the program offices of the World Wildlife Fund–Nepal Program (WWF–Nepal). Winter sun filters through stands of eucalyptus and a large sacred fig (N. *pipal*) in this calm and relatively affluent corner of the capital. The raucous cacophony of city traffic feels distant.

"Sabriya said there may be a donor who wants to support *amchi* medicine," Gyatso says as we walk toward the office.[8] Sabriya is a new WWF program officer. "Maybe it will be for more medicinal plant work in Dolpo. I hope they will consider *amchi* training courses. These have much benefit. You might need to help us write a *proposal*," my friend continues.

As you saw in chapter 1, one of my roles in working with *amchi* in Nepal has been to translate their goals and plans into concept papers, proposals, and reports. Although I've helped liaise with several donor organizations, I've had the closest relationship with WWF–Nepal. The man who would become my husband was working at the WWF–Nepal Program when we first met, in 1995. The following year, while he had a fellowship to study the impacts of Shey Phoksumdo National Park on indigenous systems of land management in Dolpo (Bauer 2004), I worked as a research assistant at WWF and helped to connect Tshampa Ngawang, whom you met in chapter 4, with an international WWF research fellowship. Over the years I've stayed connected to the organization through its support of the HAA and collaboration with *amchi* as they participated in a multiyear ethnobotany and medicinal plant conservation project in Dolpo, funded through UNESCO's People and Plant Initiative (Ghimire et al. 2001; Lama et al. 2001; Lama and Thomas 2005, 2008).

We come to a metal gate. A brass plaque bearing the famous panda bear insignia hangs beside this guarded entrance. We ring the bell. The door swings open and a familiar face greets us.

"Namaste, *amchi ji*," says the guard. After a decade of collaboration between WWF and Nepali *amchi*, he and Gyatso know each other well. Gyatso and I step into the waiting room of the large house that has been converted into this NGO's national headquarters. Posters of wildlife hang from the walls. Brochures describing efforts to combat transboundary trafficking in endangered species rest on end tables.

Sitting beside Gyatso, waiting for our meeting with Sabriya, I cannot help but think about those who died in the helicopter crash. "It feels sad here, still," I whisper to Gyatso.

"Yes," Gyatso says, squeezing my hand. I should have anticipated this wave of sadness. Now all I can do is absorb it.

Fifteen months prior to this meeting at WWF, on September 23, 2006, a fatal accident in Taplejung District, Nepal, devastated this organization. Twenty-four people died when their Russian-made craft clipped the side of a mountain, shrouded in morning fog and rain. The accident occurred near the skirts of Kanchenjunga, the third highest mountain in the world and the *axis mundi* of Nepal's newest conservation area, a project WWF had spearheaded. This happened the day after management of the Kanchenjunga Conservation Area Project (KCAP) had been handed over to local leadership, as a group of conservationists, diplomats, politicians, and researchers who initiated the project headed back to Kathmandu. Among those who died was my friend Yeshi Chödron Lama, to whom this book is dedicated.

Integrated conservation and development projects (ICDPs) such as KCAP have become increasingly popular models for engineering social and environmental change. At one level, ICDPs serve as responses to critiques of conservation, wherein *conservation* is envisioned as the preservation of wild spaces for the enjoyment of humanity, and *humanity* generally references nonnative communities. First popularized by Theodore Roosevelt and later John Muir, such models of conservation hinge on *wilderness* as a concept—a particular social construction of nature and the relationship between wild and "civilized" places.[9] This preservationist ethic came to be known as the "Yellowstone model" of conservation. While innovative in many ways, this conservation ethic also bears the legacy of having sidelined or categorically denied indigenous uses of and relations to land (Igoe 2004). Indeed, until its redefinition as "wilderness" the Yellowstone consisted of diverse Native American tribal groups.

Some view ICDPs as correctives to this exclusionary legacy. Indeed some of the most powerful efforts at providing an alternative model of conservation have emerged from the Nepal Himalayas, in no small part through the work of Mingma Norbu Sherpa and Dr. Chandra Gurung, activist-scholars who perished in the helicopter crash. Mingma and Chandra were among the first to take the stance that local people—their well-being and livelihoods, their sense of agency, their cultural identity, and their political power—are integrally connected with the fate of local ecologies. In the 1980s they launched a pioneering ICDP, the Annapurna Conservation Area Project. They both went on to work for WWF–Nepal at different points in their careers. The underpinnings of Nepal's ICDP model envisioned by Mingma and Chandra have been adapted to many other contexts, often with success. Yet ethnographies of ICDPs in action—from Indonesia (Lowe 2006; Li 2007) to Papua New Guinea (West 2006), from Madagascar (Harper 2002) to Tanzania (Igoe 2004)—show that they often spawn serious questions about the relationship between conservation and development, especially as they have fostered paradoxical linkages between environmental protection, economic growth, and consumption (Igoe and Brockington 2007).[10]

"Namaste," Sabriya greets us, her raven-black bob bouncing above the curve of her shoulders. "Sorry to keep you waiting," she says in Nepali. Like most of her colleagues, she received an advanced degree abroad and has a cosmopolitan air. I introduce myself. Sabriya leads us into her office. After we are seated, she addresses me, speaking in English. "WWF has done a lot of work in the past with *amchi*. We would like to continue this work. We understand why *amchi* are important for the local people, for the culture. But it is a problem of funding. For some time, donors were very interested in medicinal plants and ethnobotany. Now, not so much." She is poised to continue, but I ask her, in Nepali, to converse in Nepali, so that Gyatso can understand.

"Oh, of course. Sorry, Gyatso *ji.*" She repeats the preamble in Nepali. Even so, her Nepali remains peppered with English phrases. "I have been assigned to do some *follow-up* work in Dolpo," she continues, "even though we no longer have a project in the area. This is something we decided to do, after the *tragedy*. For their *legacy*. But we need to find new donors. Due to the *tragedy,* we made a request to WWF International. We told about the successes of working with *amchi* in the past, and we said we would like *continuity* in programs. Still, funds are limited." Following the latest donor trend is something at which Sabriya is undoubtedly adept, but about which she seems apologetic, if uninspired.

"What projects do donors want to fund?" Gyatso asks. "*Income generate? Culture preserve? Participate research?*" Even without much English, he has become well versed in the practice of framing what he and other *amchi* do in terms of conservation-development buzzwords. Sabriya takes these comments in stride, as if this were precisely the language she would expect from someone sitting in her office.

"These days many of the donors, especially from America, are from FBOs."

Gyatso looks puzzled. "What is *FBO?* I know NGO, INGO, CBO," he says.

"*Faith-based organization,*" Sabriya says. "They have become strong since President George Bush." These comments, spoken in English, are directed at me.

I offer a quick explanation in Tibetan for Gyatso. "FBO is like NGO, but these organizations have religious aims and views. Usually they are Christian."

"And because George Bush follows Christian *dharma*, FBO is now powerful in America?"

"Yes," I answer.

In this moment of sociolinguistic and political-economic convergence, I sense the world's smallness—what a Tibetan might call interdependent karma *(tendrel)*—as U.S. sectarian politics are helping to shape the priorities of conservation governance half a world away. A powerful conservation organization is becoming enmeshed in American philanthropic capitalism with a Judeo-Christian spin.

At the same time, WWF and other such organizations are becoming increasingly intertwined with patterns of consumption in an era that Igoe and Brockington (2007) define as that of "neoliberal conservation." In short, neoliberal conservation involves the coupling of deregulated market expansion and privatization of industry with the paradoxical desire to "save" nature, in part through novel patterns of consumption. But are these ways of buying things actually experiences of nature or its *doppelgänger?*

My colleague at Dartmouth, Jim Igoe (2010), provides several examples of neoliberal conservation. He cites the promotion of ecotourism in East Africa, on lands that have been purchased by private investors and to which local populations often lose use rights. He also mentions the promotion of "save the rainforest"–style McDonald's Happy Meals™ linked to Hollywood films that anthropomorphize the poster children of the faunal world: lemurs, whales, tigers, panda bears. Even as children consuming this fast food are drawn further into a vicious cycle of transfats and crude oil dependency, the take-home message is that by eating a Happy Meal—and perhaps even charging it on your WWF Visa card—you contribute to the conservation of real-life ecosystems.

Turning to Sabriya, I ask, "What kinds of work do these FBOs who are donating to WWF want to fund?"

"These days everybody is talking about *sacred mountain concept.*" Sabriya begins in Nepali but then switches to English. "The idea is to promote conservation through spirituality. Seeing God in nature, things like that. How you can preserve biodiversity through faith." The concept of faith-based sacred mountain initiatives in Nepal does not seem as riddled with the uncomfortable paradoxes of neoliberal conservation described earlier. However, such initiatives raise other concerns about commodification of Himalayan natures *and* cultures, and the position of people like Gyatso therein. They are also reminiscent of the ways Himalayan and Tibetan people and environments have been exoticized by the West (Lopez 1998; Dodin and Rather 2006; Anand 2008) and the ways that specific ecological nationalist narratives emerge in both Nepal and China, with respect to Tibetan places (see Yeh 2009).

The phrase *sacred mountain concept* does not translate easily from English into Nepali. This is true even though Nepal is literally and figuratively *defined* by mountains, and these mountains, in turn, are abodes of deities for Hindu, Buddhist, Bönpo, and Jain followers. The mention of this concept sparks a shift in Sabriya's discourse, back to English and to the evocation of ideas that might just as easily have been voiced by Roosevelt, Thoreau, or Muir. *What sort of God does she envision?* I wonder. Gyatso pokes my arm, prompting me to translate.

"These new Christian donors think it would be a good idea to make projects where people understand that deities *[lha]* live in mountain places. Through *dharma* we can protect the environment."

Even as I say this, the absurdity of the moment strikes me. Here I am telling a practitioner whose exemplar is the Medicine Buddha, whose training includes tantric practices by which organic matter is infused with spiritual efficacy, and who recognizes the mountains that cradle him as abodes of village protector deities and gods of place, that new funding proposals must connect religiosity to the goals of environmental conservation. I am not sure whether to laugh or sigh. This is not to say, of course, that all *amchi* or others from Nepal's high mountains treat nature with the type of reverence such a faith-based perspective might imply, or that conservation as such even remains a goal for most. However, this supposedly novel turn in donor priorities—the latest flavor of the month at the ICDP soda fountain—represents something so fundamental to Gyatso as to be nonsensical.

"Say that again," Gyatso asks. His expression bespeaks, *Did I really just hear what I think I heard?* I try the translation again.

"Is that all?" my *amchi* colleague finally offers.

"Seems so."

Sabriya says that different NGOs and bilateral agencies in Nepal might form a consortium around this theme of sacred Himalayan landscapes. "UNDP [United Nations Development Program] has allocated some money to this program idea, but nothing has gotten off the ground yet," she says in English. She goes on to explain that WWF–Nepal has a direct line to a potential Scandinavian donor who "likes Tibetans." Although she is Christian, she has traveled throughout Tibetan areas in India and Nepal and has an interest in Buddhism. "This donor may support *amchi,* but only if you can combine the goals of conservation with Buddhism and other world religions."

"Oh, so the focus is not solely on Christianity?" I ask in English.

"No. It seems most big FBOs in the States are Christian and want to promote these beliefs," Sabriya replies. "But this potential donor is talking about a small project, fifty thousand dollars or so, focused more on Buddhism. So HAA would need to figure out how to make a proposal with activities where the idea of *faith*—you know, *dharma*— is emphasized."

I find it interesting that these two words have come to stand for each other. The Sanskrit term *dharma* means literally "that which upholds or supports." It is often translated as "law," "moral duty," or "religious teachings" in Hindu and Buddhist contexts. In Buddhist philosophy *dharma* is a constitutive factor of human experience and a gloss for the teachings of Buddha. As such, *dharma* signifies ultimate reality: the interdependent nature of sentient existence, the truth of suffering caused by our penchant for attachment and desire, and the possibility of liberation from such suffering. In English *faith* references belief: in God, in the doctrines or teachings of an organized religion, and in the observance of an obligation. Faith is an abiding or theistic confidence in someone or something. It connotes not only specific religious traditions but also a sense of allegiance, trust, fidelity. The closest these two terms come to each other are when they engage a sense of morality: codes of ethics, standards of behavior.

I also note Sabriya's comment that $50,000 signifies a "small" project. Lo Kunphen scrapes together about half that annually to run a school for forty-odd students and a network of local clinics. The HAA's basic operating budget is about one thousand dollars a year, and activities are nearly all grant-dependent. Gyatso absorbs this information, as I translate, and then launches into an erudite explanation of the connections between Tibetan medicine and Buddhism, and the relationship between an ethics of medicinal resource use and dharmic principles of right livelihood, right action. Finally, he reminds Sabriya, "All *amchi* in Dolpo and Mustang, places like this, we are all lamas too."

Sabriya responds, "Yes, exactly. We should emphasize these points in a proposal. We have many sacred sites in our Nepal, but we do not have clear *criteria* for what *sacred site* means. We need to develop a *conservation perspective* for thinking about *sacred sites*. From that view, we can determine what types of project activities to propose. How is conservation *site-related?*" she goes on, her language a Nepali-English hybrid. "Westerners don't understand how connected *faith* and *nature* are in places like Nepal, for cultures of the Himalaya. We need to make this link for them very clearly."

My understanding of the situation becomes subtler. This new conceptual turn is not only about the possibility of Christian FBOs influencing global conservation in a neoliberal moment. It is also about molding one type of social ecology (that which makes a mountain or a watershed sacred according to the people who live beside it, or that which makes an *amchi* aspire to alleviate the suffering of fellow villagers) into another (that which can be accomplished through NGO monitoring and evaluation metrics). And, to become efficacious practice, this requires capitalizing on a vague primordial sense that, in the Himalayas, nature and culture are inextricably linked.

To me, Sabriya says in English, "We need to develop a full rationale for this initiative. WWF has done some other projects like this in Madagascar and Asia Pacific." She shares documents from these projects.

"If we can make connections between faith and conservation and then link this to *climate change,* this would be very good," she says, mostly in Nepali.

"What is *climate change?*" Gyatso asks.

"It is a term for the ways the weather and the environment are changing so quickly these days," I say in Tibetan.

"Like the monsoon arriving late, too much rain in Mustang and not enough snow?"

"Yes, like that."

"Climate change is really hot right now," Sabriya continues in English. I do not know if the pun is intentional. "There is also a lot of interest in water and governance but not so much for forests anymore." Sabriya is deadpan. This is not because I think the ironies here escape her, but because this is the universe in which she operates and on which she is dependent for her livelihood. I do not begrudge her this, but I do find it odd that one moment we are striving to link cosmological and conservationist understandings of the world and the next moment we are parsing up the Earth, as if forests were not connected to water or as if either could be viewed as completely distinct from the regimes of governance, both local and global, that regulate their meanings and uses.

"We understand this situation you call *climate change* in terms of the five elements," Gyatso offers. "When the relationship between the five elements changes, sometimes this can change the nature and potency of medicinal plants. So there is a strong relation between our medicine and *climate change*. It connects to what medicines we can make, what substitutions we must use."

"Good. So you should also write this in a proposal. Write about how *amchi* medicine is not only connected to *faith*, but also to *climate change*. The donor will like that."

As Gyatso and I pack up our things, the paradoxes of this meeting weigh on me. On the one hand, I am grateful for the loyalty and goodwill between WWF and *amchi* like Gyatso. They respect and support each other. On the other hand, the meeting makes me profoundly aware of the interconnections between political will and the present and future of practices like Sowa Rigpa, as well as the far-reaching effects of a vision of the world in which nature is at once deeply revered and heavily marketed.

CULTIVATING CONNECTIONS AND COCA-COLA

The Druk Air flight banks a hard left, cutting a vertiginous path to reveal Himalayan foothills, gloriously green. Those of us on the flight from Kathmandu to Paro, Bhutan, suck in a collective breath and then exhale as the runway comes into view. Many of us have traveled great distances, recruited significant resources, and endured a range of bureaucratic indignities to come to the Dragon Kingdom. Colleagues from China have had to secure special permission to travel to this country with which the People's Republic does not have formal diplomatic relations, a place where Tibetan script adorns the national currency, where Gross National Happiness is favored over the tenets of Chinese socialism, and where nationalist claims to Tibetan Buddhist culture run deep.

But never mind the difficulties of travel. Like all good pilgrims, those of us bound for Bhutan in early September 2009 have met the obstacles placed before us. We have convened as an eclectic group: more than two hundred scholars and practitioners of Asian medical systems who have come together for the Seventh Congress of the International Association for the Study of Traditional Asian Medicine. Founded in 1979 by the historian of South Asia Arthur Llewellyn Basham and the medical anthropologist Charles Leslie, IASTAM promotes the study and cross-cultural understanding of Asian medicines, in a way that embraces the difficult task of integrating the world of reflection and critique with that of engagement and practice.

In addition to anthropologists, historians, and Ayurvedic, Chinese, and Tibetan doctors, the Seventh Congress has attracted civil servants and representatives of businesses engaged in the sale of medicinal products. The motley crew includes an old hippie who runs an herbal supplements business in North America, a physicist who is the chief operating officer of a Swiss company that produces Tibetan formulas, and a representative from Coca-Cola in Beijing. The days in Thimphu pass quickly and memorably. In formal panels and discussion, and as participants feast on green chilies and red rice, connections are forged in Tibetan, Chinese, Nepali, Hindi, English, German, and lovely combinations of all these.

Gyatso and Mingkyi are among those in attendance. Many other Tibetan medicine practitioners from both sides of the Himalayas are present. The open-air corridors of the Royal Institute of Management, the congress's headquarters on Thimphu's edge, become the meeting grounds for generations of Sowa Rigpa practitioners who, by virtue of politics and geography, have rarely been afforded opportunities to interact. On the third morning of the conference, many *amchi* colleagues look particularly tired. I ask Gyatso what transpired the previous night. He tells me that Akhong Rinpoche gave an informal teaching. A senior religious figure and Tibetan medical practitioner who left Tibet in the early 1960s, Akhong Rinpoche is the organizational and spiritual head of Rokpa International, an NGO based in the United Kingdom that has helped to support the practice of Tibetan medicine in Asia and Europe (Millard 2008; Sweeney 2009).

"Rinpoche was very inspirational," Gyatso shares. "He made many important suggestions about how to cultivate medicinal plants. He encouraged us to work together, so the vast ocean of Tibetan medical knowledge does not decline." In 2007 Akhong Rinpoche sponsored a conference in Yushu Prefecture (the place later devastated by the 2010 earthquake) focusing on cultivation techniques for medicinal plants, including an introduction, in Tibetan, to Euro-American principles of biodynamic agriculture. He also stressed the problems being created in Tibetan areas of China due to environmental degradation, from the increased use of chemical fertilizer and pesticides to the impacts on human and ecological health from Chinese and multinational mining operations in Tibetan areas.[11]

"It was close to midnight when Rinpoche shared with us stories of when he left Tibet. How they had nothing to eat and they suffered blindness and severe cold. They took the leather soles of their shoes and boiled them with melted snow so they would not starve.[12] By the end of the evening, many were crying," Gyatso says.

The following morning I encounter a senior Tibetan doctor at the book display. This man spent the first half of his career in Lhasa, but went into exile in the 1980s. His voice cracks as he tells me about the encounter with Akhong Rinpoche and his delight in discovering that one of the young Tibetan doctors from China I've invited to the congress is the son of a dear friend from his Lhasa days. "This," he says, "is lineage."

The theme of the Seventh Congress is "Cultivating Traditions and the Challenges of Globalization." My colleague Denise Glover and I organize a panel on conservation, cultivation, and commodification of Himalayan and Tibetan medicinal plants. As you have already seen, medicinal plants represent pathways to healing and to profit; they remain paragons of traditional culture even as they are clinically tested for safety, quality, and efficacy according to technoscientific standards. Plants give meaning and form to a social ecology of healing. Yet their use values and exchange values are malleable and sometimes diverge. Medicinal plants embody concerns over cultural integrity and environmental protection, as well as different ways of knowing the world and the socioeconomic pressures of modern life.

Cultivation is a tricky business. During our discussions a leading ethnobotanist from the Missouri Botanical Gardens poses difficult yet crucial questions about the purpose of cultivation. She stresses that cultivation should not be viewed as a pathway to biodiversity conservation, but should be seen as linked to world economic systems and market-based activities involving medicinal plants. In other words, cultivation is not a panacea for protecting vulnerable high-altitude species like the snow lotus (Law and Salick 2005).

Aside from the difficulty of making plants grow in new environments, issues surface with regard to determining biochemical differences between cultivated and wild-crafted plants. Many practitioners, from *amchi* in the mountains of Nepal to pharmacologists in Lhasa and Qinghai, desire to compare mass spectrometry or liquid chromatography with traditional Tibetan methods of determining the potency of cultivated versus wild-crafted species. But this takes time, money, and scientific expertise that one person does not necessarily possess. Such efforts raise specters of incommensurability: Should mass spectrometry or liquid chromatographic test results trump an *amchi*'s tongue, his carefully honed ability to discern the tastes, postdigestive tastes, nature, and potency of a plant (Dawa 2011)?

These issues do not simply surface along Tibetan versus bioscientific lines. In one presentation the founder of HerbPharm, an herbal products company in Oregon, stresses the practical difficulties, time commitment, and technological resources that successful cultivation entails. Many of us stare in awe at his photographs: fields of echinacea, pistils and stamens of St. John's wort, intimate portraits of American ginseng. As he shows images that document the stable chemistry of annual harvests, he explains that although these scientific tests are useful, he can tell the quality—or lack thereof—of a crop by the sight, feel, smell, and taste of specimens. He knows if a harvest is off. When such moments occur, sometimes the scientific testing does not pick up this subtlety, or an herb simply registers within a normal spectrum. But he refuses to use a harvest when this happens.

The fact that this "hippie herbalist" does not use plants that do not meet more intuitive, organic criteria of quality but that might seem sufficiently robust by technoscientific standards provokes a range of responses. A senior Chinese botanist challenges the American, raising questions about his lack of academic training and, as such, his qualifications to make such assessments. The countercultural autodidact stands tall in his Hawaiian shirt and meditation beads, his face sun-soaked, his hands marked by decades of manual labor. "I do not need a Ph.D. to know if a plant is good or not!" he exclaims.

On the final day of the conference a representative of Coca-Cola Beijing presents on our panel. Coca-Cola Beijing kindly agreed to help sponsor this gathering (which, in itself, produced some angst within IASTAM leadership). We have an obligation to engage the global conglomerate's growing investment in Asian products, including herb-fortified teas, even though a certain skepticism prevails among those who identify Coca-Cola with a range of challenges to global health and with socioeconomic inequalities connected to multinational corporations.

Be that as it may, I listen with interest as the representative identifies Coca-Cola as an "herbal" company (think coca leaf and sarsaparilla) that is heir to a lineage of secret knowledge (think about what gives Coke® that unique taste). The representative discusses how "we" (that slippery global "we") are seeking healthier lifestyles. She emphasizes that the market turn toward natural products hinges on the modern, scientific appropriation of "ancient wisdom." This sense of primordial herbal knowledge is further linked to Chinese philosophy and medicine. She notes that, in Beijing, the company is consulting with a number of TCM councils on the formulation of new products, helping the company to distill Chinese medical knowledge into plastic bottled beverages for global distribution.

The representative acknowledges that the expansion of industry around such products necessitates new approaches to production. In its high-fructose incarnation, Coke does not rely on farmers but is more like the production of a pharmaceutical, manufactured under sterile and uniform factory conditions. Yet to produce Coca-Cola's new lines of herbal teas, the company must deal with plant suppliers. The representative reiterates many of the problems that surface with regard to commercial Tibetan medicine production: problems of determining quality but also, given the scale of this enterprise, in finding sufficient *quantities* of product to meet demands. The company is too big to address quality at the field level; it must rely on farmers who need the income Coca-Cola provides to produce high-quality raw materials. She speaks without irony but with a wealth of technoscientific knowledge about the process of meeting export quality standards.

"In India," she says, "we had too many problems with water quality. It is difficult to meet European standards." She notes that since the Coca-Cola brand is a "bloodline," the company often imposes even stricter quality measures than are required by the countries in which production is occurring. Global reputation produces extranational governance in a neoliberal era.

As I listen to the Coca-Cola representative, I think about the long-term ramifications in places like Mustang of converting fields that once grew subsistence crops such as barley and buckwheat into cash crops of commercial medicines. I am reminded of the sobering assessments given earlier in the conference by the founder of the Kathmandu-based company Wild Earth, which is committed to sustainable sourcing and income generation through production of soaps, essential oils, and related products. She discussed a practical limitation of medicinal plant cultivation. Using the example of *tigta / gyatig (Swertia* spp.) used in Tibetan and Ayurvedic formulas, she spoke about the glutting of markets with key species for commercial production, which might throw other local agricultural systems and economies into rapid, unpredictable change—even as such work might be viewed as a "successful" project outcome by ICDP standards (see Subedi 2006; Saxer 2010a).

In a parallel fashion, I imagine Coca-Cola contract farmers producing herbs that will be processed into fancy teas, even as they use cash earned by these enterprises to buy Coke and Fanta—signs of modernity and social capital in their own right—or to purchase other necessities: rice, medicines, cooking oil. I also note medical problems associated with shifts away from local whole foods toward processed commodity foods (Dickerson et al. 2007). In the margins of my notebook I scribble thoughts about the problematic concept of tradition. Why is it that "ancient wisdom" required to produce Coca-Cola's novel commodities resides within people who might prefer to drink Coke and who cannot afford the herbal-infused concoctions their labor produces? Where, in this multinational mess of social-ecological interconnectedness, does "health" reside?

WILDNESS AS VALUE, SUBSTITUTION AS METHOD

"Medicine is like food," says Gyatso. "Everyone wants it to be good. Not everybody knows how to prepare it. The more you try to cook at one time, the less likely it will be tasty, even though it might stop the thunder in your stomach. If you give the job of cooking to someone you do not know, then you cannot always trust the results. It could be fine. But it could also be poison, like McDonald's in your country." Gyatso lets out a boyish, high-pitched laugh. "Or those tins of food that come over the border from China into Mustang these days. Or the very strong *chemicals* and *drugs* people like to inject into their veins," he goes on, serious now.

Gyatso makes these comments as we are sitting in the back of a Bhutanese taxi, winding our way toward the National Institute of Traditional Medicine (NITM), the state-supported institute for Sowa Rigpa. These thoughts are his response to a question I have posed about the quality of ready-made Tibetan medicines, such as those produced at NITM, for distribution to health posts in rural Bhutan. His answer, by way of metaphor, continues.

"Even more than for making good food, we need the best and most potent ingredients to make medicines. In my view, the medicines they make here in Bhutan are good. Better, probably, than medicines from India or China. Part of what makes them good is that they do not produce too much, and they are able to get very excellent ingredients right here, in Bhutan. They know the sources. The quality is clear. And they have done a good job protecting the forests, so there are plenty of medicinal ingredients, even rare ones like musk *[ladzi]*."

"But musk deer are protected by the government, right? Just like in Nepal. Musk still must be difficult to find, even if the animals are more plentiful."

"Government rules are one thing. Making potent medicine is another. I know there is good quality musk here," Gyatso answers. "Finding some for sale is not difficult, if you have money." Just the day before I read in an Indian daily that the Indo-Tibetan Border Patrol had suspended two of its officers for allegedly smuggling red sandalwood *(Pterocarpus santalinus)* in Himachal Pradesh. According to the Border Patrol, the two officers allowed trucks to cross the border carrying approximately 1.5 tons of this rare, precious timber used in many Asian medicines.[13]

Preliminary estimates suggest that over one hundred species of medicinal plants in Nepal are under great pressure of overexploitation due to the expansion of herbal trade; among them about fifty species have been labeled as "highly threatened" (Shrestha and Joshi 1996; Ghimire 2008). National and international laws now protect many medicinal plants utilized in Sowa Rigpa production. For example, the government of Nepal has imposed restrictions on the collection of nineteen forest products, including medicinal plants. The HAA has its own list of twenty-eight critical species; other practitioners have come up with similar lists.[14] Yet Tibetan medical production continues to rely on threatened and endangered species, some of which are included in the appendices published by the Convention on International Trade in Endangered Species of Wild Fauna and Flora (CITES) and on the "red list" compiled by the International Union for Conservation of Nature (Ghimire et al. 2001). Besides plants, endangered and threatened animal products—including musk, bear's bile, ivory, tiger bone, and rhinoceros horn—are used in Tibetan and Chinese medicines (Sung and Yi-Ming 1998; Ghimire et al. 2010). These are often nonlocal commodities rather than locally available ingredients. Trade in such animal products between countries in the Himalayan region and beyond has a long history. However, as the industries surrounding these medicinal products grow, risks associated with overharvesting are redoubled. Beyond these risks, the globalization of Sowa Rigpa will encounter increasing difficulties as such formulas come up against food and drug regulations in places like the European Union, where regulations stipulate that herbal products must not contain any animal-based ingredients, even honey (Schwabl 2011).

Member countries of CITES have called for promotion of viable species substitutes, and a number of medically acceptable substitutes for threatened or endangered plant and animal species have been proposed. For example, China is promoting the bone of a common type of mole rat as a substitute for tiger bone. The WWF pamphlet *Alternatives to Tiger Bone Medicine* lists nearly twenty plant-based, medically acceptable substitutes for this rare ingredient, including evening primrose and Chinese star jasmine (Ghimire 2010). Similarly a medicinal ingredient used to dissolve gallstones is being made synthetically from cow bile as a substitute for bear's bile. Recent studies have also proposed pharmaceutical substitutes derived from common floral and faunal species for endangered and threatened taxa (Zschocke et al. 2000; Ghimire 2010). These examples are both hopeful and problematic, in that they are useful alternatives that still might be viewed as inferior to their rare counterparts. The ingredients embody wildness. With this comes a use value that posits such ingredients as more potent than domestic, cultivated, synthetic substitutes; the fact of their wildness increases their exchange value.

Gyatso and I arrive at the grounds of the NITM. A sign indicates this facility has received support and attention from the WHO and the United Nations Development Program.

"What about using a substitute, *tshab*, for musk?" I ask Gyatso, as we walk through an exhibit of medical *thanka*. "You know, a plant that by its nature and quality could be used instead of musk?"

"If I could not afford musk, then I would use a plant substitute. But this is only one meaning of *tshab*. Sometimes you find substitutes because of the environment where you live. Like if you have only one kind of *tarbu [Hippophae rhamnoides]*, but maybe you are supposed to use another variety, according to medicine texts. This type of *tshab* changes a lot from place to place. It is a common form of substitution. Plant for plant. The other kind of substitution is for things like *domtri* (bear bile), which is difficult to find and expensive. It has always been this way." One set of substitution practices accounts for the ecological diversity and trade patterns; another form has to do with specific substances that have not only become rare as a consequence of commodification and the growth of the industry, but that, for centuries, have been highly valued trade items.

Gyatso knows of what he speaks. For several years now, since after our meeting with Sabriya, he and other Nepali *amchi* have worked with a leading Nepali botanist on a project funded by WWF's Critical Ecosystems Partnership Fund. The project built on work my friend Yeshi began before her death to explore *amchi* knowledge about medicinal substitutions in Dolpo and Mustang, Nepal, and Sikkim and Darjeeling, India. The project catalogued substitution species, recorded *amchi* knowledge about specific patterns of alternative resource use, and translated an extant medical text about substitution from Dolpo; it also explored the relationship between *amchi* medicine-making and prescribing practices and their knowledge of substitutes for key ingredients they can neither afford to purchase nor access (Ghimire 2010).

Results from this work have revealed that while one can trace geographic and lineage-based knowledge through both oral and textual sources, patterns of substitution are not necessarily standardized. This points to larger issues regarding the problematic assumption that standards can or should serve as a proxy for determining efficacy. Part of what produces efficacious Sowa Rigpa formulas, for either individuals or populations, is the capacity to incorporate substitutes and adapt formularies based on a range of factors, from a patient's need to an *amchi*'s means, from the constraints of particular ecologies to the nature of an illness. Even so, finding viable substitutions for crucial yet endangered ingredients remains a pressing challenge.

"Have you heard about schemes to raise musk deer as you would raise sheep, so more musk can be sold without endangering the wild animals and people can make money from raising the deer?" I ask Gyatso as we walk around the Bhutanese institute.

"Yes, I have heard such things. From one point of view, it is not a bad idea, so the musk deer does not die out. But if you grow musk deer like you would sheep, it also means maybe killing more sentient beings than if you just harvested musk from the wild." Gyatso pauses for a moment. I absorb the Buddhist logic at work here. "Besides, even if people raise musk deer, I would still prefer musk that comes from wild animals. They have survived in the mountains. Their essence is more potent."

"So would you buy musk from a source that comes from the wild, even if you know it is harvested illegally? Or would you buy it maybe for less money but from deer raised by people?"

"If I were wealthy?"

"If you were wealthy."

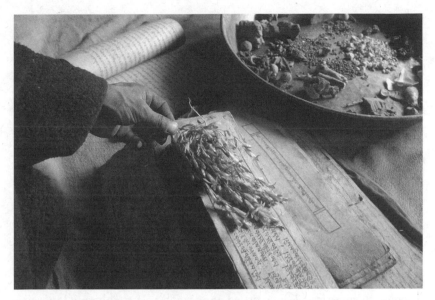

Tibetan medical texts, recently gathered medicinal plants, and a plate of *materia medica*, including plant, animal, and mineral products, Kathmandu, Nepal, 2005. © Thomas Kelly

"I would buy the wild one. I would only need a small amount to make potent medicines."

"Even if you knew the musk came from an animal that is being killed too often, that may not exist in the future because of too much hunting?"

"Yes, even so. I know it is not the right attitude when we think about *sung kyob,* conservation. But as an *amchi,* I also have to think about what will make the best medicine." A long history of involvement with conservation projects, an understanding of the dangers of resource depletion, and a knowledge of protective laws and trade bans are not enough to stop Gyatso from flirting with the use, albeit theoretical, of threatened and endangered species in medicines. At times the desire to serve patients with the best quality medicine possible clashes with a conservationist ethic.

Beyond issues of legal and illegal trade, Gyatso's comments reveal a distinct valuation of wildness. This value is not only about the environment from which particular *materia medica* are harvested—the top of a mountain, for instance, or the gall bladder excretions *(gi-wang)* of an Asian elephant or an ox—although it may be connected to relative difficulty in sourcing. Wildness can become a metonym for efficacy. The value of wildness can be symbolic—alchemical even. An *amchi* might use what can most aptly be described as an *emblematic* amount of a precious substance if he does not have sufficient quantity. A drop of musk in an ocean of herbs, so to speak. Yet this infusion of wild potency can, in some instances, be sufficient to create strong medicine. Wildness and its inverse, that which is cultivated, represent correlates to other powerful dialectics anthropologists have explored: the raw and the cooked (Lévi-Strauss 1964), the sacred and the profane (Douglas 1966).

The consistent skepticism, if not direct resistance, I encounter among *amchi* and others working in the Tibetan medical industry when I ask about using cultivated varieties as alternatives to wild-crafted ingredients points to an association of that which is wild with that which is potent, and that which is potent with that which has the best chance of healing or otherwise producing a desired effect. Another common response to questions I have posed about wild versus cultivated ingredients has to do with the five elements *(jungwa nga)* and their place at the heart of medical theory. Part of what lends a Himalayan poppy or a snow lotus medicinal value is the air, earth, and water that nurture it, the heat from the sun it absorbs, and the space in which it grows. An ecologist might concur with this sensibility, even if she were to employ a different vocabulary to describe it, one that references soil conditions and pH levels instead of the elements as such.

Many people I have interviewed agree, in theory, that medicinal plant cultivation is necessary. However, this does not necessarily quell the equally pervasive sense that medicines made with *ex situ* cultivated alternatives will never be as efficacious as those made with wild ingredients. Notably the *materia medica* that most fully embody this paradoxical relationship between wild and cultivated are not necessarily those ingredients unique to "precious pills." Substances such as alchemically purified mercury, gold and silver, pearls, turquoise, and coral are all subject to other dynamics of value, at once cultural and economic. With these ingredients, the greater concern is distinguishing real specimens from imitations and making sure impurities and other forms of contamination have been removed (Sallon et al. 2006; Dawa 2011). Rather, when it comes to wildness, the *materia medica* in question often refer to odorous plants and animal products: things associated with raw virility, with perfume and incense, things that embody, in materiality and metaphor, the spice of life. Consider camphor and sandalwood, saffron and musk.

The complexities of this dynamic are perhaps most clearly illustrated by *yartsa gunbu*. This caterpillar fungus confounds categorization; at one point in its lifecycle it seems most clearly animal, yet at another point it becomes mycological. It is also quintessentially wild in terms of where it grows. *Yartsa gunbu* surfaces in high-altitude alpine pastures where particular soil types and precipitation patterns support the life cycle of the caterpillar moth (Winkler 2005). Phallic in form, it is ascribed a range of social and pharmacological attributes that address virility, vitality, and even the ability to counteract autoimmune disorders, as we saw in chapter 5. Due to *yartsa gunbu*'s market value, it is an indicator of economic potency as well as something that can conjure social capital when given as a gift. In *yartsa gunbu* we can observe not only an indigenous penchant for valuing wildness, but also the ascription of these qualities to Himalayan and Tibetan landscapes. At the same time, we witness the association of wildness—the blessings and the burdens of being *uncultivated*—with socially produced and politically inflected visions of *Tibetanness* produced by Tibetans and non-Tibetans alike (Yeh 2007). Yet *amchi* I have interviewed rarely claim that *yartsa gunbu* is a crucial substance for meeting the needs of their patients, unless of course you count its ability to function as the equivalent of hard cash with which one might purchase other medicines, either Tibetan or biomedical, or afford an urgent operation. In this sense, *yartsa gunbu* becomes a potent means of substitution in its own right.

Let us consider one last illustration of social ecologies and wildness. It is August 2001, and I am with Lama Namgyal, an *amchi* and HAA member you met in chapter 3. We are on the eastern edges of Dolpo, the Nepali district that includes Nepal's largest national park, Shey-Phoksundo.[15] The region is known for its snow leopards, the highest-flying butterfly in the world, and more than 280 species of plants with ethnobotanical importance (Lama et al. 2001). The beauty of Dolpo—west of Mustang, bordering the TAR to the north—is indeed dramatic. But beauty is not all there is to see. The district hospital is a week's walk away for many in Dolpo. Women routinely die during childbirth; most families have lost children under age five.[16] Indeed Namgyal recently lost a son. Few educational opportunities exist in this region. Those that do are supported by foreign NGOs, augmented by local patronage.[17] Despite its claims to this territory, the government of Nepal feels far away here. However, the presence of the national park as well as the annual appearance on Dolpo's high hills of *yartsa gunbu* means that various outsiders—lowland Nepalis, Tibetans from across the border, and foreigners—see a certain kind of possibility in Dolpo, in its remoteness and its bounty.

Namgyal reaches down to inspect a flower. I watch him carefully uproot this specimen and place it in a canvas sack. The flower's cerulean petals are soft and slightly mottled, like raw silk, with golden pistils and stamen. This gorgeous specimen emerges from a craggy outcropping. Wind howls through the Himalayan landscape in which the flower blooms. High-altitude sun beats down on this vast and rugged place. The flower seems, if not impervious to these elements, then at home in them. Its spiny leaves and relatively short stature are adaptive here. Three heads emerge, hydra-like, clustered in close proximity along the main stem. This is a Himalayan poppy (*Meconopsis* spp.). Even though the species can bloom red, it is often called a blue poppy, a name that mirrors its Tibetan counterpart, *üpal ngonbo*, wherein *ngon* means "blue." The poppy blooms in the saddle between mountain passes, at about 16,000 feet. Patches of snow cling to north-facing slopes, even though it is summer. Usually only the flower is used to make medicines, but due to its relative scarcity, the plant's leaves, seeds, and stems may also be used (Dakpa 1997: 273). According to Tibetan medical theory, the flower's taste is sweet and bitter; it has a cooling and heavy nature. It is compounded in medicines that address fevers as well as bile- and liver-related disorders.

As we walk, the *amchi* speaks in his own language about climate change, gesturing toward retreating glaciers, motioning to a place on his thigh to show how deep the snow used to be, telling me that plants are moving farther up the mountains. Namgyal pulls out his digital camera, GPS unit, altimeter, and his notebook and pen to record this specimen as part of a plant survey with which he is involved and for which he is being paid by an international conservation organization. The money he earns in this capacity, and in forays to Taiwan, helps him to afford the 100,000 rupees ($1,400) or more he spends each year to purchase medicines he cannot gather locally, but which are integral to his ability to make medicines.

"If it were not for conservation patrons, *sung kyob jindag*," he quips, "I could not afford to make medicines and treat patients." Like many other Nepali *amchi* with whom I work, Namgyal wonders what will happen to his clinical practice once the current round of conservation-development funding ends. He neither receives governmental support for his practice, nor does he set prices for his medicines. Yet, as you have already learned, the costs of purchasing and transporting essential lowland ingredients are on the rise.

I've seen images of the blue poppy imbedded within English and Chinese text that touts the high-mountain purity of Tibetan medicines. I've seen this image positioned beside pictures of black-necked cranes, under a banner that exhorts people to make tax-deductible donations to a conservation organization's annual campaign. I've even seen the poppy's image beside text that tells the story of this prized flower's "discovery" by nineteenth-century Western adventurers and botanists traveling through high Asia, and how it became, in the words of Vita Sackville-West, "the dream of every gardener" (Terry 2009). But this is the first time I've seen a blue poppy in situ. I am humbled by its presence, here at the end of its life.

SUMMARY

In previous chapters I've used medical anthropology's focus on health and illness and its concerns with "upstream" causes and conditions of human suffering—poverty, structural inequality, political repression—to discuss the central issues of this book: how and why a medicine works, who gets to make such calls, and what the social-ecological impacts are of these relations of power. In this chapter I've explored the intersections of medical anthropology and political ecology by examining ways the Himalayas and Tibet exist not only as natural spaces but also as deeply social and political places, and how this bears on the future of Tibetan medicine.

The work of political ecology encourages us to question our presumed understandings of nature and culture and to critically examine how we use resources. We can see examples of political ecology in the work of writers and public intellectuals like Wendell Berry, Bill McKibbin, Barbara Kingsolver, and Michael Pollan, whose work asks fundamental questions about how we sustain ourselves and what it means to value nature. In academic circles, political ecology has explored the eviction of indigenous populations from landscapes they have stewarded for decades, if not centuries, and on which they depend, in the name of "conservation." This includes a critical engagement with the creation of national parks and protected areas and the way "scientific" rationales formulated around concepts such as desertification, overgrazing, and overstocking of animals can justify evictions, resettlement, and land grabs from indigenous inhabitants. Often these claims are connected to governmental or extraterritorial desires to use land in different ways: for mineral extraction, ecotourism, or to control nomadic populations.

Political ecologists also examine the reinscription of group identities around ideas of indigeneity and land-based claims to ethnic heritage. To paraphrase the anthropologist Tim Ingold (2000), political ecology aims to understand ways of dwelling in the world and to investigate how human lifeways, including the medicines we make and how we address suffering, are enmeshed in relations of power. Such relations of power can produce what Agrawal (2005) has dubbed "environmentality." Following Foucault's concept of "governmentality," this is one way of saying that nature does not just exist sui generis, but is produced by human perceptions and actions, in the ways we govern, use, map, and conserve such spaces. Such dynamics extend from imperial projects to postcolonial nation building and global conservation campaigns.

As I shared stories of traveling with three generations of Sowa Rigpa practitioners in Yunnan, you've seen how their experiences dovetail with and depart from conservation-development agendas, as articulated by the Chinese state, international conservation organizations, even ethnobotanists. As you've watched a Nepali *amchi* navigate a meeting with a conservation international NGO in Kathmandu, you've see Buddhist ideals of protection and the pragmatic ethics of a Sowa Rigpa practitioner intermingle with faith-based funding channels from Europe and the United States in an era of neoliberal conservation. Through ethnography from Bhutan and Dolpo, you've glimpsed the paradoxes of commodification from the perspective of plants as opposed to products, and gotten a sense of the cultural and economic power behind wild things.

In the final chapter of this book I piece together this social-ecological mosaic of Tibetan medicine with the biography of one formula, from its mythohistorical origins in the thirteenth century to its transformation into a study drug used in a Randomized Controlled Trial.

CHAPTER 7

The Biography of a Medicine

You could keep some remnant of it, a talisman that would become rare and fine, worn over time into something familiar. It would naturally become more thin and precious the more the air wore it out, like the bones of a saint. After all, it was only an object in the physical world, not something more potent, like something in the mind: memory.

—Susan Brind Morrow, *The Names of Things*

RECOLLECTIONS OF THE BIRTH-HELPING PILL

The women's inpatient ward at Mentsikhang smells of disinfectant and butter tea. Nurses in cool pink frocks and doctors in white lab coats talk with patients and family members in the building's corridors. Unlike other hospitals in Lhasa, Mentsikhang is known for providers with good bedside manner and a willingness to treat patients regardless of their ability to pay.

One morning in late 2002 I arrive at Mentsikhang with one of the Principal Investigators (PIs) of the NIH-funded project with which I am involved as a research coordinator and ethnographer. She is a midwife with a Ph.D. in public health, with a long list of successful research across Latin America, the Middle East, Africa, and South Asia under her belt, and is now helping to redirect our project toward a hospital-based clinical trial. In earlier meetings between U.S. and Tibetan collaborators various ideas were proposed. We could study anemia, for instance, or the effects of micronutrient deficiencies on birth outcomes. Or we could focus on Postpartum Hemorrhage (PPH). Of the approximately 380,000 to 500,000 women who die each year from complications related to pregnancy and childbirth, a full quarter of these deaths are due to obstetric hemorrhage (World Health Organization 2005b; Hogan 2010).

We are met by the director of Mentsikhang's Inpatient Women's Division, a middle-aged woman with a moon-shaped face and freckles.

She was recruited to start this division from a hospital in Shigatse Prefecture, where she worked for many years. Although she is a biomedical physician, she hails from a lineage of Sowa Rigpa practitioners.

"Welcome to Mentsikhang," says the director, nodding toward the PI. Over the next few minutes we visit patient rooms where mothers-to-be wait to be examined and the postpartum recovery rooms where swaddled newborns grope for their mothers' nipples and aunties pour endless cups of butter tea. The Tibetan OB leads us to a delivery room, a clean space of narrow delivery beds, metal stirrups, trays of stainless steel instruments, and cabinets of medical supplies. As a skilled clinician who made her early career attending home births in the United States, the PI looks over the room. Perhaps she is contemplating the visceral experience of what it would mean to work here.

"Standard protocol for a woman who hemorrhages is oxytocin, correct?" she asks her Tibetan counterpart, referring to the synthetic version of a hormone the body naturally produces that helps to contract the uterus. Oxytocin is used to induce and augment labor and to manage PPH.[1] My colleague Pema's wife, a young doctor who works under the director and whose medical English is competent, translates, with assistance from me.

"Yes," the director replies. "We also massage the woman's uterus and sometimes give other medicines." The PI nods, noting the presence of magnesium sulfate, a treatment for eclampsia.

"What is this?" asks the PI, pointing to a sepia-colored bottle whose label is handwritten in Tibetan.

"That is *zhijé 11*," answers the director. "It is a Tibetan medicine—the only Tibetan medicine we use for delivery here, actually." This piques the PI's interest.

"The only one? What is it used for?"

"We call it the 'birth-helping pill' *(kyesu rilbu)*," the Tibetan physician answers. "It is used to help aid and speed delivery. It helps to expel the placenta and stop the bleeding after birth."

"So it is like a uterotonic?"

"Yes, but we still use oxytocin if the woman is bleeding too much."

"When do you give it? What is in it?"

"We give it to many women who are proceeding normally through delivery. We do not give it if there are complications. We give it if contractions seem slow, and then sometimes when a woman begins to sweat—you know, when the baby is about to come. This helps to bring out the placenta and also stop blood after delivery."

"So you give it at transition, to help the woman not bleed too much after delivery?" the PI queries, referring to the third stage of labor, when a woman's cervix is dilated and she is about to push. The Tibetan physician nods.

"I am not a Tibetan doctor," she continues, "so it is difficult for me to tell you exactly what is in the medicine, but it has ingredients that help the downward-expelling wind *(thursel lung)*. This is part of why it is effective."

The Mentsikhang doctor takes the brown glass bottle off the shelf and pours out several *rilbu* into her palm. They are about one centimeter in diameter and smell faintly of ginger. She explains that the pills are crushed and swallowed with boiled water. Dosage is determined by examining a woman's progress during labor and her physical stature. The pills are made at the Mentsikhang factory, not in a GMP facility but in the part of the factory that produces only for clinical use.

The PI rolls the pills around in her palm, considering them. After a pause she says, "We have talked about different possibilities for a clinical trial. If this medicine is really used to help stop women from bleeding after birth, if it is also used to augment labor, then it could be a possibility. Misoprostol might be a good comparison." The Tibetan physician has only vaguely heard of this drug, branded as Cytotec and known here as "miso."

"Would you be interested in doing clinical research on this Tibetan medicine?" the PI queries.

The Mentsikhang doctor seems cautious as she frames her answer. "We want to learn more about research," she begins. "I think it could be good. But there are many issues to consider. We use this medicine at Mentsikhang. It is the only Tibetan medicine we use regularly during delivery. The other hospitals don't use Tibetan medicines. Maybe they won't believe it works." She references Lhasa Municipal Hospital and the Maternal-Child Health Hospital. Leading clinicians from Mentsikhang and these two hospitals, as well as several other experts, constitute the Research Committee, a body working closely with the PI and other researchers to develop and implement this project.

"Those are all good points. Things we should talk about with the others. But do you think it is worth exploring this idea?" asks the PI.

"I believe in this medicine," the Tibetan doctor says, by way of an answer.

The other members of the Research Committee are open to the idea. All are eager to learn more about Randomized Controlled Trials (RCT), the "gold standard" of biomedical research. As one member of the committee put it, "RCT, this is how you get taken seriously." Some feel that picking a Tibetan medicine is a good idea. Others are unsure about how to design such a study.

"How will we tell women at our hospital that they might be given a Tibetan medicine?" asks a physician from Lhasa Municipal Hospital. "What will happen if the trial shows *zhijé* 11 does not work," asks another committee member. Both optimism and caution are warranted. The committee decides we should learn as much about *zhijé* 11 as possible before making a decision.

Mingkyi is a member of the Research Committee. She and I are tasked with interviewing women and Sowa Rigpa practitioners about the medicine. Samples of *zhijé* 11 are also sent to one of the PI's home institutions, where it will be tested for toxicity and its chemical composition will be analyzed. We begin our inquiries into *zhijé* 11's story with an exploration of language.

"What does *zhijé* mean? I thought it was a term of religion, not medicine," I say, as we sit in the program office. "Isn't *zhijé* something to do with pacification or appeasement of suffering?"

"This is correct, but not only that," Mingkyi answers. "*Zhijé*, this idea comes from the Padampa tradition of the twelfth or thirteenth century, I think. *Zhijé* is what he taught, the names for his teachings. It is a big tradition, like the teachings of Je Tsongkapa.[2] But it is not just this. This *zhijé*, it is about making suffering stop. This is the Buddhist understanding. So it is a good general name for medicines, since medicines pacify physical suffering."

"This is interesting," I say, getting back to the task at hand, "But what do doctors or lay women mean when they say *zhijé* 11 is a 'birth-helping pill,' or the 'quick pill' *(gyok ril)*, as some people have called it? How have they heard of it? When do they use it? Do they think it is beneficial or not?" These questions guide our initial work into the social life of *zhijé* 11.

One afternoon Mingkyi and I arrive at Mentsikhang to conduct interviews. A young woman from a farming village has just delivered a healthy girl. Her mother feeds her postpartum daughter bone soup. We ask these two generations of women if either has heard of *zhijé* 11 or the birth-helping pill. The younger woman shakes her head no.

"Do you remember if you were given a Tibetan medicine when you were in labor?" I ask.

"I don't really remember. I was in so much pain," she admits. Her mother picks up the conversation.

"Oh yes, she wailed! Even though the doctors told her not to." The older woman pauses. "I have not heard of *zhijé* 11, but I have heard of the birth-helping pill," she goes on. "When someone is having difficulty birthing a child. If you give the mother this medicine, then it will help deliver the baby."

Another woman adds, "This medicine makes deliveries faster, easier. It has benefits when doctors are not around. It acts like a woman's friend." I note the younger woman's inability to identify the medicine, and the fact that her mother knew the medicine only by one of its colloquial names. This is a theme across many interviews. Of the newly postpartum women who do not know the medicine, more than half of their attending elder female relatives have heard of it, and in many cases have used it themselves. A woman in her early forties has just emerged from her ninth delivery, although she has only seven living children.[3] "I have taken the birth-helping pill. This medicine helps get the placenta out," she offers. "Only *amchi* call it *zhijé* 11. With all my other children I gave birth at home. I took this medicine with every other pregnancy. I think it works well."

A woman in her fifties who is here attending a younger relative tells us, "I have taken this medicine three times out of six pregnancies, all of which I delivered at home, only with the help of my husband. It worked well, but the overall effectiveness decreased with every delivery. I am not sure why. It just seemed to be less powerful in my body. Was this a result of the medicine or my condition?" This woman tells us the benefits of the medicine are its low price, the fact that you don't have to go to the hospital to take it, and that it helps women with labor. I notice that *zhijé* 11 is a medical intervention that seems to help in the case of an otherwise nonmedicalized pregnancy and delivery. What we are learning about *zhijé* 11 is a kind of "authoritative knowledge" about childbirth (Davis-Floyd and Sargent 1997), but knowledge operating outside the boundaries of conventional medicine.

By asking about women's knowledge of *zhijé* 11 we also learn about their familiarity with PPH. More than two-thirds of the approximately forty women we interview have known a woman who has experienced "too much bleeding after delivery." Some died. Most of these women link such deaths to a combination of social and structural factors: a dearth of emergency transportation services, lack of funds to pay hospital fees, poor quality and availability of health services, and the general conditions of life for women in a rural Tibetan village (see Pinto 2008; Berry 2010).

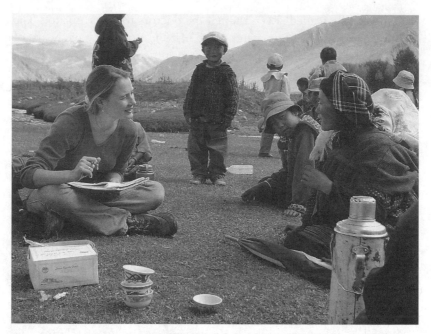

The author interviewing a rural Tibetan woman about her experiences of pregnancy and childbirth, Lhasa Prefecture, Tibet Autonomous Region, China, 2003. © Sienna Craig

When we ask women what causes "too much bleeding," most do not know. Those who offer an explanation cite prolonged labor or a woman's general "weakness." Few mention nutritional deficiencies. Some say demanding physical work can deplete a woman, rendering her vulnerable during delivery. When asked if *zhijé 11* can be helpful once a woman has already lost a lot of blood, most say they don't know. Several offer an opinion. "I don't think so," says one woman who has just given birth to her fifth child, while on pilgrimage in Lhasa. "At that point maybe only Western medicine is strong enough. But even then, if the woman's life force *lung* has declined, then maybe even Western medicine is not useful." Such comments reveal women's perceptions of Tibetan medicine as opposed to biomedicine, as it is available in rural China, and about cultural and economic conditions that contribute to the high rates of home births and maternal, newborn, and child deaths in Tibetan communities (Adams et al. 2005b; Craig 2009, 2011c).

Mingkyi and I ask Dr. Sangye,[4] a senior Mentsikhang physician, more about *zhijé 11*. "In old times, *amchi* would give one *zhijé 11* pill to women to keep in their home as their delivery time drew near. We use it still because it has beneficial effects for a normal delivery. *Zhijé* 11 is a good medicine, but it can be strong. Before using this medicine you need to consider the situation of the baby and mother."

"What you say is true," replies Mingkyi. "When I worked at Nagchu Prefecture Hospital, once a woman was having a difficult delivery. She was given *zhijé* 11 and some other medicines. She bled more, not less. Eventually she died. Some wondered if *zhijé* 11 had been harmful, but I think it was more complicated than that. The woman was in bad physical condition. She had high blood pressure."

Sangye responds, "If a woman is not healthy, you should not give this medicine. Even with a healthy, strong woman, with powerful contractions sometimes a woman does bleed more at first. But *zhijé* 11 can shrink the uterus quickly. Women bleed for many reasons during delivery, also from rips and tears. *Zhijé* 11 does not help this kind of bleeding. With medicines like oxytocin, we know how it works, when to give it, and how much to give. But with *zhijé* 11, it is sometimes less clear. We do not have numbers or laboratory tests to know it works, but I trust this medicine."

In listening to Sangye, I am struck by this issue of evidence. When people like her or Mingkyi speak about research that has been done on Tibetan medicine, they understand it to be "evidenced-based" in that it is empirical. Much of the research done at Mentsikhang is conducted without the same assumptions about reproducibility, control populations, or statistical significance that structure biomedical research agendas in places like the United States (Adams 2002a; Adams and Li 2008). Yet the desire and necessity to study Tibetan medicine through a new kind of evidentiary lens is increasing, as generations of Tibetan medical practitioners grow more accustomed to and reliant on biomedical diagnostic methods, etiology, and drugs, and as the state continues to increase its jurisdiction over the standards by which Tibetan medicines are produced, as you saw in chapter 5. Sangye has been administering *zhijé* 11 for many years. When faced with the possibility of using it in an RCT, however, she worries about how to quantitatively account for its efficacy and questions her own understanding of the mechanisms by which it works.

"*Zhijé* 11 is used for other reasons too. It can be given if a woman's period is irregular," Mingkyi adds, "and it can be used to end a pregnancy in the first months of gestation." This is the first time I hear of *zhijé* 11's abortofacient qualities, but given its relation to both uterine contractions and downward-expelling *lung,* this indication does not surprise me. Other doctors mention this indication, often with ambivalence. During a meeting of our Research Committee, one member explains that women still come to the Mentsikhang and ask for the pill. "Unless we can see the woman is pregnant," she says, meaning beyond her first trimester, "we are careful about selling it."

Abortion can be a heated a topic among Tibetans. Consciously ending a fetus's life can be viewed as sinful in a Buddhist sense. Abortions are readily available through the Chinese health care system. However, in the Tibetan context, religious injunctions, combined in some instances with forced sterilization campaigns in Tibetan areas or political concern about survival of Tibetans as a people, make it a problematic proposition (Goldstein et al. 2002; Adams 2005a: 230–31; Childs 2008: 208; Schrempf 2012). We are working in the politically fraught context of Tibet *and* under a U.S. administration firmly against abortion (the George W. Bush administration). As such, this revelation about *zhijé* 11's varied indications worries me. How might this multiplicity of indications be addressed as we move forward?

Interestingly, misoprostol, the biomedical drug we are considering using alongside *zhijé* 11, has a similar profile. Like *zhijé* 6, a simplified version of the *zhijé* formulary, misoprostol was first designed to treat gastrointestinal problems, specifically gastric ulcers; it is indicated for early abortion, to treat miscarriages, and to induce labor. The drug is on WHO's List of Essential Medicines for labor induction. Some argue that its ability to "ripen" the cervix as well as its quick bioavailability make it more effective than other drugs for inducing labor.[5] We might note parallels with how Tibetan women talk about *zhijé* 11 as a pill that "aids and speeds" delivery. Misoprostol's utility in preventing and treating PPH has been clinically tested, and it was approved as part of WHO's list for this purpose in 2011, but its history is not free from controversy. It has been connected to increased rates of uterine rupture and was slow to be approved by the U.S. FDA due to its abortofacient nature, only gaining approval in 2002.[6] Furthermore studies have shown that it has more side effects and is, overall, less effective than oxytocin for the prevention of PPH. However, it has been argued that these issues are counterbalanced in "resource-constrained" settings since misoprostol is produced in pill form, which is usually cheaper and safer to use than intravenous oxytocin (Villar et al. 2002; Bradley et al. 2007). Whether this social history of misoprostol is reflective of medical "best practices" or politics is a point of debate. The controversies surrounding both *zhijé* 11 and misoprostol are uncannily parallel.

LOST MEDICINES AND FOUND HISTORIES

The biography of *zhijé* 11 is bound up with the pharmacological and social lives of other Tibetan medicines. Tibetan doctors Mingkyi and I interview about *zhijé* 11 mention other formulas that seem practically, if not etiologically, related to *zhijé* 11. *Gur gum* 8 and 13, both saffron-based, are used to stop bleeding from lacerations that can occur during birth. Several doctors speak of a medicine called *gyaru* 30. Known from textual sources to assist in labor and delivery, it is rarely produced today because its key ingredients are endangered species: musk *(ladzi)* and the horn of a Himalayan ungulate, preferably, that of the endangered Tibetan antelope. When prepared correctly and given properly *gyaru* 30 is said to reduce postpartum blood loss. Like *zhijé* 11, it is an abortofacient.

Over a lunch of MSG-laden spinach, fried mutton, and rice, I speak with Dr. Gyaltsen about *zhijé* 11.[7] Gyaltsen is the director of a county-level Maternal and Child Health program. He served as a Barefoot Doctor and received some Tibetan medical training during the Cultural Revolution years.

"In my experience, *zhijé* 6 and another type of *lung* medicine, *sokdzin* 11, are used during delivery more than *zhijé* 11," says Dr. Gyaltsen. "Sometimes *agar* 20 or *agar* 15 are also used or used instead of *sokdzin* 11. These medicines will be given first, if she is weak or past due. Once labor has begun, then *zhijé* 6 will be given. *Zhijé* 6 and 11 both contract the uterus and hasten delivery." He confirms that *zhijé* 11 is sometimes used for its ability to produce spontaneous abortions.

"Doctors used *zhijé* 11 often in the old society," Dr. Gyaltsen continues, "but I don't see this medicine as much today, at least not at the county hospital. We mostly use oxytocin. This is not unique to *zhijé* 11, though. We don't use much Tibetan medicine at the county hospital anymore." This was true in many areas I visited across the TAR—one of the effects of health care reform that has included more fee-for-service models and has often left counties with supply budgets and fewer subsidies, particularly for Tibetan medicine (Tibet Information Network 2004; Hofer 2008).

Tsultrim is an ex-monk and a graduate of the Tibetan Medical College.[8] At the time of our interview he is directing a medical education program funded by an international NGO. Tsultrim and I discuss the indications of *zhijé* 11 and the properties of its ingredients. He compares *zhijé* 6 and 11, concluding, "*Zhijé* 11 is the stronger of the two formulas.

This could be good, but also potentially more harmful." As he describes it, a medicine's strength and potency is revealed not as a fixed measurement but rather along a continuum from benefit *(phentok)* to harm *(kyön)*, manifest in a particular healing encounter; efficacy arises when a doctor's ability, a patient's condition, the innate power of specific medicines, and the social-ecological circumstances of treatment are positively aligned. The fact that both Gyaltsen and Tsultrim view *zhijé* 6 as interchangeable with *zhijé* 11 also reveals gendered differences. Female doctors with whom I speak do not view these two medicines as equivalent, but most male doctors I interview do.

Tsultrim is generally supportive of the idea of research, but he cautions against comparing only one Tibetan medicine to one biomedical drug. "You should also use other formulas, and move away from the idea of one medicine for one problem. This is a Western approach, not a Tibetan approach." This comment reveals an interesting bias by this Tibetan doctor, in that biomedicine also relies on multiple approaches to therapy. He assumes biomedicine acts monolithically, while Tibetan medicine is more "sensitive" or contingent in its approach. These comments are observant, yet I also note that PPH is caused *specifically* because the uterus fails to contract after birth. It is a clear medical event with consistent symptoms, at least from a biomedical perspective.

"*Zhijé* 11 *is* related to the uterus contracting," Tsultrim goes on, "but to say this is the overriding condition is not entirely correct, at least according to Tibetan medicine. We can't just say 'postpartum hemorrhage' without considering how *lung* and blood are related. What does this 'blood loss' mean? It is not only because the uterus doesn't contract. This is a reason from Western medicine. We must also know the patient's unique condition, her economic situation, how she is giving birth, even her karma. If you want a research project that considers Tibetan medical theory when measuring results, then the definitions need to be different from the start."

Other doctors with whom I speak echo this view. These comments are valuable, but sometimes difficult to reconcile with the medical practice I observe at the women's division of Mentsikhang (see Adams 2001a)—the only hospital in Lhasa that uses *zhijé* 11 regularly—or the comments of women who have used this medicine during home births. In these settings considerations of *lung* may sometimes be voiced, but the medicine is referred to more often in a "folk etiological" perspective (Nichter 2008) that emphasizes "speeding up" delivery and acting as a "woman's friend." Neither an erudite understanding of Tibetan medical theory nor a grasp of labor and delivery reflective of evidence-based biomedical obstetric practices consistently guide *zhijé* 11's practical use.

Perhaps in this disjuncture we can gain a more holistic understanding of Sowa Rigpa. Maybe we can acknowledge moments when private, lineage-based, and often male physicians differ from their male and female colleagues who have received other training—or differ from the knowledge of laboring women themselves. However, it remains difficult to reconcile the richness of lived experience with the realities of a multidisciplinary, cross-cultural research project beholden to two medical bureaucracies. Given this, I return to Mentsikhang to speak with an elder female *amchi* about *zhijé* 11 and this clinical research in an effort to clarify, if not reconcile, the different information Mingkyi and I have collected.

Dr. Palden,[9] the most senior female *amchi* on staff at the outpatient facility, greets us with paper cups of steaming jasmine tea. It is late spring 2003, but the hills surrounding Lhasa are still snow-capped. I give the senior *amchi* a brief overview of the idea of a clinical trial of *zhijé* 11, most likely compared with misoprostol.

"We have asked many doctors and women patients about their use and knowledge of this medicine," I begin. "We have questions about how and why *zhijé* 11 is effective during deliveries, and how we might use it in a clinical research project."

The aging doctor has a beautifully lined face, sharp eyes. Her hair is pulled back in a low bun, and she wears a fine wool *chuba* underneath her white coat. "First, many other Tibetan medicines are used during labor and delivery. *Zhijé* 11 is best for helping to have a quick and less painful delivery. Other medicines help to control blood loss, both Western and Tibetan medicines. But," continues Palden, "when *zhijé* 11 is used during delivery, it must be considered in relation to the patient's *lung* and also with medicines that are specifically for blood, medicines like *thangjé* 25 and *gurgum* 8, or a new medicine we are making called *trakshö lepchok*." This novel formula translates as "excellent for stopping blood loss."

"We are making this new medicine in capsule form at the factory," Palden continues. "But I should be clear: this new medicine is good for blood, but it does not contract the uterus. *Zhijé* 11 *does* contract the uterus. It is mostly beneficial for women who do not have strong enough contractions at the beginning of labor. It helps to expel the placenta and shrink the uterus after delivery. These functions are related to the condition and strength of the woman's downward-expelling *lung*. Medicines such as *agar* 20 also help the downward-expelling *lung*, which makes it possible for the woman to have the strength for her uterus to close after delivery. *Zhijé* 11 aids this process, but *only if* the downward-expelling *lung* is sufficiently strong and balanced in the woman. Otherwise there can be a risk to the mother in using *zhijé* 11. Therefore we often give *zhijé* 11 along with other *lung* medicines, such as *agar* 8 or 20."

Palden recounts the ideal timing for giving these different medicines. "Women should be given *thangjé* 25 in the morning, or when they first start to have weak contractions. This is followed by our new medicine or *gurgum* 8 in the afternoon or a few hours later, followed by *agar* 20 or 8 in the evening, or as contractions increase and quicken. Then they are given *zhijé* 11 if the doctors feel it will be beneficial for a quick and less painful delivery, around the time the cervix is dilated." This exegesis of Tibetan best practices is fascinating, but it is difficult to reconcile with the fact that many Tibetan women labor at home alone, or with a friend or relative, without access to this or any other health care (Adams et al. 2005b; Gyaltsen et al. 2007; Craig 2009).

Palden raises other issues. One of the reasons we have assumed *zhijé* 11 is the only Tibetan medicine used during delivery at Mentsikhang is simply because it is given *in the delivery room*. We have not checked to see what Tibetan medications, if any, are being given to women at other times. Nor have we fully investigated the relationship between the inpatient division at Mentsikhang, where biomedicine dominates, and the outpatient division, where Tibetan medicines are ubiquitous. These issues are profound in what they say about assumptions on which the narrow edifice of a clinical trial can be built.

We talk more about the idea of a comparison between *zhijé* 11 and misoprostol. Palden voices concerns about how such a comparison will be structured. Although she confirms what we have learned about *zhijé* 11's indications and uses, she emphasizes, "You must understand: these are brief explanations. If you really want to ask questions about *zhijé* 11 and other medicines, we need a long time. We cannot expect Tibetan medicines to have the same kinds of functions as Western medicines. Research is important. We have a lot to learn from Western science. But we need to help all of you think about which medicines to study and how to study them, if we want to do *your* kind of research on *our* Tibetan medicines. It is a good idea to work on blood loss after delivery, because many Tibetan women suffer from this. But we need to go slowly on which medicines to use and how to make this comparison."

As I thank Palden and prepare to leave, I hope the PIs will be interested in the perspective she has shared. Yet I know it may be impossible to retrain their expectations of the seemingly perfect fit of *zhijé* 11 for this clinical trial in order to recast our research protocol in a way that takes into account other Tibetan medicines and the clinical context in which *zhijé* 11 is normally given, at least at the Mentsikhang. Years later I learn that this might have been possible using whole system research methods, as mentioned in chapter 2, but for now it seems beyond the pale.

Later that afternoon I send off a lengthy email to the PIs describing the concerns Palden and others have raised about picking only one Tibetan medicine, as opposed to looking at a more comprehensive Tibetan medical protocol for labor and delivery. The responses of the PIs are kind, if firm. Designing an RCT with multiple Tibetan therapies will be impossible, they say. It will be difficult enough to structure a meaningful comparison between *zhijé* 11 and misoprostol. It is likely that each will be compared to a placebo rather than directly compared with each other—what medical researchers refer to as a "two-arm" study—for ethical and practical reasons. The PIs also remind me of the circumstances at hand: Mentsikhang, our primary institutional collaborator, is already using *zhijé* 11 as a routine part of their obstetric care; it is the only Tibetan medicine our ethnography has uncovered that seems to have roughly equivalent uterotonic qualities to misoprostol. This, coupled with the complexities of satisfying both the U.S. and Tibetan agencies sponsoring this research and the demands of Institutional Review Boards, leads the PIs to conclude that *zhijé* 11 will be the only Tibetan medicine we will engage in the clinical trail.

Some weeks after my visit with Palden, Mingkyi rushes into our program office, flush-faced and smiling. "I've found more about the history of *zhijé* 11," she says. "It was first made by a woman!" Despite the theoretical basis for a Tibetan medical vision of women's health as described in the *Fourfold Treatise* and other texts, social reality has kept many *amchi* uninformed about obstetrics and gynecology; they often play a distant role during births (Adams et al. 2005b; Craig 2009; Gutschow 2010; Pordié and Petitet in press). Knowing this history, Mingkyi feels her findings about *zhijé* 11's gendered origins are important. They help to validate the choice of *zhijé* 11 as a focus of the RCT. Mingkyi and I sit down, and she reads from her notes about the woman who was said to have invented *zhijé* 11:

In a chapter from the *Collected Treasury of Divine Nectar,* the author Diumar Geshe Tenzin Phuntsok says the first person to make *zhijé* 11 was a woman, named Jomo Menmo.[10] According to *A Recounting of the History of Accomplished Women in the Land of Snows,*[11] it is said that Jomo Menmo was born in a place called Zarmo. Today we do not know this exact location. Jomo Menmo's father was called Dorje Gyalpo. He was associated with a *kagyü* lineage. Her mother was called Pema Paldzom. Jomo Menmo was born in the fourth sixty-year cycle, in the earth monkey year (1212 C.E.).

Jomo Menmo grew up as a shepherdess. Once, while she was watching the herds, she uncovered a treasure text *(terma)* in a Guru Rimpoche cave on the tenth day of the month.[12] The name of this treasure text was *The Dakini Heart Essence of the Buddhist Doctrine.*[13] After this, she stayed in meditation and came to a state of realization based on the teachings in this text.

Later Jomo Menmo went to a place in what is today Lhoka Prefecture to have an audience with a tantric householder teacher named Guru Chöwang, and later to receive teachings from him. She became his consort. After much tantric practice and accomplishment by the lama and his consort, Jomo Menmo reached a state of all-pervading awareness *(yéshe).* The practice of these two devout practitioners had benefits for all sentient beings.

When Jomo Menmo reached the age of thirty-six, in the fifth sixty-year cycle (1248 C.E.), on the tenth day of the sixth Tibetan month, she climbed to the top of a mountain, along with her consort and their son, to make offerings to the female tantric deities (T. *kandro,* Skt. *dakini*). While they were performing this ritual, each of the three beings flew like birds up into the sky, into the Buddha realm.

Mingkyi finishes reading. "We are lucky to have picked a medicine made by such a person," she says.

I agree, but I also wonder about the details of Jomo Menmo's life. This text does not mention her training as an *amchi.* The specifics of *zhijé* 11 are cited in another section of the text, but Diumar (b. 1672) couches these within extensive commentary. The female adept's fragmented biography raises questions about the place of women's health within Sowa Rigpa praxis, as well as the nature and qualities of *zhijé* 11. From the hagiographic account of Jomo Menmo's life, we learn she is a woman of spiritual accomplishment, but also that she enters the Buddha realm at the age of thirty-six. Although the text alludes to her passing as a willing ascension, I wonder about the less metaphorical circumstances under which she "passed on." The text mentions a son. Did she die during childbirth? Did someone else attribute this recipe to Jomo Menmo after she died? Perhaps the compassionate act of making *zhijé* 11 arose from Jomo Menmo's bearing witness to the suffering of other women. There is no way to know.

This account of Jomo Menmo mentions her medicine but does not reveal any specific Sowa Rigpa training. Her teacher and consort could have been an *amchi,* but with what the text leaves us, it is impossible to know. Was she instructed in the *Fourfold Treatise?* Did she apprentice to a relative who was an *amchi?* What of Jomo Menmo's name? *Jomo* has two distinct, though related etymologies: *jomo* is a generic title given to noblewomen, often of spiritual accomplishment; it literally translates as "woman of the *dharma.*" Both titles can refer to nuns.[14] *Menmo* literally means "female medical practitioner." In Jomo Menmo we have an archetypal female medicoreligious figure, perhaps a historical person, perhaps not.

I ask Mingkyi these questions, but my friend is unable to answer them—and relatively uninterested. Instead she focuses on what we know of Jomo Menmo's legacy: the medicine itself. From Mingkyi's perspective, the relevant details of Jomo Menmo's biography are that a recipe was revealed—itself an expression Sowa Rigpa truth—and that this revelation was the work of a woman who upheld the moral duty of the *dharma,* whose medical knowledge could be trusted. Mingkyi reads these fragments of a woman's life almost as an allegory for the beneficent origins of medicine. I read it as an anthropologist or historian might: wondering what is being left out of this text, what does it not say.

BRINGING A RECIPE TO LIFE

Mingkyi creates a document that describes *zhijé* 11's history and ingredients and provides a Tibetan medical explanation for the more general causes and conditions of blood loss after delivery. Building on the comments of Tsultrim, Palden, and other colleagues, she and I hope the English translation of this text will show the PIs the history of this medicine and the social-ecological context into which this clinical trail is being inserted. As we translate the document, I notice that after months of intense work Mingkyi has come to see *zhijé* 11 as *associated* with the biomedical understanding of PPH. She describes PPH as a result of *lung* and blood imbalances along with a medical "complication" resulting from weak uterine contractions and/or prolonged labor. Connections between *zhijé* 11, oxytocin, and misoprostol inch toward each other.

Even so, Mingkyi's essay reveals a more comprehensive Tibetan medical understanding of what biomedicine calls PPH. The notion of honing in on a single medicine, she writes, is contrary to basic tenets of Sowa Rigpa theory. But this does not mean such an approach is incommensurable with the realities of clinical practice in Tibet or in other contexts in which Tibetan medicine is used. As at Arura and even in private clinics in Nepal and China, technological crossovers between Sowa Rigpa and biomedicine are common. Mingkyi thinks pharmacological points of connection between *zhijé* 11 and misoprostol can help build methodological bridges between biomedicine and Sowa Rigpa. She agrees with others who argue against the equation of Tibetan medical terms with loose biomedical equivalents, but she is also realistic about the constraints of RCT methodologies. In her essay she describes each of *zhijé* 11's ingredients: their tastes, potencies, postdigestive tastes, and pharmacological uses. The ingredients in *zhijé* 11 include the five ingredients in *zhijé* 6 (in bold below).

TIBETAN NAME	LATIN NAME	COMMON NAME
Manu	*Inula racemosa Hood;* *Inula helenium*	Elecampane
Gakya	*Zingiber officinale Rose;* *Hedychium spicatum Ham*	Asian ginger; galanga
Arura	*Terminalia chehula Retz*	Chebulic Myrobalan
Chumtsa	*Rheum palmatum L*	Chinese, Turkish, or East Indian rhubarb
Jongshi	*Calcitum*	Calcium; calcite
Bultog	*Trona*	Sodium bicarbonate; soda ash
Tarbu	**Hippophae rhamnoides L**	**Seabuckthorn**
Drulsha	**Zaocys dhumnades Cantor**	**Black snake meat**
Gyatsha	**Sal ammoniacum**	**Salt of sulfur**
Digzin	**Potamon yunnanense kemp**	**Freshwater crab shell**
Olmosé	**Sinopodophyllum hexandrum Royle**	**Himalayan or Chinese mayapple**

"I am happy with what we are discovering about *zhijé* 11," says Mingkyi, "but there are problems with this information, and how Western science will understand it. There are also problems in the way texts from the old society are interpreted to make factory medicines today.

Diumar's text says Jomo Menmo first made *zhijé* 11 and mentions the five ingredients that are added to *zhijé* 6. It doesn't list the *amounts* of ingredients to be used. It only lists the names. Diumar's text was written in the eighteenth century, but Jomo Menmo lived in the thirteenth century. We don't know what happened in between."

This absence of specific preparation guidelines for Tibetan medicine is not unusual. Crucial details such as ratios of ingredients can vary based on a healer's experience and training, local ecology, the price of raw materials, and sometimes the specifics of a patient's condition. This aspect of pharmacological knowledge has, historically, been passed down through oral tradition. This is a clear example of how scientific knowledge—indeed science as a category—is culturally constituted and negotiated. This is not to say, however, that such tailoring of medicines to a patient is absent in biomedicine. Indeed the whole idea of varying dosages based on a patient's physiology and/or medical history has a long history in biomedicine; the age of genomic medicine brings this issue to light in new ways.

Mingkyi explains that the root medicine *(tsawé men)* of the five ingredients that transform *zhijé* 6 into *zhijé* 11 is *olmosé*, mayapple. In a moment of scientific convergence, chromatography and toxicology reports from the United States as well as Western pharmacological literature report that mayapple has chemical signatures with uterotonic properties. When Mingkyi hears this news, she is excited but not surprised. We are sitting side by side in front of our office computer, reading an email sent by one of the PIs. Mingkyi types a few characters into her Chinese-English pocket translator.

"You know *Periodic Table?*"

"Yes," I answer. "Why do you ask?"

"Well, this Periodic Table is useful for scientific research with Tibetan medicine. Periodic Table and our *jungwa nga* are both about *elements*, right?" Mingkyi uses the English term *elements*.

"Yes," I say. "The table represents the weights and properties of things like oxygen, calcium, and silver, different elements that make up our world, according to the laws of chemistry."

"Ah! Then they are like our elements!" answers Mingkyi. "Only the names and divisions are different. Or maybe it is better to say what we in Tibet have known as the Five Elements helped to make the Periodic Table. In Western chemistry they try to know the element's function and properties. It is the same with us, though we use different words to define these things."

I am intrigued by Mingkyi's efforts to create a scientific bridge across cultures. This translation is a moment of accommodation and recontextualization, to be sure, but it is also a reminder of Tibetan medicine's empirical basis. To Mingkyi, the possible equivalence between the Periodic Table and the Tibetan five elements might serve as a possible foundation for other comparisons between Sowa Rigpa and biomedicine. Yet many practical questions remain. Would isolating *zhijé* 11's active ingredients contradict or confirm what we know about mayapple and the other *materia medica* that, as Mingkyi so eloquently puts it, "encircle" this root medicine? Mingkyi compares recipes for *zhijé* 11 as it is being made at Mentsikhang and several other factories. She discovers the amounts of mayapple and other ingredients added to *zhijé* 6 to make *zhijé* 11 are small compared to the dominant six ingredients that constitute the more common medicine.

"This is a problem," Mingkyi says. "If we use *zhijé* 11 as it is being made at Mentsikhang, it will not have as beneficial an effect as it could on postpartum bleeding."

"But Mentsikhang uses pills as they are made at the factory now," I respond.

"These work, yes, but there could be more benefit if it were made differently," Mingkyi challenges. "Most factories that produce *zhijé* 11 use the ratios from Khyenrab Norbu's book, *Setting Out Medical Treatment with Medicine and Astrology*." To remind you, Khyenrab Norbu was a Chagpori-trained monk-physician instrumental in founding the Mentsikhang in 1916.

"In his version of the medicine, the final five ingredients are just added on top of the original six. There is not much consideration of function," Mingkyi continues. "*Olmosé* is used in very small amounts, as is seabuckthorn and the animal ingredients. But each of these medicines has an important relationship to downward-expelling *lung*. In Western terms, these ingredients help the uterus contract. In the case of *olmosé*, it is now confirmed with chemistry."

"Could there be other reasons why these five ingredients are used in smaller amounts? Are they harder to get? The recipe calls for crab shells and snake meat. Certainly these are not easy to find," I comment.

"Some are more rare than those in *zhijé* 6. But none are *very* rare. This might be a reason why a poor *amchi* living in a remote place might have used *zhijé* 6. But it can't be the reason why someone like Khyenrab Norbu would write a recipe in this way. No, I think this reflects a lack of attention to women's problems, not a shortage of ingredients. He was a very good doctor, but he was also a monk.

"For our study," Mingkyi continues, "we should make our own *zhijé* 11. Then we can really determine quality—get the best possible ingredients, the right varieties of each, and the right quantity. The recipe says to use *manu*, but there are eight different types of *manu*. For *jongshi* there are male and female varieties. *Bultog* should be of a certain age. There are many different kinds of *tarbu*. At the big factories, care in choosing sources and selecting specific varieties is often not taken. Now people care more about GMP."

Mingkyi argues we should create a special version of *zhijé* 11 with respect to what a clinical pharmacologist would call "bioavailability": how easily the medicine is absorbed into the body.

"We have the problem of timing and strength," she continues. "Tibetan medicine works more slowly than Western medicine. In a clinical trial this creates a disadvantage for our medicine. We have an opportunity to change the strength of *zhijé* 11 so it will be more comparable to misoprostol. But we must also change the *form* of the medicine into a powder and put this into capsules so the amount is always the same. Powder is more easily and quickly digested than pills." When we discuss this issue with the PIs and the Research Committee, they agree this is a good idea. Powder in capsules will allow for a placebo-controlled RCT, whereas it would be nearly impossible to create a traditional Tibetan placebo pill.

You have already seen that pharmacological variation in Tibetan medicines is common. Yet Mingkyi's suggestion that we alter a formula so that it might better "compete" with a pharmaceutical in a clinical trial seems novel. She does not doubt the inherent healing capacities of *zhijé* 11, but she knows it will not perform as well as it could within the constraints of a clinical trial unless it is made differently, attentive to the biomedical indications under study. This suggestion raises questions about the basis by which drug safety and efficacy are determined. As you've read in chapter 5, these are issues not only of pharmacology but also of governance and culture.

Mingkyi compares notes with other *amchi* on tastes, potencies, and varieties of ingredients in *zhijé* 11. She discusses sourcing and preparation methods with Mentsikhang factory executives. Mentsikhang agrees to produce a special batch of *zhijé* 11 for the RCT. The PIs focus less on this issue of reworked ratios, and more on the need to produce one standardized *batch* of the medicine made in one location, in line with NIH quality assurance regulations. The relative invisibility of this work on the specific recipe for *zhijé* 11 to be used in the trial, when compared with the development of our research protocol, data collection instruments, and baseline data collection, illustrates that which was considered "cultural" as opposed to "scientific" in planning for the trial.

One of the eleven ingredients, snake meat *(drulsha)* continues to trouble Mingkyi. According to compendiums of Tibetan *materia medica,* different snakes are used in preparations. Interviews and cross-checks with Tibetan-language pharmacopeia (Dilmar and Tashi 1970; Chöpel 1993; Dash 1994; Dorje 1995; Norbu 2004) reveal inconsistencies. As you learned in chapter 6, this issue of contradictory nomenclature in Tibetan medicine is not unique to snake meat. But snake meat is the only ingredient in *zhijé* 11 that requires a detoxification process before it can be compounded. Snake meat is a key ingredient in *zhijé* 11's formulation because its functions include helping to deliver the baby and placenta. As a result, we attempt to seek out clarity from a herpetologist at Tibet University and, when that doesn't pan out, from Gawai Dorje, the author of *Pure Crystal Mirror of Medicinal Plants* (1995). Although this conversation proves edifying in many respects, we leave Gawai Dorje's office no clearer on which type of snake meat to recommend. Mingkyi is left to make this judgment, in discussion with the pharmacologists at Mentsikhang.

At our next Research Committee meeting, Mingkyi announces that she hopes to have the reformulated recipe prepared in the coming weeks. To all but one of the members of the committee, this news is not significant. They've known of and approved of this work. Likewise Mingkyi has already received approvals for the alteration to this recipe from the Mentsikhang factory, which will ultimately produce the drug. To Yangkyi,[15] the single nonclinician on the committee, this announcement of new ratios comes as a surprise. A key person at the Tibet Drug Administration, Yangkyi is incredibly busy. Her appearances at our meetings have dwindled of late, since her department has been charged with preparing all TAR factories to meet GMP standards by 2004, in accordance with the 2001 Drug Administration Laws, as discussed in chapter 5. But Yangkyi's support and approval for this part of the project are essential.

"What is this about a new version of *zhijé* 11?" she queries. Mingkyi summarizes her work on the topic, handing her a copy of the research document and draft recommendations for new ratios. "This raises some issues," Yangkyi says, stoic. "First is the question of Mentsikhang. Do they want to apply for a drug registration number for *zhijé* 11? If so, they will need to apply with the standard recipe. If you make a new version, this complicates things."

"But what if the medicine will work better now, especially for PPH?" asks Mingkyi.

"I am not a doctor. I can't answer questions about how the medicine works. But I can tell you that government rules on drug production are becoming stricter. Before, it was easier to get approvals for Tibetan medicines. Now it is more difficult for everyone—factories, doctors, hospitals. Before, Tibet was just at this basic level. People didn't know how to do proper standardization. The government didn't expect this. Now, as Tibetan medicine develops, we need to follow national standards."

Mingkyi responds, "Mentsikhang can apply for a drug registration number if they want. But how should we make *zhijé* 11 for our clinical research? This is the most important question."

Yangkyi answers, "Yes, but we have to consider the *results* of research. Now *zhijé* 11 is not registered, not made for commercial sale. If good results come from the study, then Mentsikhang will maybe want a drug registration number." She blows the thin buttery film from her cup of tea and takes a delicate sip before continuing. "These are more issues of money and of"—she turns toward me—"what you call *intellectual property*" (Pordié 2005, 2008a; Saxer 2010a). These are real, pressing issues, I think, and yet they presume a market logic over a biocultural logic that might not recommend the commercial production of *zhijé* 11 for a range of reasons, from giving this medicine in the presence of a birth attendant to issues of its abortofacient qualities. "As for changing the way the medicine is made," Yangkyi refocuses on Mingkyi, "explain why this is necessary."

"Mentsikhang *zhijé* 11 is being made according to ratios from Khyenrab Norbu's book. These guidelines do not consider specific conditions. For our research, we must consider the specific causes and conditions that produce PPH."

"You say ratios are 'general,' but I'm not sure what this means. All recipes must be made according to factory and national standards."

"True, but these regulations are new, and the recipes are old. The official Tibetan medicine compendia list specific amounts of ingredients, but there should be allowance for the patients, the types of conditions, the medicinal ingredients available. This is how Sowa Rigpa should be used." The document to which Mingkyi and Yangkyi refer here is the *Drugs Standards of the Ministry of Public Health of the People's Republic of China–Tibetan Medicine*, which was published in 1995. Unlike the well-regarded and frequently updated *Chinese Pharmacopoeia,* which has been in play since the state's efforts beginning in the late 1950s to standardize Chinese medicine, the Tibetan version is highly criticized by those most knowledgeable to do so: Tibetan medical scholar-practitioners (Saxer 2010a: 67).

"I have heard this criticism from many doctors. But this way of thinking does not allow for *quality control,*" Yangkyi says in English, "for making sure medicines are safe. That there are not *counterindications.*"

"These are Western concepts, *Gen la,*" Mingkyi volleys back.

"Even so, these are the regulations. We must abide by them. Besides, if you remake the medicine, how will you ensure this new recipe is safe?"

"*Zhijé* 11 is an old medicine and it can be beneficial for many purposes," Mingkyi answers obliquely. "We are focusing on postpartum blood loss. So we need to pay attention to how the medicine works for this purpose."

Different layers of negotiation occur in this dialogue. Yangkyi is trying to do her job according to a set of regulations derived from a biomedical model. Although she is not a clinician, she has sincere concerns about drug safety and takes to heart the purposes behind standardization and manufacturing procedures as a way of protecting patients from unnecessary harm. What if this new, untested version of *zhijé* 11 causes more or different complications in laboring women? What if it is too strong? Mingkyi understands Yangkyi's position and is resigned to the realities of China's drug regulations. However, she does not see the redefining of ratios as a breach of these rules. Rather she indicates a Tibetan way of doing science (Adams, Dhondup, and Le 2010) and points out the dearth of RCT evidence about recipes for most Tibetan medicines. Finally, she relies on a biomedical model of illness to explain the necessity of creating a version of *zhijé* 11 tuned to PPH and that can be given within a hospital-based clinical trial.

"I can't give you a final answer on this issue," concedes Yangkyi. "Go see Dr. Kelsang at the Drug Standardization Department.[16] If he agrees, then you will have my permission."

A few weeks later Mingkyi and I arrive at Dr. Kelsang's office. He is a tall man with glasses and neatly cropped hair, graying at the temples. He wears a rumpled suit, with cigarette ash on the thighs. After introductions Mingkyi synopsizes our work. In so doing she stresses the novelty of the RCT as method here in Tibet, as well as its place of esteem within international medicine and pharmaceutical fields. It is important that Dr. Kelsang understands our work not only as powerful, in that it is connected to U.S. institutions, but also as innovative, something that represents "progress" toward the goals of "modernizing" Tibetan medicine. Mingkyi sets a tone of confidence. She has told me prior to this meeting that if she shows any lack of resolve, it will be easy for Dr. Kelsang to dismiss her research on *zhijé* 11 and, with it, the hope of a reformulated recipe. Mingkyi summarizes *zhijé* 11's pharmacology, points to evidence of conflicting ratios, and indicates the need for a changed formula. Here Mingkyi does not express this most crucial point with any reverence for Sowa Rigpa history and practice; rather she stresses the need to move away from "secretive" models of knowledge transmission inherited from the "old society," toward collective efforts necessary to develop Tibetan medicine. These conscious rhetorical moves are a way of negotiating within the political constraints of Tibet, as well as within biomedical models of research.

"Please describe more about the function of this medicine," responds Dr. Kelsang. "I am trained in Western medicine. Understanding the uses of Tibetan medicine is difficult." For a man of power, he seems humble, open.

"*Zhijé* 11 is like the Western drug called misoprostol, *miso*," she replies. "Maybe you have heard of this?"

"Yes. It is used for labor and delivery, like oxytocin."

"Exactly. *Zhijé* 11 has a similar overall function. The main property of this medicine is to encourage delivery of baby and placenta; it helps to increase uterine contractions." As Mingkyi speaks, I note her strategy of translation and accommodation. To a different audience, she might have focused on the *differences* between *zhijé* 11 and misoprostol. She would have mentioned downward-clearing *lung;* here she does not.

"Western medicine works more quickly and is usually stronger than Tibetan medicine, even though Tibetan medicine has fewer side effects," Mingkyi continues. Dr. Kelsang listens intently, puffing on a string of cigarettes. Mingkyi's presentation is strategic, if also stereotypical.

"But we must think about this medicine *specifically* for the goals of this clinical trial. This is why we came to see you. *Zhijé* 6 is the base of *zhijé* 11. Five extra ingredients have been added to make *zhijé* 11, but without the overall ratios changed from the original *zhijé* 6. This does not account for *why* those five ingredients are added—why the medicine is made only for women and how it works to reduce bleeding after delivery."

Dr. Kelsang interjects. "You have done careful research. But are you saying the recipe we use is wrong?"

"The main issue is to change the *ratios* of ingredients, not to change the recipe. The recipe is not wrong, but for PPH it is not as beneficial as it could be. We need to reconsider the balance between the first six and last five ingredients. We need your permission to make these changes. Mentsikhang will make the medicine to these standards, if your office approves."

Dr. Kelsang studies the ratios for *zhijé* 11 as they are written in the official government compendium of Tibetan medicines, as they are listed in Khyenrab Norbu's text, and as they are used at Mentsikhang and two other factories. He compares these recipes to Mingkyi's proposed ratios.

"It would be good to make the medicine in a way that helps guarantee an efficacious product," he says after a time. "If the medicine does not show good effects during the research, it will be a problem for the future, for the reputation of Tibetan medicine." To Dr. Kelsang, success or failure is connected not only to drug safety, but also to scientific "face," even prospects for profit within the Tibetan medicine industry.

Dr. Kelsang reviews the recipes again. "I am not a Tibetan doctor, so it is difficult for me to evaluate the changes you are proposing. We must think about patients. Your reasons for changing the recipe are clear, but there could be risks. I will approve using these new ratios, based on your research—we have to use traditional knowledge in this way—but before finalizing the plans for the RCT you should do a comparison between the old *zhijé* 11 recipe and the new one." This suggestion of such a pilot study seems crucial, not only from the perspective of determining drug safety, but also to evaluate the impacts of pharmacological change on dosage and timing of drug administration, so these practices can be finalized for the RCT protocol. It is a suggestion that the Research Committee and the PIs readily take up.

"Thank you," says Mingkyi, as we prepare to leave. "It is important to describe the exact effects of our medicines. It is always said that Tibetan medicine can help only small problems or old diseases but not emergencies, because it works more slowly. But in doing this work, we are trying to show through one example how Tibetan medicine can also benefit patients quickly. We still have work to do, but altering the recipe is the first step."

As we drive back to our office, I replay Mingkyi's final comments to Dr. Kelsang. Not only is this project revealing the social-ecological contexts in which clinical research is conducted and efficacy is produced, but it is also challenging stereotypes about the ways Tibetan medicine is *perceived* to work, what it is thought to be "good for."

MEDICINE AS PERFORMANCE

Mingkyi makes her final recommendations for the reworked medicine, with approvals from the Drug Standardization Department, the Research Committee, and the PIs. We finalize arrangements with Mentiskhang for the production of this special batch of *zhijé* 11. Well before ingredients have been mixed, compounded, and poured into capsules, the RCT begins to seem more and more like a performance, a space in which *materia medica* and types of knowledge play well-defined roles. Medicine production is a complex choreography of meaning, method, and market price. The stage is being set. We hone in on a final study protocol: our script.

Since *zhijé* 11 and misoprostol are given at different points in labor, we can design a two-arm study in which a woman will either receive *zhijé* 11 and placebo or misoprostol and placebo. No woman will receive only a placebo, and any woman who begins to hemorrhage will be treated with the "standard of care" of IV oxytocin.[17] The props are made: Mentiskhang produces *zhijé* 11 for use in the trial. No longer formed into *rilbu*, the study drug is a powder in green capsules, identical to other green capsules that Mentsikhang fills with potato starch for the placebo. Players are cast and rehearsals begin. We complete an analysis of baseline hospital data (Miller et al. 2007b), finalize data collection forms, and train participating clinicians in how to use them as well as the tapered plastic sheets with calibrated ends that will be placed under delivering women so postpartum blood loss can be measured and recorded.[18] Permissions are put in place. The study protocol is approved by IRBs at three U.S. institutions as well as the Tibetan IRB. We determine eligibility and exclusion requirements and also pilot, review, and finalize an informed consent process (Adams et al. 2007; Miller et al. 2007a).

Finally, an important dress rehearsal is conducted. As intimated by Dr. Kelsang, issues regarding dosage and timing in administering new *zhijé* 11 remain to be determined, when compared with the old version in traditional pill form. Practitioners at two of the three hospitals will be administering Tibetan medicines for the first time. Dosage and timing depend on how fast the new version of *zhijé* 11 becomes bioavailable. The only clinical data we have are from the old *rilbu* formulation at Mentsikhang, the pills the Women's Division director showed one of the PIs many months ago now. For these reasons we execute a small pilot study of new versus old *zhijé* 11 at Mentsikhang.

If the pilot study results are positive, the Research Committee may proceed with more confidence in *zhijé* 11 and clinical research, as well as the methods employed by Mingkyi to alter the pharmacological formulation of the medicine. Yet if *zhijé* 11 fails to perform well in the pilot, this would cause a range of setbacks. The biomedical hospitals might refuse to participate; the Chinese Health Bureau or the U.S. agency could reject the project as ethically unsound. Certainly this entire research endeavor illustrates how Tibetan ways of doing science can inform biomedical methods and not simply the reverse. Yet at least as far as final RCT protocol is concerned, *zhijé* 11's clinical effectiveness will still be determined by a singular performance: its ability, compared with misoprostol, to reduce the amount of blood women shed during and immediately after delivery.

The pilot study includes eighty-eight women. Results indicate that the new version of *zhijé* 11 *does* reduce blood loss better than the old version, and that it takes effect, on average, ten minutes quicker than the old version. These data are further compared with baseline statistics on normal rates of blood loss in all three participating hospitals, and protocols for the dosage and timing of drug administration are adjusted accordingly. A random sampling of the new *zhijé* 11 capsules reveals standard doses and stable chemical formulation of the ingredients. The historical, ethnographic, and pharmacological research on *zhijé* 11 finds its place in our *Manual of Operations,* and is used by the PIs to justify our choice of study drug. However, the *rationale* for changing the *zhijé* 11 formula—an aspect of this research project that initiated a dialogue between Tibetan medical praxis, biomedical conventions regarding good clinical practice, and RCT design—is hidden backstage.

By June 2004 the start of the clinical trial draws near. The capsules of *zhijé* 11 and the placebo equivalents are produced and safely stored; we await shipments of misoprostol and its sugar-tablet double. As one phase of our work on this project ends and another is about to begin, Mingkyi, our Tibetan staff, the Research Committee, and I contemplate, and eventually plan, a final significant event. We decide the medicine should be consecrated through a *mendrup* ritual. According to Tibetan tradition, *mendrup,* or the "alchemy of accomplishing medicine" (Garrett 2009), perfect and ritually activate medicines. Religious specialists recite a specific text and perform offerings to the Medicine Buddha, in

the presence of emblematic or symbolic amounts of compounded medicines and/or medicinal ingredients. As mentioned in chapter 5, *mendrup*
were curtailed in Tibet by the Chinese government during the worst
years of political repression, but have been reinstated since the 1980s,
even at state-supported institutions like Mentsikhang.

Some of my Tibetan colleagues feel compelled to sponsor this *mendrup*. They have no control over whether *zhijé* 11 will be proven effective
in biomedical terms, according to the RCT. They can, however, ensure
that the first Tibetan medicine to be tested in such a manner in the TAR
is vested with another type of efficacy, sourced not only from the potency of herbs and minerals, proper production methods, and skillful
clinical practice, but also from the syllables of *mantra* properly spoken.
Also, although Research Committee members understand the rationale
for using placebos to make the research scientifically robust, most are
not convinced that using placebos at all is ethical. Given these issues,
sponsoring the ritual seems worth the risk. My colleagues decide not to
inform the PIs or our government partners in Lhasa about this ritual.
They are worried these authority figures may not approve—that it
could be seen as a waste of time or, worse, as an act that marked this
otherwise "scientific" endeavor with the stigma of religion. Although
mendrup are now performed in state and private factories, religion remains taboo in relations between Tibetans and foreigners working in
official capacities. This reality gives my colleagues pause—initially. As is
often the case in China, they reason it will be easier to ask for forgive-
ness afterwards than permission prior to such a ritual.

We prepare for the *mendrup*. We sweep and purify the office with
incense. Our data manager brings fresh blocks of tea and white butter.
Our project manager fetches a large bag of *tsampa* flour that the monks
will use to shape ritual *torma* offerings. While the monks make *torma*,
Mingkyi and I find offering bowls and butter lamps, filled with *ghee*
and sprouting new wicks. The monks have brought an offering pitcher
and a peacock feather with which to sprinkle blessed water over a symbolic sample of the medicine, along with other ritual implements and
their copies of the text they will read while performing this ritual. One
of the monks asks if we have an image of the Medicine Buddha. From
in between the Tibetan, Chinese, and English medical reference manu-
als, and the data collection forms that occupy our shelves, I remove a
book of Tibetan medical paintings, the front cover of which depicts the
Medicine Buddha. I place the book on the altar. One of the monks positions a box of *zhijé* 11 alongside it. The desk that is usually cluttered

with thermoses and a humidifier in the shape of a green plastic bunny now becomes an altar.

Now all we need is the lama. The two monk attendants run downstairs to fetch their teacher. Each grabs one fleshy forearm, and the triad spends the next ten minutes climbing the stairs. Like many Tibetan lamas I have encountered, Tashi Rinpoche suffers from hypertension and arthritis, perhaps the net result of spending years with his legs crossed and being plied with thick butter tea and fried yak meat in thanks for his ritual services.[19] He struggles for breath.

"I . . . must . . . rest . . . tea . . . please," he says, by way of introduction. The lama settles into the carpeted seat of honor we have prepared for him. He takes a sip of tea. His enormous yet delicate hands unwrap his copy of the *Yuthog Heart Essence* text, his scepter, and his bell. In today's Tibet it is difficult to find a lama considered by fellow Tibetans to be an authentic, knowledgeable religious practitioner and deemed politically correct by state authorities. Tashi Rinpoche is such a character. He suffered during the 1960s and 1970s, but now can move between his rural monastery and an office in Lhasa. Within his rotund and labored being, he balances political expedience with Buddhist practice.

"So, where are the medicines?" Tashi Rinpoche asks Mingkyi, who met the lama on several previous occasions and has arranged the day's event.

"Here," she answers, pointing to the cardboard box. "But there is only one medicine."

"Only one? Usually when I do a *mendrup* it is for many medicines—a whole year's supply for a factory or clinic."

"I know. But this *mendrup* is just for one medicine, called *zhijé* 11. We are doing a research project about this medicine. This box is from the batch we will use in hospitals. *Zhijé* 11 will be compared to a Western medicine. Both are used for women's problems, to help with the delivery of babies and to stop bleeding after birth. As you know, many women in Tibet die while giving birth."

Tashi Rinpoche nods. "What you say is true. It is also more difficult to find good quality Tibetan medicines in the countryside, or good doctors. We have the herbs, for now, but many people don't know how to use them anymore."

Mingkyi agrees. "Tibetan medicine is becoming more famous in the world, but without proof that it works according to Western methods, it will be difficult for Sowa Rigpa to help more people in the future. With research, maybe more people will trust our medicine."

"But why only test one medicine?" asks Rinpoche. "There must be others used to help delivery and help stop bleeding."

"Many *amchi* have also suggested this. It would be my wish too. But according to Western science research methods, it is too difficult to tell what medicine does the work of healing if there are many being given to the patient. So we are using only *zhijé 11*."

"Why have you not just gotten *zhijé 11* from Mentiskhang, where they already do empowerments? Are these special pills?"

"Yes," answers Mingkyi. "We made a special batch of this medicine to make sure that all the medicine that will be given to patients in the study is exactly the same, to meet the Western standards. We changed the ratios of ingredients used, to quicken the effect of the medicine and make it stronger, more like the Western medicine. The factories just add five more ingredients in small amounts to change *zhijé 6* into *zhijé 11*. They do not consider the reasons *why* each ingredient is added—the real function and potency, how they help women during childbirth. We also had to change the form. "Do you know *jao nang?*" Mingkyi uses the Mandarin word for *capsule*.

"Like the Western medicines for infections?" Rinpoche asks.

"Yes, exactly. People are making Tibetan medicines in this new form, so we decided to try. This is partly because our Tibetan medicine has to work more quickly, to compare with Western medicine. So we put *zhijé 11* powder in the capsule. But the change is also because of Western research methods. This kind of research is called 'blind.' This means neither the doctors nor the patients know what medicine is being given. The only way to make sure the doctor does not know which medicine she is giving is to change the form, so both *zhijé 11* and the *anweichi*, the placebo, look the same." Mingkyi relies on the Mandarin word for *placebo*. Indeed the ability to translate the goals and structure of this research project between English, Tibetan, and Mandarin requires a degree of multilingualism and code-switching that has as much to do with language itself as it does with translating ideas of science and research across cultural and medical boundaries (Adams et al. 2005a).

"What is *anweichi?*" asks the lama.

"In Tibetan we say *semso men,*" Mingkyi answers. Literally this means "medicine to heal the mind" and implies a substance that helps patients "not to worry."

"According to the teachings of the Medicine Buddha, every substance on Earth has the potential to be medicine. If this no-medicine

medicine puts the patient's mind at ease, then how is it not medicine?" he asks.

Ironically the PIs made similar comments upon hearing the Tibetan translation of the term *placebo*. "We have to change the wording," they insisted. "Otherwise the IRBs will think we are telling subjects the placebo is some sort of anti-anxiety medication." Tashi Rinpoche speaks from a very different sociolinguistic place than the PIs. However, this question about what sorts of substances in what forms can be considered medicinal remain critical to the lama as he prepares for the *mendrup*.

"From a Tibetan view, the placebo *is* a medicine, a mind medicine," answers Mingkyi. She has been preoccupied with these issues for months now. "But according to Western science, we can't think of it as a medicine, because the material inside the capsules is just potato flour. The substance's nature has no medicinal qualities—at least none we know of."

"Rinpoche, let us show you the medicine," interjects our project manager. He pulls out two packets of identical green capsules, one of *zhijé 11* and one of the placebo, and removes an individual capsule from each. He then empties the contents of the two capsules on the table in front of Tashi Rinpoche. In so doing he reveals the physical difference between them. The opaque green shell of the capsule masks the *zhijé 11*, a fawn-colored powder that smells of ginger and salt, and the white, odorless placebo powder.

"I see," says the lama. He clears his throat and takes a sip of tea. "So, do you want me to bless *only* the *zhijé 11*, or should I empower the *anweichi*, this no-medicine medicine, as well?"

My Tibetan coworkers and I look at each other. We had discussed this question earlier and had reached an agreement. Mingkyi speaks, "We would be happy for you to bless both. That way we will be giving the patients some benefit from the medicine *and* the placebo because any substance that has been empowered will have some effect and will bring some benefit."

"This is my feeling too," answers the lama.

For the next several hours we watch Tashi Rinpoche and his attendant monks perform the ritual. Time is marked by soundings from the lama's bell, the baritone resonance of his voice. His massive hands slice through air as if it were water. His ability to ritually imbue these medicines with power and potency is something he acquired through textual study, oral instruction *(lung),* and empowering initiations *(wang)* conferred by master practitioners. Unlike the much more elaborate *men-*

drup held at factories each year, this ritual has been pared down to its most basic elements.

Ritual complete, Tashi Rinpoche's attendants dispose of *torma* on the roof, casting out impurities or defilements that might have been present in the medicines.

As the patrons of this ritual, my colleagues and I fill three envelopes with crisp renminbi notes, in denominations that are respectful though not extravagant, wrap the envelopes in *khatag* offering scarves, and give them to the lama and his attendants. We then retire to the hotel garden for lunch and conversation. The entire procedure takes a morning, no more. By midafternoon all remnants of the ritual are cleaned, polished, and put away. Yet through this ritual we see the ways that Tibetan medicine is engaging biomedical science. The ritual also puts into relief some of the cultural assumptions embedded within RCTs. Consider the placebo as form and as method (see Kaptchuk 2002). Tashi Rinpoche's initial confusion over the term *semso men* reflects larger concerns about what can be classified as an "inert" substance. The dialogue between this Tibetan lama and Mingkyi points to the types of blinders required of an RCT: what counts as data, what it means if study cohorts who are given placebos respond to treatment in clinically significant ways.

Even though the lama and my Tibetan colleagues are quick to acknowledge the material differences between the *zhijé* 11 capsules and their placebo equivalents, the idea of inert medical substances is called into question, not only by the performance of *mendrup*, but also by the perceived need, according to RCT protocol, for a "medicine to heal the mind" of patients who will participate in this study. As Moerman (2002: 10–11) notes, the etymology of the word *placebo* is filled with layers of meaning, from "I shall please [the Lord]" (likely an ancient mistranslation of Hebrew by way of Greek and Latin), to the medieval English connotations of "someone out to please others with artifice rather than substance," to more contemporary translations in the biomedical context, which pivot around ideas of the "inert." This history is a useful reminder of how the supposedly distinct fields of religion and science are deeply implicated in each other in Western medical traditions as well. None of this complexity is expressed in the official language of the RCT protocol. In that context the need for placebo control in the study is taken as given. But we can see the ways that this "gold standard" of research methods is also an imperfect cultural product (Kaptchuk 1998, 2001).

The discussion about whether to bless the placebo echoes more extensive debates about the ethics of placebo use that took place during this project (Adams et al. 2005a: 280–81). In turn, these conversations reflect broader concerns within both social and clinical sciences about the ethics of conducting clinical research in low-income and/or "treatment-naïve" settings (Petryna 2009). Both Tibetan medicine's moral epistemology and my colleagues' understanding of the socioeconomic constraints that many potential "study subjects"—pregnant women in Tibet—face in accessing health care make the idea of "control" populations difficult for them to justify. They remain uneasy about the need for placebos at all, despite the fact that *zhijé* 11 and misoprostol are being given as prophylaxis against PPH, and even though, according to the RCT protocol, any woman who begins to hemorrhage will be treated with the standard of care in each of the three participating hospitals. The *mendrup* ritual and surrounding conversations about the purpose of clinical research and the nature of placebos encourages a reevaluation of normative bioethical assumptions and definitions of efficacy.

In addition, in the act of ritually blessing both *zhijé* 11 and the placebo, different beliefs about the benefits of clinical research and the measurement of efficacy are presented against prevailing ideas about the source of a medicine's curative power and the nature of a control group. Although it was a practical impossibility at the time of the *mendrup,* because the boxes of misoprostol had yet to arrive in Lhasa, my colleagues also discussed the potential benefit that could have come from blessing misoprostol. Had these pills arrived in time for the *mendrup,* they would likely have been ritually blessed. In other words, the purpose of the *mendrup* ritual was not exclusively to imbue the Tibetan medicine with the best chance of performing well in this trial. The *mendrup* was also an effort to overlay onto the clinical trial an element of potential benefit to participants that is at once socially valued and yet completely absent from the list of risks and benefits explained to women who became study subjects, as part of the enrollment and consent process. In this sense, the *mendrup* echoes the strict and circumscribed procedures that trials of study drugs must follow, procedures that hinge on narrow definitions of a medicine's safety and efficacy. Like procedures to ensure such standards within biomedicine, the *mendrup* represents practitioners' concerns about remaining accountable to the lives of study participants, even as its performance reproduces particular hierarchies of cultural and scientific knowledge within a particular social ecology.

Enrollment for the clinical trial began in 2005 and concluded in 2007. More than nine hundred women participated in the study. The objective of the study was to compare *zhijé* 11 to oral misoprostol for prophylaxis of PPH. Postpartum blood loss was measured using a calibrated plastic collection drape that was tucked under women delivering vaginally. The design hypothesized that misoprostol would have a greater overall effect in the reduction of postpartum blood loss than *zhijé* 11. The PIs and other researchers write, "The primary combined outcome was incidence of PPH, defined as: measured blood loss (MBL) of greater than 500mL, administration of open label uterotonics, or maternal deaths" (Miller et al. 2009: 133). The hypothesis was that misoprostol would reduce postpartum bleeding more effectively than *zhijé* 11, a hypothesis borne out by the study's conclusions. The frequency of PPH was lower in the misoprostol group than the group who received *zhijé* 11. However, mean and median blood loss was very similar between the two groups; rates of PPH fell over the duration of the study in both groups, when compared to baseline data; and there were no maternal deaths among study participants. The rate of the combined outcome was lower among the misoprostol group (16.1 percent versus 21.8 percent for *zhijé* 11; $p = .02$), but those in the misoprostol more commonly experienced side effects, with fever occurring at statistically significant rates (Miller et al. 2009: 133, 138). There were no significant differences in MBL greater than 1,000mL or mean MBL between the two groups. Given the overall scope of the data, the question of which medicine had a greater capacity to produce the desired outcome—which one worked better in this context—was arguably not so clear.

In the article in which the PIs and other clinical researchers summarize the trial results, they stress the methodological rigor and sheer number of participants, as well as the combined qualitative and quantitative research that led to the creation of the study protocol. They emphasize the need to make available to women in Tibet a "reliable, safe uterotonic that is culturally acceptable and inexpensive," and to encourage future research aimed at testing the efficacy of traditional obstetric medications against allopathic preparations (Miller et al. 2009: 139). In a subsequent study of *zhijé* 11's efficacy and mechanisms of action, researchers associated with this project further suggest "potential for both allopathic and continued traditional use of [*zhijé* 11] as a uterotonic, with further research warranted to understand the underlying mechanisms of action and synergy between ingredients" (Coelius et al. 2012: 8).

Through other channels, I know that rural health workers and SBAs in Lhasa Prefecture are now geting training in misoprostol use. We do know, however, that the new *zhijé* 11 formula is still being used at Mentsikhang, to positive effect, and that it is now called *zhijé khatsar,* which literally translates as *zhijé* "on the fringes" or "on the edge." This choice of names was apt, indicating the still marginal space that the sort of methodological innovation Mingkyi spearheaded occupies at Mentsikhang, but also indicating a sensibility that this is indeed a special type of Tibetan medicine, tuned to a biomedical condition.

Within the official record of the RCT, the *mendrup* is invisible. Had the fact of the ritual been shared with the PIs, it would likely not have raised any scientific concerns because the RCT protocol did not include a way to measure the difference between ritually consecrated and non-blessed medicines. Materialist methods are hard-pressed to evaluate what could be considered metaphysical acts. Yet the *mendrup* was a pivotal moment in the RCT process and in its social analysis. It helped give voice to ethical concerns about the use of placebos and the power of study drugs; it integrated lay conceptions about the power, value, and efficacy of medicine with that of "religious" ritual and Tibetan medical pharmacology. In this sense the ritual's invisibility—or rather the maintenance of certain epistemological boundaries between aspects of biomedical and Tibetan medical culture through the exclusion of the *mendrup* from official RCT protocol—is also a *source* of its efficacy.

The fact that the *mendrup* and the official clinical trial protocol are never put into direct dialogue illustrates one of the most fruitful lessons to emerge from this research project. An integration of medicosocial systems is not forced. Nor is there an attempt to institutionalize complementarity between a traditional Tibetan practice and the strictures of modern science—circumstances that can subordinate nonbiomedical praxes. Instead both the ritualized acts of the *mendrup* and the RCT occupy distinct spaces, deepening the process of inquiry into what makes a medicine "work." In part because the *mendrup* stood on its own, we can see more clearly how the RCT also is a cultural product, invested in its own ways of ensuring ritualized efficacy. After all, the next ritual to which the green capsules would be subject was the randomization process, in which hundreds of envelopes would be marked with computer-generated numbers and filled, according to this statistical divination, with either *zhijé* 11 or potato starch, later to be repeated with misoprostol and sugar pills. This ritual process of randomization helped to ensure that the RCT would produce clean data and sound results. Results from the RCT would not be valuable if such ritualized acts were not performed with precision and care.

This clinical trial, inclusive of feasibility studies, baseline data collection, ethnographic research, related work in research ethics and methods, and institutional development, broke new ground in many ways. Those involved remained committed to working collaboratively, across divides not only of culture and language but also of power and influence in the work of global clinical trials research. Yet despite this goodwill, the process of envisioning, planning for, preparing, and executing this RCT was neither simple nor smooth. We were able to be innovative, yet we were also forced to compromise. We did not always take advantage of opportunities to redefine how clinical research is done on traditional medicines in ways that account for their social histories and the epistemological systems in which they are embedded. However, we were able to appreciate some of the invisible blessings that can come from not forcing integration of medical and cultural systems at all levels, but rather allowing some spaces in which different systems of meaning and knowledge production could retain distinctive claims or domains of authority.

But what if the *mendrup* had not been invisible? What if not only the Tibetan medicine and its placebo but also misoprostol and the sugar pill had been empowered? What if this fact had been shared with study participants? Might these factors have influenced the outcome of the trial, or even the willingness of eligible women to consent and enroll in the study? Would such measurements have produced statistically significant results? What might the results of the clinical trial have shown if we had been able to record patients' conditions according to Tibetan medical theory? What might we have learned about Sowa Rigpa empiricism *and* biomedicine were this to have been the case? These are questions I cannot answer, but they are no less important to pose—particularly in considering how future clinical encounters at the frontiers of Sowa Rigpa and biomedical sciences are structured.

To this end it is worth noting a few lost opportunities. Despite our innovative research on *zhijé* 11's pharmacology, history, and clinical use, the research protocol ultimately did not reflect any of the Tibetan medical theory underlying how and why *zhijé* 11 works. References to downward-expelling *lung*, for instance, were absent from the study documents and likely would have been meaningless to the NIH. Similarly, data points such as pulse diagnosis of women at different stages of labor and delivery in the two arms of the study could have been collected, especially at Mentsikhang, but data collection instruments were limited strictly and exclusively around biomedical parameters. Had we had the vision, previous experience, financial and institutional support, and time, we might have done well to consider designing the entire project according to a whole systems methodology, or perhaps conducting a pragmatic trial instead of the RCT as it was eventually carried out (see Ritenbaugh et al. 2003; Witt 2009). Such a choice would have brought with it other areas of compromise and different obstacles, but it could have set a benchmark for this sort of research on Tibetan medicine and, in the process, helped to address the methodological, ethical, and epistemological challenges to conducting meaningful clinical studies on Tibetan medicine (Witt et al. in press).

While ethnographic research was a crucial component of the feasibility stages of this trial, an opportunity was lost in not extending such ethnographic research through the execution and data analysis of the RCT itself. Practical limitations of time, human resources, and money posed potential barriers to such work, but they needn't have been ultimate barriers. In most cases, ethnographic research is far less expensive to conduct than a clinical trial, and our team included well-trained and well-positioned anthropologists who could have collected observational and qualitative data during the clinical trial. This could have further documented a range of issues that were of central concern in the development of the protocol, including how the informed consent process actually worked in practice (in addition to the recall testing for comprehension that was completed, using survey and structured interview methodologies). Unfortunately it was as if the utility of social science research methodologies ended when the RCT began—that the "cultural" work had been done and now the work of "science" could begin. However, I argue that such ethnographic work could have augmented clinical trial work, contributing to social studies of science and an anthropology of biomedicine. Such work might have also revealed extremely valuable methodological lessons for future clinical research projects that seek to engage Tibetan medicine.

SUMMARY

The value of a material object is neither fixed nor objective; it is a mutable judgment by the people who encounter, trade in, work with, and make use of it. Social analyses of material culture have long been a focus of anthropology. We can find resonance with what Appadurai (1986) has called the "social life of things" in some of the most iconic anthropological studies. Bronislaw Malinowski and Marcel Mauss, for instance, were interested in kula exchange not simply because shells and armbands circulated around islands in the Pacific. They were interested in how, through the circulation of *kula,* people created and maintained enduring social relationships, and how these objects became imbued with value—material and symbolic, utilitarian and economic.

Scholars have built on these fundamental interests in materiality and patterns of exchange to consider areas of inquiry as diverse as Mintz's (1986) social history of capitalism and colonialism through the lens of sugar, to Myers' (2002) study of postcolonial identity, indigenous rights, the invention of tradition, and what he calls "differential regimes of value" through the lens of Australian Aboriginal art. As Appadurai writes, "Focusing on things that are exchanged, rather than simply on the forms or functions of exchange, makes it possible to argue that what creates the link between exchange and value is *politics,* construed broadly. This argument . . . justifies the conceit that commodities, like persons, have social lives" (1986: 3). Narrating the biographies and social lives of medicines demands that we pay attention not only to a medicine's pharmacological value but also the cultural context in which it is used: how it is ingested, how much it costs, where it is accessed, why people use it, and how they experience its effects.

As the final chapter in this book, the story of *zhijé* 11 recapitulates themes from the previous six chapters. This biography exemplifies how efficacy is produced within specific social ecologies, even if these social ecologies include diverse fields of scientific knowledge and practice. The story of *zhijé* 11 reveals dynamics of lineage and legitimacy, not only in how this medicine is made and prescribed, but also in how its creator is remembered. When women speak about pregnancy and childbirth, and the place of *zhijé* 11 therein, the social ecology of women's health and suffering on Tibetan ground becomes apparent. *Zhijé* 11's characteristics and qualities, its tastes and potencies illustrate the biocultural value ascribed to this eleven-ingredient compound as it acts on Tibetan women's bodies *and* acts across medical, social, and scientific worlds.

To tell the story of this one Sowa Rigpa formula is also to write a social history of science and healing in a Tibetan context. This in turn reveals a lot about what it means to say a medicine "works" because it demonstrates points at which this capacity to produce desired outcomes is facilitated or undermined by the parameters established to measure such results. In this biography of *zhijé* 11 you've witnessed the ways pharmacological practices and clinical research paradigms can raise important questions about the shifting borders between religion and science, tradition and modernity. You've seen how use values and exchange values can be very distinct, even when what is being exchanged is not money exactly, but the currency of medical knowledge. You've also witnessed how objects can at times defy exchange just as words can resist translation. Certainly this story of *zhijé* 11's transformation into an RCT study drug shows how Tibetan medicine is becoming increasingly dependent on Western science for validation (Adams 2002b), and how this is neither a monolithic nor unidirectional process (Adams, Schrempf, and Craig 2010). In the biography of this one medicine we can see more clearly the future domains in which Tibetan medicine and biomedicine might continue to interact and, in the process, transform each other.

Conclusion

We are never as steeped in history as when we pretend not to
be, but if we stop pretending we may gain in understanding
what we lose in false innocence. Naiveté is often an excuse
for those who exercise power. For those upon whom that
power is exercised, naiveté is always a mistake.

—Michel-Rolph Trouillot, *Silencing the Past*

Hair cropped short, monk-like, Kalden meets me squarely, head-on. I had
just been calling his cell phone as he pushes through the double doors of
the Himalayan Yak Restaurant in Jackson Heights, Queens. Autumn air
blusters in behind him, and with it the metallic clatter of the Manhattan-
bound 7 train.

"Demo," we greet each other Amdo-style, though neither of us is sure
on which language to land. When we spoke on the phone over the previous year, his Amdo dialect had, for all its crispness, eluded me. I had
been reticent to speak Lhasa dialect, knowing that this doctor from Qinghai Province feels a strong allegiance to the northeastern Tibetan Plateau. To him, Lhasa remains important, if far from the center of his
world. I know Kalden not only as the long-term research assistant of
several friends, but also as the student of a famous Qinghai doctor renowned for his finely compounded medicines, especially remedies for
liver and gall bladder disorders, and his penchant for eschewing the
newly minted forms of profit created by the Tibetan medical industry.
After a few moments, now face-to-face in New York, we find a comfortable rhythm between English, his Amdo *gé*, and my Lhasa Tibetan. Distance and dialect are bridged across a simple table, mugs of sweetened
coffee, an afternoon.

By way of introduction, I share with Kalden that the eldest son
of Tshampa Ngawang manages this restaurant. Tshampa, the *amchi*
from Mustang whom you met in chapter 4, had initially hoped his son

Jamyang would inherit his lineage and medical practice. However, this young man, who goes by the name "Jimmy" in America, had other designs. He is now a successful entrepreneur, selling Mustang-style curries and dumplings to a diverse clientele and opening up this restaurant for Nepali karaoke nights and meetings of the New York Mustang Association, as needed.

Kalden tells me about his practice. "I work with a Chinese woman doctor in Manhattan," he explains. "She is a fertility specialist. She left China because she says there is no *real* Chinese medicine left in China anymore. Only concern for money, with no shame. She is a compassionate person. Here she does good business but also helps many people. All those women who work too hard and wait until they are old to have children . . . and people who have been harmed by *gya men*," he says, referencing biomedicine.

I ask Kalden how he is finding life in New York. He smiles broadly. He is in the midst of an immigrant's tale. His lawyer, whom he refers to as "my pro bono," is arguing Kalden's case for asylum. Unlike this Tibetan's facile explanation for his Chinese boss's decampment from the Motherland, his reasons for leaving are more opaque. Years of work in China have schooled me not to ask Kalden for more details about his own passage to the United States.

"How do you practice here?" I ask. "I mean, legally."

"Right now I work under the Chinese woman's license." This is an arrangement I'd heard about from several other Tibetan medical practitioners in the United States. "But I am thinking about a program for acupuncture and OMD, *doctor of Oriental medicine*," he continues, signaling a path to legal status by way of enrolling in an American institute for Oriental and integrative medicine in the Northeast. "The tuition is expensive, though." Kalden does not disagree with some of his Tibetan medical colleagues who are also making a life in the United States who have put forth the possibility of lobbying for recognition and the right to practice *as Tibetan doctors* in this country, but he does not see it as a practical option.

"This path will not come to fruition," he says. "It is too costly, too political, and Tibetan medicine is still too small." Instead Kalden sees the benefits of practicing in the shadows of Chinese medicine, as it is recognized in this country.

"What about medicines?" I ask.

"This is not so difficult, at least for now. I have medicines sent from Qinghai and from friends in Lhasa." He pauses. "But I also make some myself, here." He then describes his visits to Chinatown and South Asian markets. Pungent scavenger hunt, this search for herbs. Kalden speaks of the Six Excellent Ones *(sangbo druk),* key ingredients in the Tibetan pharmacopeia, and how they "just call them spices here." He has found high-quality saffron, green and black cardamom, cloves, nutmeg—five of the six. Even bamboo concretion, the last of these ingredients, can be found sometimes in stores tucked into the folds of New York, off Canal Street. He's come across acceptable *arura* at an Indian grocery in Jackson Heights. True to his innovative and entrepreneurial spirit as well as his exposure to Chinese medicine, he has begun compounding medicines from these simple raw materials in individual batches, for specific patients.

These medicines are compounds of words and things, as healing elements are made real beyond Tibetan territory. I do not ask, but I imagine how he might have turned a Cuisinart or a marble mortar and pestle, both sourced from among the porcelain bowls and dumpling steamers in Chinatown shops, into the service of his growing list of patients. I am reminded that to a Tibetan doctor, this *menjor,* the act of compounding, is never solely local, but local still, even in a tenement kitchen. Kalden is nimble in his new home, making efficacious medicines within a social ecology of possibility and loss.

As we have seen, Sowa Rigpa is adaptive. It has never been exclusively a local tradition, either with respect to the *materia medica* it employs, the relevance of its possibilities for healing, or the settings in which knowledge is passed down. Yet in recent generations, the circumstances under which most practitioners make medicines, transmit knowledge, and treat patients have changed dramatically. History has shown us that the teaching and practice of Sowa Rigpa have been adopted to suit many different social institutions, from individual households to monastic colleges, from state universities to private schools. This adaptability has fostered certain tensions and social inequities over time, particularly around issues of gender and class, with respect to who has access to Tibetan medicine and who can train as an *amchi.* This adaptability has also helped to ensure the survival of Tibetan medicine(s) through many moments of intense transition in a variety of national contexts.

Yet the quest for national and international legitimacy for Sowa Rigpa is filled with points of contradiction and compromise. The shift toward institutionalized forms of knowledge transmission, modernized spaces in which Tibetan medicine is practiced, and standardized, commoditized formulas produced according to technoscientific parameters is fundamental. At the same time, remedies made with rare, wild ingredients and endowed with religious blessing or other forms of ritual efficacy are also actively sought by culturally Tibetan people across High Asia and beyond (Janes 2002; Craig and Adams 2008).

These dual desires illustrate the ways Tibetan medicine is at once *process* and *product:* material substances, repositories of meaning, forms of practice, objects of value. In Nepal and Tibetan areas of China there remains a sense that seeking state legitimacy for Sowa Rigpa is necessary not only because its practitioners are often in the front line of providing health care in rural and urban settings, but also because the support of Sowa Rigpa represents a wider validation of Tibetan and Himalayan culture and history within the context of nation-states that, for distinct reasons, have marginalized or overtly persecuted their culturally Tibetan populations. Even so, state recognition and the different forms of support this engenders are not always a positive experience for practitioners or a simple proposition. For many *amchi* with whom I've worked, the defense and transformation of Tibetan medicine is an ethical imperative. And yet, as we have seen, there is often very little consensus at the ground level about how to achieve the abstract goals of "developing" *(yargyé tang)* Sowa Rigpa and guarding against its "decline" *(nyam)*. Tensions exist between practitioners at various levels. Elite, institutionally trained doctors sometimes scoff at the more earthy local knowledge of rural *amchi*. Practitioners from the same regions can cooperate with each other, but they can also harbor bitter local rivalries, occasionally going back generations.

As we have seen, different regimes of value (Myers 2001) are emergent, with respect to the social and political efficacy of Tibetan medical training, practice, and production. Some see the incorporation of *amchi* medicine into state-supported health care, collaboration between Tibetan medicine and biomedical theory and clinical research, or engagement with pharmaceutical industries as antithetical to the ethics of Sowa Rigpa; others are more pragmatic about this conjoining of medicines, markets, and traditions. Some embrace forms of institutionalization such as that which emanates from centers of learning such as the Tibetan Medical College in Lhasa or the Men-tsee-khang in Dharamsala; others see these institutions as limited in what they can teach, beholden to political and economic agendas rather than fundamentally concerned with good medicine. While a government-issued diploma or license does not replace the invaluable imprimatur of a virtuous local reputation or connection to a root teacher, these models of legitimacy sometimes escape each other. Practitioners are compelled to navigate within and between these domains.

Tibetan medicine's entrance into regional and global marketplaces and medical imaginaries has required shifts in how and for whom medicines are produced. In turn, this prompts questions about the ways in which the quality, safety, efficacy, and value of these medicines are determined. In this ethnography you have seen how such issues have been linked to standards derived from biomedicine, international in scope yet tooled to specific national contexts and associated with commercial markets as well as more hegemonic "traditional" medical systems, Ayurveda and Traditional Chinese Medicine in particular. In Nepal this is occurring in concordance with a rise in the number of *amchi* being trained in institutions and the changing gender composition of students. In China the lucrative business of producing commercial Tibetan medicines hinges, in part, on navigating a maze of licensing and regulatory structures for drug administration and the phenomenon of large, for-profit Tibetan pharma producers consolidating patents and market shares.

Recent accolades for Tibetan medicines in China and the 2009 decision by the Indian government to recognize Tibetan medicine as an "Indian system of medicine" will continue to put socioeconomic pressure on small-scale producers and on the environments from which *materia medica* is sourced. These shifts engender points of scientific and cultural incommensurability about how a medicine's quality and safety are determined, what it means to produce efficacious formulas, at what cost, and for whom.

Parallel trends toward the evaluation of Tibetan medicines through clinical research, along with legal and political jurisdiction over such formulas through national drug administration regulations, are not only impacting how Tibetan medicines are produced, prescribed, and consumed in China and Nepal (Saxer 2010a). They are also altering how *amchi* living in places such as the United States and Europe are able to access their pharmacy and treat patients (Sweeney 2009; Schwabl 2011)—an area for further inquiry, beyond the scope of this book but implicated in its trajectory and conclusions. By virtue of the theoretical flexibility yet practical strictures of regulations such as Good

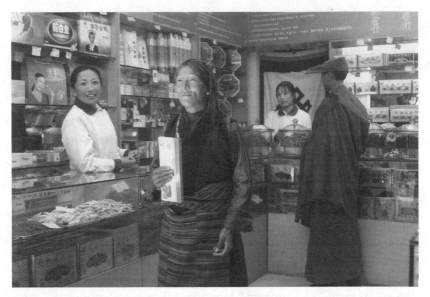

A Tibetan woman buying a ready-made Tibetan pharma product, the main ingredient of which is *solo marpo (Rhodiola rosea),* from a retail shop in Lhasa, Tibet Autonomous Region, China, 2004. © Thomas Kelly

Manufacturing Practices or methods for producing medical evidence such as Randomized Controlled Trials, power relations within and between nations are revealed. Hierarchies of scientific and cultural knowledge can become entrenched through their implementation.

Shifts in Sowa Rigpa practice, production, and consumption include not only trends toward standardizing formulas and making mass-produced medicines, but also new pharmacological innovations. This is the case even as efforts to conserve, cultivate, and sustainably harvest medicinal plants, animal products, and minerals have begun in some areas and are challenged in others. These changes are impacting noninstitutional *amchi* from Nepal, India, and China, by which I mean people who gather ingredients themselves or oversee the harvesting and regional trade or exchange of medicines; who produce medicines they prescribe; who treat primarily local populations; and who are committed to passing on their expertise through apprentice-based modes of knowledge transmission. Some argue that such practitioners and culture brokers are as "critically endangered" as the plants on which their medicine depends (Blaikie 2011). Indeed their fates have become intertwined, in part through conservation-development projects and the reconfiguration of Himalayan and Tibetan nature this requires.

In conventional terms, the phrase *translational science* connotes a way of thinking about the value and utility of biomedical research. Translational science seeks a mode of engagement wherein venture capital, academic medicine, and Big Pharma become invested in moving innovations from "bench to market" or "bench to community." Sometimes this is done to bring out new drugs more quickly and efficiently, with the hope of increasing positive health outcomes, although this is not always or necessarily the case. A net effect can also be the increase in the drug industry's profit. As such, *translational science* is a term filled with possibility and paradox. In its most narrow definition, it fails to capture the ethical ambiguities, political risks, and social-ecological impacts of defending and transforming a "traditional medicine," particularly given the ways moral economies and market economies interact with each other in today's world.

When considered more broadly, however, this entire book chronicles types of translational science. What occurs when a Tibetan medical text is transformed into a state-approved curriculum? How might an RCT protocol account for ritual efficacy? What happens to the potency of a medicinal plant when it is cultivated instead of wild-harvested? Does this, in turn, translate into changes in pharmacology or therapeutic process? How are Tibetan idioms of "protection" and natural resource management encompassed by, or occluded through, conservation-development programs?

To this end, I propose we expand not only our understanding of efficacy, as this book has argued, but also our conceptualization of the term *translational science* such that it might account for the social ecologies in which the work of science, healing, and knowledge transmission occurs. The potential of translational science is compelling for anthropology because, at its most catholic, this idea speaks to the structures, expectations, and parameters we put in place to judge whether or not a medicine, a therapy, or a social practice "works"— whether or not it has the capacity to produce desired outcomes. Given the ways the conventional concept of translational science is implicated in neoliberal late capitalism and what my colleague Vincanne Adams (2011) has called the "evidence economy," the concept seems expansive enough to include these forces as they work in, on, and through Tibetan medicine.

I hope this book will contribute to understandings in the social and medical sciences of what we mean when we speak of efficacy: how it is determined, by whose standards, and what the stakes are in these transactions. For the stakes are high. Year by year *amchi* colleagues in Nepal and China note the deaths of senior practitioners, those teachers and "living treasures" about whom I've written. My interlocutors speak of rapid, unpredictable, and sometimes devastating changes in the High Asian environments from which they hail. They also speak of the pressure to earn cash, the push-pull factors edging their children into urban centers at home and abroad, and the problems they face in making medicines and treating patients. The increasing drive to bottle and buy Himalayan and Tibetan nature and to wrap it up in culture is palpable, from Kathmandu to Lhasa and beyond.

As I bear witness to these transitions, I am more convinced than ever of the need to imagine different possibilities for the realization of medical pluralism across modern places—and to do so in ways that are honest about global health inequities and the social-ecological and political-economic price of commodifying traditional medicines as well as the sincere desire to at once honor currents of tradition and innovate in ways that are meaningful. I hope my work will help us—scholars, practitioners, and consumers as well as, simply, sentient beings who strive for wellness but who inevitably suffer—move toward more truly collaborative, respectful domains within which distinctive yet mutually constituted medical worlds and social ecologies might interact.

Back with Kalden in New York, one hour turns to two. We plan for what we hope will be our next meeting, in Kathmandu, where we will come together with *amchi* and *menpa* from Ladakh, Nepal, and China as well as several of my anthropologist colleagues for a week of collective medicine making, ritual practice, and conversations about what it means to make efficacious formulas.[1] We will be in the company of elder *amchi*, listening to their sensibilities about taste and potency, toxins and antidotes, new recipes and old, immersed in that organic substrate we call tradition. This gathering, a temporary space for knowing, represents a fragile alliance, shot through with personal fissures yet buffered by sincere concern for what this medicine is, and what it will become.

Outside our small workshop in Nepal's capital, we will hear echoes of recent self-immolations—Tibetans setting themselves on fire in protest over the fraught, constrained realities under which they live in China[2]—and the heavy boots of Nepali armed police, a new border patrol for this

Himalayan nation, flush with millions of dollars in Chinese military aid. What would we hear, I wonder, if plants could speak?

In this vein of beginnings and endings, being and becoming, I turn to one of Rainer Maria Rilke's last poems:

> The space the birds go hurtling through is not
> The form-intensifying space you trust.
> Out there in the open, you deny yourself
> And disappear without returning.
>
> Space reaches out from us, translating things.
> To realize the inner being of a tree
> Project your inner space around it.
> Surround it with awareness.
> It will not be confined.
> Only its reconfiguration
> Within your emptied mind
> Can make it fully tree.

In New York, Kalden and I part ways. Concrete and a cool November sky lead him back to his apartment, where a patient awaits. His gait is measured, as if this sidewalk too were a pulse to read.

Glossary

Phonetic Transcription	Transliteration According to Wylie (1959) for Tibetan	English Translation/Definition
C. *anweichi*		Mandarin for "placebo"
arak	*a rag*	Distilled grain alcohol
akar kara	*a dkar ka ra*	*Anacyclus pyrethrum*
amchi	*a mchi*	Mongolian-derived word for medical doctors widely used in Tibet and across the Himalayas
Ari	*A ri*	United States of America
arura	*a ru ra*	"King of Medicines," *Terminalia chebula*
N. *bandh*		Strike
barché	*bar che*	Obstacles
bardo	*bar rdo*	In between realm between death and rebirth
béken	*bad kan*	"Phlegm"; one of the three *nyepa* or "humours" in Tibetan medicine

N. *bhote bhasa*		Lit. "language from the culturally Tibetan people of Nepal's high mountains" "Bhote" carries some derogatory connotations in Nepal
N. *bikas*		development, as in socioeconomic development
bö	*bod*	Tibet
bömen	*bod sman*	Tibetan medicine
bön	*bon chos*	Collective term for many pre-Buddhist religious traditions in Tibet; today also acknowledged as one of the main schools of Tibetan Buddhism
bongkar	*bong dkar*	*Aconitum* spp.
bönpo	*bon po*	A practitioner of the *Bön* religion
bu	*bu'*	Bug, microorganism, insect
bultog	*bul tog*	Sodium bicarbonate or water containing this substance; also known as Trona
bumshi	*bum bzhi*	*Bön* medical text equivalent to the Buddhist *Gyüshi*
chang	*chang*	Fermented barley beer
chang tser	*byang tser*	*Morina nepalensis*
chikgya	*phyi rgyal*	Foreigner, stranger, outsider
chimagyü	*Phyi ma rgyud*	*Last Tantra*, the fourth volume of the *Four Tantras*
chi men	*phyi sman*	Lit. "outsider medicine"; used to refer to Chinese-style biomedicine; also called *tangmen, gyamen/jermen*
chinlap	*sbyin slab*	Ritual blessing
chitsok Nyingpa	*Spyi tshogs rnying pa*	"Old Society," term used to refer to pre-1959 Tibetan society
chö	*chos*	Religion, Buddhism (Skt. *Dharma*)

chökhang	*chos khang*	Buddhist chapel
chö kyi khorlo	*chos kyi 'khor lo*	Dharma wheel; Skt. *Dharma cakra*
chöten	*chos rten*	Buddhist cairn or reliquary; Skt. *stupa*
chöyon	*chos myon*	Priest-patron relations
chu	*chu*	Water, river; one of the "five elements"
chuba	*chu ba*	Tibetan style dress
chumtsa	*Lcum rtsa*	*Rheum palmatum*
chu ser	*chu gser*	Lit. "yellow water"; term used to translate synovial fluid
depa	*dad pa*	Faith
digpa	*sdig pa*	Sin
domtri	*dom mkhris*	Bear gall bladder
döndre	*gdon dre*	Nefarious spirit
drib	*grib*	Lit. "shadow"; references spiritual defilement and pollution
drulsha	*sbrul sha*	Snake meat
drumbu	*'grum bu*	Joint disorder often associated with rheumatoid arthritis
duk sum	*dug gsum* (i.e. *'dod chags, zhe sdang,* and *gti mug*)	Lit. "three poisons" (Skt. *klesha*) of attachment/desire, hatred/aversion, and ignorance; another way of referring to *nyépa sum*
durapa	*bsdus ra ba*	Degree in Tibetan medicine, comparable to a bachelor's degree within the modern Tibetan medical education system
dutsi	*bdud rtsi*	Nectar, divine nectar, associated with production of medicine
dzong	*rdzong*	District capital, fortress, citadel
gangla metog	*gangs lha me tog*	*Saussurea medusa/laniceps*

Gelug	*Dge lugs*	One of the main schools in Tibetan Buddhism; lit. "the virtuous ones"; the *Gelugpa* School was founded by Tsongkhapa Lobsang Drakpa
gek	*gegs*	Obstacles
gen/gen la	*rgan lags*	Honorific personal address, meaning "sir" or "teacher"
giwang	*gi wang*	Elephant or ox gall bladder excretions
C. *guanxi*		Mandarin for "connections"
gur gum/kache gur gum	*gur gum/ kha che gur gum*	Safflower/saffron
gyalmo, N. *rani*	*rgyal mo*	Queen
gyalpo, N. *raja*	*rgyal po*	King
gya men/Jer men [Amdo pronounciation]	*rgya mi'i sman*	Lit. "Chinese medicine" but refers usually to Chinese-style biomedicine
gyu	*rgyu*	Primary causes, reasons
gyü	*rgyud*	Numerous meanings, including: tantric treatise, thread, string, character, consciousness and life, continuity, connection, lineage
Gyüshi	*rgyud bzhi*	*Four Tantras, Fourfold Treatise*; core texts of Tibetan medicine
honglen	*hong len*	*Lagotis*, spp.
N. *janajati*		Ethnic politics/political movements in the Nepali context
jangchub sem	*byang chub gyi sems*	Bodhisattva mind, Skt. *Bodhicitta*
C. *jao nang*		Mandarin for "capsule"
jindak	*sbyin bdag*	Patron or sponsor, literally "master of the gift"

jinden	*byin ldan*	Ritually consecrated pills
jomo	*chos mo*	Female religious practitioner
jungwa nga	*byung ba lnga*	"Five elements," "five phases," or "five agents": earth, air, fire, water, and space/consciousness.
kachupa	*bka' bcu ba*	A degree in Tibetan medicine, comparable to a master's degree in the modern Tibetan medical education system
Kagyü	*Bka' brgyud*	One of the schools in Tibetan Buddhism
kandro	*mkha' 'gro*	Female tantric deity, "sky dancer"; Skt. *Dakini*
kanjenpa	*bka rjen pa*	A degree in Tibetan medicine, comparable to a health assistant degree in the Nepali state education and vocational training system
kathag	*kha btags*	Offering scarf
khäldram	*mkhal gram*	Kidney-related disorder
khogpa natsa	*lkog ma nad*	Throat disorder/illness
kora	*kho ra*	Circumambulation
Kudrak	*sku drag*	Nobility, member of the upper classes
kuma	*rkud ma*	Thief
kyen	*rkyen*	Secondary causes, reasons
kyön	*skyon*	Harm
la	*bla*	The subtle life-essence or "soul," also one of the five factors in Tibetan astrology
La chö	*la chos*	Buddhism, *dharma*
ladzi	*la dzi*	Musk
laglén	*lag lan*	Practice
Lama	*bla ma*	Tibetan term for a spiritual teacher or mentor (Skt. *Guru*)
Lamenpa	*bla sman/bla sman pa*	Personal physician

lang na	*glang snga*	*Pedicularis* spp.
lé	*las*	"Action," the law of cause and effect (Skt. *Karma*)
lha	*lha*	God, deity
lhaje	*lha rje*	Honorific term for Tibetan medical practitioner
lu	*klu*	Serpent spirit; Skt. *naga*
lü	*lus*	The physical body
lung	*Rlung; lung*	Air, wind; one of the "five elements" and the three humours; oral instruction
N. *madhesi*		Groups of indigenous people who live along Nepal's southern border with India
manu	*Ma nu (pa tra)*	*Inula racemosa*
mé	*me*	Fire, flame; one of the "five elements"
C. *mei guo*		United States of America
menaggyü	*man ngag rgyud*	*Oral Instruction Tantra,* the third volume of the *Four Tantras*
mendrup	*sman grub*	Medical empowerment ritual
menjor	*sman byor*	Act of compounding medicines
menpa	*sman pa*	Physician, doctor; equivalent to *amchi*
menpé gyü	*sman pa'i rgyud*	Doctor lineage, medical lineage
menrampa	*sman ra ba*	Degree that used to be awarded at Chakpori Medical College after nine years of study
mentsikhang	*sman rtsi khang*	Lit. "house of medicine and astrology"; with or without the "*rtsi*" term for clinic, hospital, or pharmacy
métsa	*me btsa'*	Cauterisation therapy
mi chö	*mi chos*	Way of humans, a Tibetan medical ethics

mi kha	*mi kha*	Gossip
C. *minzu*		Minority nationality or ethnicity in the Chinese context
misé	*mi ser*	"Common people," used widely in Tibet's pre-1959 society to refer to people of low social class, still used today in referring to rural people
mo (sho mo, treng mo)	*mo (sho mo, phreng mo)*	Divination, prophecy
moné	*mo nad*	Women's illness
mopa	*mo pa*	Diviner
Skt. *mudra*		Ritual hand gesture
nakpa	*sngags pa*	Tantric practitioner; lit. "someone practising mantra"
namkha	*nam kha*	Sky, space; one of the "five elements"
netsang	*gnas tsang*	Fictive kin or trading partners; relationships often passed through generations
ngobo	*ngo bo*	Nature
nö	*nod*	Harm or injury
norbu	*nor bu*	Precious jewel
nüpa	*nus pa*	Potency, effect; sometimes a gloss for strength of a medicine
nyam	*nyams*	Decline, deterioration
nyen	*gnyan*	Type of earth spirit
nyépa/nyépa sum	*nyes pa gsum*	Commonly translated as "three humors," these are the three faults or dynamics corresponding to wind, bile, and phlegm
nyingjé	*snying rje*	Compassion
Skt. *nyingma*	*rnying ma*	"School of the elders"; one of the Tibetan Buddhist sects
nyingné	*snying nad*	A disease/illness of the heart
nyomba	*snyom ba*	Crazy, mentally unstable

olmosé	*ol mo se*	*Sinopodophyllum hexandrum Royle*
pångtse	*spang rtsi do bo*	*Pterocephalus hookeri*
peja	*dpe cha*	Tibetan-style book in which loose pages are held together between two boards made of wood or paper, wrapped in a piece of cloth
pentok	*phen thogs*	Benefit
N. *pipal*		Sacred fig tree
putsé	*pu tse*	Quality
rabchampa	*rabs 'byams pa*	An advanced degree in Tibetan medicine
rangzhin	*rang bzhin*	Inherently existing
rigné chu	*rig gnas chu*	Ten-fold system of the Tibetan sciences derived from the Indian system of *vidyāsthāna*
rikné nyingba	*rig gnas nyingba*	Old systems or traditions
rilbu	*ril bu*	Tibetan medical pill
rinchen rilbu	*rin chen ril bu*	Precious pills
rinpoche	*rin po che*	Lit. "precious jewel"; honorific title given to Tibetan religious teachers, and a category of precious and semi-precious gems used in Tibetan medicinal compounds
ro [druk]	*ro drug*	[Six] tastes
rongba	*rong pa*	Tibetan term used by highland Nepalis of Tibetan cultural backgrounds to refer to lowland Nepalis, usually Hindu in cultural orientation or background
rü	*rus*	Bone, also refers to father's side of one's lineage or biological inheritance

rulba	*rul ba*	Rotten, expired
ruta	*ru rta*	*Saussurea lappa*
sa	*sa*	Earth, soil, land; one of the categories of ingredients used in Tibetan medical compounds; one of the "five elements"
Sakya	*sa skya*	One of the schools of Tibetan Buddhism; a place name in Central Tibet
C. *San Daolu*		Three Roads Policy
Sangbo druk	*bzang po drug*	Six Excellent ones, inclusive of bamboo pith, saffron / safflower, green and black cardamom, cloves, and nutmeg
Sangye Menla	*sangs rgyas sman lha*	Lit. "Master of Remedies," Medicine Buddha (Skt. *Bhaisajy-aguru*); common shortened versions are *Menla,* and *Sman lha*
sap dak	*sab dag*	Type of earth spirit
sem	*sems*	"Heart/mind"
semchung gépa	*sems chung dge pa*	Virtuous Mental Factors (Skt. *Kusalacitta*)
sem sangpo	*sems bzang po*	A pure heart/mind
semso men	*gsem gso sman*	Placebo
ser khab	*gser khab*	Tibetan golden needle therapy
sha	*sha*	Flesh; also used to refer to the mother's patrilineage
shabjé	*shabs rje*	Footprint of a Buddhist holy person
shégyü	*bshad rgyud*	*Explanatory Tantra,* the second volume in the *Gyüshi*
shindre	*shi 'dre*	Particular type of nefarious spirit
sok lung	*srog rlung*	Lit. "life-force wind humour"; a category of disease in Tibetan medicine

solo marpo	*Sro lo dmar po*	*Rhodiola crenulata*
Sowa Rigpa	*gso ba rig pa*	"Science of Healing," one of the five "major Tibetan sciences"; one of the terms used to refer to "Tibetan medicine"
sukpo	*gzugs po*	The corporeal body
Sungkor; sungdu	*srung 'khor; srung mdud*	Amulets; protection cords
Sung kyob	*srung skyob*	Conservation, protection
surjé	*zhu rjes*	Post-digesetive taste
tang men	*tang sman*	A code-switching word that combines the Chinese term for "communist [party]" with the Tibetan word for "medicine"; a reference to Chinese-style biomedicine
tarbu	*starbu*	*Hippophae rhamnoides*
tendrel	*rten 'brel*	Interdependent karma
terma	*gter ma*	Lit. "treasure," refers to hidden texts, which are revealed in later times and under more favorable conditions
thanka	*thang ka*	Tibetan-style scroll painting
thob wang	*thob dbang*	Rights
thursel lung	*thur sel rlung*	Downward expelling wind
tianku	*bri yang ku*	*Dracocephlum tanguticum*
tigta/gyatig	*tig ta/rgya tig*	*Swertia* spp.
torma	*tor ma*	Ritual barley cake offering
trak	*khrag*	Blood, female reproductive substance
treng	*'phreng*	Rosary, prayer beads
tripa	*mkhris pa*	"Bile"; one of the three *nyepa* or humours
tsa	*rtsa*	"Channels," often translated as veins, arteries, or nerves, depending on context

tsakar	Rtsa dkar	Lit. "white channels"; often refers to a particular type of disorder
tsagyü	rtsa rgyud	Root Tantra, the first volume in the Gyüshi
tsa lung	rtsa rlung	Lit. "Channel wind"; relates to circulation in the body and a particular group of meditation instructions
tsampa	tsam pa	Roasted barley flour, the staple food in Tibet
tsang ma	tsang ma	Clean, free from defilements
tsawé lama	rtsa ba'i bla ma	Root lama, one's principal teacher
tsawé men	Rtsa ba'i sman	Root medicine
tsen	btsan	Type of earth spirit
tséwang	tshad dbang	Power; long life rituals; also a proper name
tshab	mtshabs	Medicinal ingredient substitute
tsothal	btso thal	Mercury-sulfide ash, a purified form of mercury used in Tibetan medical formulas
tulku	sprul sku	Reincarnate lama
u chen	dbu can	Tibetan print
upal ngongbo	u pal sngon po	Meconopsis spp.
wang	dbang	Empowerment or consecration
C. Xizang		Mandarin for "Tibet"
yartsa gunbu	dbyar rtswa dgun 'bu	Lit. "summer grass-winter insect"; Ophiocordyceps sinensis
yenlak dün	yan lag bdun	Seven limb procedure in the Fourfold Treatise for preparing medicines
yeshi	Ye shes	Gnosis
yijé	yid byed	Belief
yönten	yon btan	Abilities, aptitudes, qualities

C. *Zang yi*		Tibetan medicine
zhijé 6 or 11	*Zhi byed* 6 or 11	Tibetan medical formula
C. *Zhong yi*		Chinese medicine
zimbu	*zim bu*	*Allium przewalskianum,* type of wild chive found in northern Nepal

Notes

1. I use the term *nyépa* instead of *humors*, as it is often translated in English, following Yonten Gyatso's (2006) arguments arguing against the word *humors*.

2. I capitalize Traditional Medicine to refer to the vast array of nonbiomedical systems and practices that are lumped together under this rubric by organizations such as the World Health Organization, as well as to bring attention to the ironies of defining such a term so broadly. The WHO defines TM as follows: "The sum total of knowledge, skills and practices based on the theories, beliefs and experiences indigenous to different cultures that are used to maintain health, as well as to prevent, diagnose, improve or treat physical and mental illnesses. Traditional medicine that has been adopted by other populations (outside its indigenous culture) is often termed alternative or complementary medicine. Herbal medicines include herbs, herbal materials, herbal preparations, and finished herbal products that contain parts of plants or other plant materials as active ingredients (www.who.int/mediacentre/factsheets/fs134/en/).

3. In political-economic theory, particularly in Marxian economics, use value signifies the utility of a good, service, or labor product, while exchange value signifies an object's commoditization and/or the price it fetches within a system of exchange.

4. See Saxer (2010a) and Kloos (2010) for uses of this phrase to examine how Tibetan and Buddhist concepts regarding ethics, behavior, and benefit have become enmeshed in the creation of Tibetan medicine industries and institutions in China and India.

5. The Unites States dollar equivalents for local currency throughout this book are rendered approximately, according to current rates of exchange at the time the fieldwork was conducted.

6. Barefoot doctors were a hallmark of Maoist socialist ideals, put into health care policy and rife with practical problems and contradictions. In many cases, people recruited to become barefoot doctors—whose charge was to provide rural Chinese populations with basic primary health care—were young, inexperienced, and given only between three and six months of training, and very limited medical supplies. In other cases, traditional doctors whose practices were suspect, by virtue of political ideology, recast themselves or were recast by state authorities in this role of barefoot doctor.

7. Bön refers to the pre-Buddhist or indigenous religious traditions of the Tibetan cultural world. See Snellgrove (1967) and Karmay (1998) for an overview. Bön is now recognized by the Tibetan government-in-exile as a fifth school of Tibetan Buddhism. The *Bumshi* is the Bön equivalent of the *Gyüshi*.

8. In discussing the history of women and gender relations in Tibetan medicine, Fjeld and Hofer (forthcoming) make an important argument about the role that "medical houses" and household-based knowledge have played in the transmission of Tibetan medicine, in contradistinction to an exclusive focus on lineage, either as patrilineage or as articulated in medico-religious master-disciple relationships.

9. See Kloos's (2010) ethnography of the Men-tsee-khang in Dharamsala.

10. Unani medicine is Greco-Arabic in origin and often associated with Islam. It is recognized by the governments of India, Bangladesh, Pakistan, and Sri Lanka.

11. Export of Tibetan medicines to countries outside of China is a relatively recent phenomenon (China Tibet Information Center 2007a); however, Tibetan medicinal products produced by GMP-certified factories in China are available for purchase over the Internet. They have also begun circulating through the tourism industries in Tibetan areas of China. In the United States such products are marketed as "nutritional supplements." See Adams 2002b; Janes 2002; Prost 2008: 99; and Kloos 2010.

12. The final section of chapter 2, which takes place in an English-language class, actually occurred two days after the rest of the events recounted in the chapter, but for the sake of narrative structure and the importance of its content, I include it.

13. The interviews in Mustang ($n = 39$) were conducted with a modified version of the McGill Illness Narrative Interview (Groleau, Young, and Kirmeyer 2006, also see Craig, Chase, and Lama 2010). Other interviews were conducted in one primarily agricultural county ($n = 23$) and one primarily nomadic county ($n = 24$) in Qinghai Province, China; these interviews were adapted from the MINI but included a more explicit focus on the economics of health care decision making and the relationship between Tibetan medicine, biomedicine, and forms of ritual healing.

14. Notable exceptions include Harper 2002; Petryna 2002; and McElroy and Townsend 2003.

15. I note the work of scholar-activists like Vandana Shiva and public intellectuals and ethnobotanists Michael Plotkin and Wade Davis.

CHAPTER 1

1. Day care centers were instituted in the region in the early 2000s, with support from the Lo Gyalpo Jigme Foundation and the American Himalayan Foundation. These centers offer early childhood education, promote a daily schedule (class time, naps, snacks, etc.) and an introduction to basic health and hygiene for children ages two to six years. These centers were created as a response to shifting labor demands, changes in family structure, and several unfortunate incidents in which young children drowned in local rivers due to lack of available adults or adolescents to watch them during the busy summer and harvest seasons.

2. Established in 1992, the Annapurna Conservation Area Project encompasses 7,629 square kilometers.

3. *Tsampa* is roasted barley flour, a staple among Tibetan communities.

4. When upper Mustang was initially opened to foreigners in 1992, the government of Nepal promised that 60 percent of the then $70/day fees would be returned to upper Mustang's people so that they might direct their own community development and environmental protection projects. This promise was not kept, resulting in the threat of a ban on foreign tourists in the autumn of 2010 and the subsequent written governmental declaration that, beginning in 2010–11, this rightful percentage of royalties would be paid. See Craig 2008a, 2010b.

5. For comparative perspectives on such questions in Ladakh and Spiti, India, see Besch 2007; Pordié 2007, 2008b; and Blaikie in press.

6. See www.kinoe.org.

7. See Bode (2006, 2008), Banerjee (2009), and Cameron (2009) for discussions of Indian and Nepali commercial Ayurveda industries.

CHAPTER 2

1. Current practice in many culturally Tibetan areas of China is to call such institutions of Tibetan medicine either *bö menkhang*, as described shortly, or *bö lug menkhang*, wherein *lug* means "system," "mode," or "way."

2. See Larsen and Sinding-Larsen (2001) for a comprehensive study of Tibetan architecture.

3. "Tibetan Medicine in the Modern Era," *China Perspective*, October 10, 2006.

4. "Enterpriser Devoted to Tibetan Medicine Preservation," *CRIEnglish. com*, August 26, 2010, http://english.cri.cn/6909/2010/08/26/1881s591264.htm. Accessed January 6, 2011.

5. See Saxer (2010a) for more in-depth discussions of Arura's institutional history.

6. A pseudonym.

7. See www.oneheartworld-wide.org and Craig (2011b) for a discussion of this organization.

CHAPTER 3

1. *Madhesi* are native people of Nepal from the southern plains. The word is often used in contrast to *pahadi*, people from the hills.

2. The Nepal Homeopathic Medical College in Biratnagar offers a five-year course, following an Indian curricular model, with Nepali government accreditation. The Bhaktapur Homeopathic Clinic (BHC), which follows a similar model of certification, was established in 1995, with European support. Under the leadership of Dr. Bharati Devkota, a homeopath and psychiatrist, the BHC now has a three-year homeopathic health assistant program geared toward extending homeopathic expertise and clinical care to remote Nepal. This model has provided inspiration for the HAA and their hopes for the *kanjenpa* and *durrapa* programs.

3. In recent years, and with increasing intensity since 2008, the Nepali state has aligned closely with the PRC's "One China Policy." This has included suppression of peaceful protests by Tibetans in Kathmandu against human rights abuses in China, holding representatives of the Tibetan government-in-exile under house arrest, curtailment of public celebrations in Kathmandu of events such as the birthday of His Holiness the Fourteenth Dalai Lama, and even turning back newly arrived Tibetan refugees from the mountains of Nepal at the border to the TAR, where they face imprisonment or other forms of state persecution.

4. The process of achieving this CTEVT accreditation cost 500,000 rupees ($7,000) for initial approval of the *kanjenpa* curriculum. Lo Kunphen incurs annual fees for examinations and program evaluation. The development and approval of the *durapa* curriculum is ongoing, and will be an additional expense.

5. MBBS stands for Bachelor of Medicine, Bachelor of Surgery. Modeled on the British educational system this is the most common equivalent to an MD degree in many countries, including India and Nepal. The degree often requires five years of study.

6. Comparable dynamics exist with respect to nonstandardized and state-sanctioned Ayurvedic practitioners in Nepal. See Cameron 2008.

7. A pseudonym.

8. There is scholarly and practitioner-oriented debate about Yuthog Yonten Gompo. Some Tibetan medical historiography speaks of an Elder and a Younger Yuthog. The Elder, said to have lived in the eighth century, is credited with having overseen a great meeting of medical practitioners from throughout Eurasia, at the behest of King Trisong Detsen, as well as the initial compilation of the *Fourfold Treatise*. The Younger, said to have lived in the twelfth century, is credited with writing a range of supplementary works on the *Fourfold Treatise* and codifying it into its present form. Yet as Meyer (1995: 114) notes, "Their biographies evoke mystical tales of highly realized tantric masters, and their similarities suggest that they might refer to a single historical figure." See Yangga 2010. For a biography of the two Yuthogs, see Rechung 1973.

9. The thirteenth-century the Tibetan scholar and ruler Sakya Pandida (1182–251) developed the India-derived classification system into a tenfold system *(rigné chu)* of Tibetan sciences. These included five major and five minor sciences, of which the major included the "inner science" (Tibetan Buddhist philosophy), epistemology and logic, grammar, medicine, and arts and crafts. The minor sciences included poetry, astrology, lexicography, the performing arts, and language.

10. See Kohrt and Harper (2008) and Craig, Lama, and Chase (2010) for a discussion of disease categories, including *gyastric,* in Nepali contexts.

11. See Pordié (2007) and Kloos (in press) for related discussions of Buddhist ideals and social dynamics among *amchi* in Ladakh.

12. See www.agiftforthevillage.com/.

13. See Millard (2002) for a study of this school.

CHAPTER 4

1. Comparatively most American general practitioners are allocated fifteen minutes per patient visit.

2. Samuel (1999, 2006) makes this point with reference to his study of Tibetan medicine in Dalhousie, India; Gerke (2012) discusses these issues in Kalimpong and Darjeeling, India.

3. In China one often hears *tang sman,* which is a combination of the Chinese word for "party," as in Communist Party, and the Tibetan word for "medicine." In Nepal *rongmen* is heard; *rong* connotes lowland Nepalis.

4. See www.who.int/inf-new/tuber4.htm for an overview of tuberculosis in Nepal.

5. See World Health Organization (2008) for an illustration of this perspective.

6. Such fear reflects a general awareness in the global traffic in human organs, as described in recent scholarship by Scheper-Hughes (2000).

7. Biomedical literature and the results of my own fieldwork and that of others reveals that hepatitis B is a particular problem in Tibetan communities, with both behavioral and genetic implications. See Shrestha et al. 2002; Clift et al. 2004; Xu et al. 2005.

8. Diemberger's (2005) discussion of oracles in modern Tibet provides a similar example of such dynamics.

9. We see illustrations of this discussion of the social lives and values ascribed to medicines (van der Geest and Whyte 1989) and in the relationship between subjectivity and pharma (Biehl 2005; Carpenter-Song 2009).

10. This, in turn, involves reaffirming village domains by walking around the physical borders of the settlement with sacred texts on one's back and expelling spirit-caused obstacles from the place using dough effigies, fire offerings, and other devices.

11. See Millard (2007) for a comparative discussion of psychological illnesses with Tibetan medicine in Nepal and the United Kingdom.

12. See Huber (1991, 1997) for discussions of problematic assumptions that can follow from the idea that Tibetans are somehow *inherently* "ecological" or environmentally minded.

CHAPTER 5

1. Pema and the other names in this chapter are pseudonyms.

2. See Hsu 2009 and Langwick 2010.

3. See Fischer (2005, 2008) for analysis of employment patterns in Tibetan areas and Chinese migration.

4. Drug registration numbers are in some ways akin to patents, but correspond more directly to which factories have the authority to produce specific named formulas. Three phases of clinical testing (chemical toxicology, animal testing, and testing on humans in a clinical trial) are required to procure a new drug registration number. Processes differ slightly for medicinal compounds that are viewed as old (e.g., that are referenced in Tibetan medical texts) versus new formulas. Introduced in the mid-1990s, drug registration numbers are proprietary; they also contribute to the rising costs of Tibetan pharmaceuticals. See Saxer (2010a) for a detailed discussion of this process.

5. The China Tibet Information Center (2006) reported nineteen GMP-certified factories in Tibet. However, this raises questions about what qualifies as a Tibetan medical factory. Some Chinese pharmaceutical companies produce several drugs that they label "Tibetan," while there are also several small to medium-size Tibetan enterprises that produce some Tibetan formulas, as well as incense. My research did not focus on such enterprises, but they do figure into how such statistics are generated.

6. In chapter 5 of his dissertation, Martin Saxer discusses China's administrative protection scheme for traditional medicine, which eventuated in a legal dispute over the right to produce "precious pills."

7. The term *potency (nüpa)* designates both particular qualities of medicinal substances, which constitute their therapeutic properties (the eight *nüpa*), and their therapeutic effect (Boesi 2006: 2).

8. See Aschoff and Tashigang 2001: 45–46.

9. Factories sometimes underreport revenue. Statistics vary widely, and it is never clear how they are calculated. The figures presented here are cited in Chinese media sources (*China Daily* 2004; Xinhua News Agency 2004) and China Tibet Information Center reports (2006, 2007b, 2007c).

10. An important strategy for the regional government and business is foreign direct investment. Total FDI in 2000 was $160 million in the TAR, involving investment in 125 enterprises, loans to seven projects, and financial support of forty-nine programs. The major investor countries were the United States, Japan, Germany, Hong Kong, Malaysia, Nepal, and Macao. Of these, the first four have sustainability indexes. Furthermore, in recent years small Tibet-focused social capital organizations have appeared in these same countries. While interest in FDI has increased in recent years, accessibility is limited. Opportunities for Himalayan businesses to meet potential business partners and investors, dialogue and analysis to plan business strategies, and motivation for cross-cultural business, scientific, and environmental understanding are all limited (www.arunamgyal.com/5W/Industry/people.htm).

11. The WHO has also developed various collaborating centers for Traditional Medicine, the goal of which is often to "integrate" or "harmonize" traditional or alternative practices with conventional medicine. However, these centers often espouse policy, in line with the WHO Traditional Medicine strategies, often equate such "harmonization" with "modernization" and "Westernization" in a very uncritical way. See Hofer (2006) for a discussion of one such conference. The

full conference report and other relevant information can be found on the website of the International Association for the Study of Traditional Asian Medicine (IASTAM), www.iastam.org.

12. In some English translations of this term, it is written Shongpalhachu. I have chosen to follow the transliteration established by Saxer (2010a) here, Shongpalhachu, as it reflects more closely the Tibetan spelling of this name.

13. By 2007, in follow-up interviews in the TAR, industrial microwave ovens were considered state-of-the-art drying technology. In practice, however, they were rarely being used because of producers' wariness about the effects of radiation on *materia medica*. Saxer (2010a) devotes much of his chapter 3 to a detailed comparison of the *Seven Limb Procedure* and the strictures of GMP production, emphasizing areas of innovation, incommensurability, compatibility, and confusion. This includes a detailed treatment of the microwave oven issue.

14. The vice director of Mentsikhang factory said in an interview (August 29, 2007) that funds for GMP compliance were garnered through the Bank of China. The interest rate was paid for a period of time by the "concerned with poor people department" *(min zong wei)* and the "Training for needy people department" *(nong mu ting)*. The cost of building the new Mentsikhang factory was 40 million renminbi ($5 million at the time). In contrast, a senior administrator at the Tibetan Medical College factory, also a state-run institution, said the factory retrofitting cost 1.3 million renminbi ($162,500). This difference also reflects the range of size and scale within this industry.

15. Also see China Tibet Information Center (2006) and Hofer (2008a). Many people I interviewed indicated that GMP implementation had contributed to increasing costs of medicines. There is internal contradiction and dissent, however, in the data on this point. Health Bureau and Tibet Drug Administration regulations officially fix prices for Tibetan medicines, a practice that is also connected to the state health insurance regulations. Some people have indicated that regulations on production and distribution were creating more barriers for state-owned factories to turn a profit (M. Saxer, personal communication, January 2009).

16. Chapter 5 of Saxer (2010a) includes a discussion of knowledge and intellectual property as it relates to patents, "precious pills," "old" and "new" formulas, and Randomized Controlled Trials.

17. See Olsen and Larsen (2003) and Olsen and Bhattarai (2005) for a discussion of trade patterns and livelihoods.

CHAPTER 6

1. "Wangdu" is a pseudonym.

2. "Gawa" and "Samphel" are pseudonyms.

3. See Glover (2006) for an overview of Tibetan medicine in Gyalthang.

4. See Litzinger (2006) for an example of this dynamic in relation to the Critical Ecosystems Partnership Fund in Northwest Yunnan.

5. See Saxer (2010a: chapter 4) for a discussion of sourcing from the Nepal Himalayas to Tibetan medical factories in China.

6. See www.bbs.com.bt/Lingships%20not%20interested%20in%20herbal%20collection%20anymore.html (accessed March 19, 2012) for an example of this dynamic.

7. Mycologist and Tibetologist Daniel Winkler provides an extensive discussion of many of these issues on his website: www.danielwinkler.com. In a highly publicized murder case, a Nepali high court convicted nineteen villagers of the murder of local farmers in Manang District, in conjunction with *yartsa gunbu* trade. Similar clashes were reported in Qinghai, China (ENS News Wire 2005).

8. "Sabriya" is a pseudonym.

9. Parallel cultural constructions of the dichotomies between wildness and barbarism, on the one hand, and cultivation and civilization, on the other, are not a product of conservation in the twentieth-century sense of the term. Such distinctions can be observed at many moments in history, across a range of human communities. The relationship between successive Han and Manchu dynasties in China and the Mongols is emblematic of this division, as are the general and widespread stereotypes held about nomadic versus farming communities (Williams 1996). Often these divisions play out over vertical and latitudinal axes as well, with those dwelling up-mountain considered less "civilized" than those living at the valley floor (i.e., those relying more exclusively on agricultural production for subsistence and the generation of wealth).

10. See *Antipode* 42(3), 2010, edited by James Carrier, for more studies of the relationship between conservation, development, and capitalism.

11. M. Cuomu, personal communication, November 2009.

12. This story of boiling the leather soles of shoes for sustenance is commonly referenced in stories of the Tibetan Resistance Army. See McGranahan 2010.

13. *Press Trust of India*, September 9, 2009 issue.

14. See Craig and Glover (2011) for plant lists that were shared at this conference in Bhutan.

15. Formally gazetted in 1984 and nominated as a UNESCO World Heritage site in 2000, this park contains the turquoise-colored Phoksundo Lake, the deepest in the country.

16. Figure based on UNICEF World Summit for Children Indicators (2001) for Nepal, a preliminary assessment of MCH in Dolpa District carried out by Dr. Bernhard Fassl, as part of OneHEART Worldwide, and qualitative data from my own fieldwork.

17. These schools include Tapriza (www.tapriza.org), the Crystal Mountain School sponsored, in part, by Action Dolpo (www.actiondolpo.com), the Kula Mountain School supported by several foreign NGOs and local patronage (www.drokpa.org/education.html#kula), among others.

CHAPTER 7

1. PPH was defined as more than 500ml blood loss, or 1,000ml following a cesarean section. The standard of care was intravenous oxytocin.

2. Tsongkapa a fourteenth-century Tibetan Buddhist master, founded the *gelukpa* school of Tibetan Buddhism.

3. Readers may notice that these figures for numbers of children far exceed China's One Child Policy. Under this policy, minority nationalities are officially allowed two to three children, depending on their residence (urban vs. rural). However, many Tibetans living in rural areas continue to have more than three children. See Schrempf (2012) for a discussion of state family planning policies and their impacts on Tibetans.

4. A pseudonym.

5. See Goldberg, Greenberg, and Darney (2001) for an overview of the uses of misoprostol in pregnancy.

6. Misoprostol can be used in conjunction with mifepristone (RU-486, or the "morning after" pill) to induce early abortion. See Gynunity (2006) for an example of misoprostol use for abortions in Brazil.

7. The name is a pseudonym.

8. The name is a pseudonym.

9. A pseudonym.

10. Aschoff and Tashigang (2001: 33–34) give a brief biography of Diumar Geshe Tenzin Phuntsok *(bstan 'dzin phun tshog dil dmar dge bshes)*.

11. Reference is from folio XX of this text. [[insert pg. number]]

12. In the Tibetan calendar the tenth day of the month is reserved for prayers and offerings to Guru Rimpoche.

13. According to the Tibetan Himalayan Library, text is by Dudjom Jigdrel Yeshi Dorje *(bdud 'joms 'jigs bral ye shes rdo rje, 1904–89)*.

14. I use the *jomo* spelling throughout, following Mingkyi's original notes. Although *jomo* is often translated as "nun," this is not entirely accurate, as many such figures are often consorts to tantric masters, often associated with the *nyingma* school of Buddhism, or Bön. *Jomo / chömo* is often substituted for *ani*, which means both "nun" and "maternal aunt," although the latter is more closely associated with a life marked by formal vows of celibate monasticism in an institutional setting. See Shneiderman 2008.

15. The name is a pseudonym.

16. The name is a pseudonym.

17. Research Committee members were initially concerned about the ethics of what they viewed as "withholding" medicine that may be beneficial or decrease suffering, specifically prophylactic doses of oxytocin, which, we discovered, routinely happens at our three participating Tibetan hospitals even though this is not "evidence-based" practice according to the American PIs. These concerns helped to propel all of us to envision a two-armed study.

18. These plastic drapes had never before been used in Tibetan hospitals or rural clinical settings. Normally postpartum blood loss was collected in a bucket placed at the edge of the delivery bed, and a provider would estimate the amount of blood loss. During our research project in Tibet, the drapes were simultaneously used in India on another NIH "global network" project.

19. The name is a pseudonym.

CONCLUSION

1. Unfortunately, he was unable to attend, but the workshop was held from December 5–12, 2012. See Blaikie, Craig, Gerke and Hofer 2012 for a summary of this event.

2. Since 2010, more than thirty Tibetans, most of them under thirty years of age, have set themselves on fire in ethnically Tibetan regions of China. Discussions of these self-immolations can be found in a special on-line issue of *Cultural Anthropology* (www.culanth.org/?q=node/431) and in a *New York Times* article from March 23, 2012 (www.nytimes.com/2012/03/23/world/asia/in-self -immolations-signs-of-new-turmoil-in-tibet.html?_r=1&emc=eta1).

Bibliography

Adams, V. 1998. "Suffering the Winds of Lhasa: Politicized Bodies, Human Rights, Cultural Difference and Humanism in Tibet." *Medical Anthropology Quarterly* 12(1): 74–102.

———. 2000. "Women's Health in Tibetan Medicine and Tibet's 'First' Female Doctor." In *Women's Buddhism, Buddhism's Women: Tradition, Revision, Renewal*. Ed. E. B. Findly. Cambridge, MA: Wisdom Publications, 433–50.

———. 2001a. "Particularizing Modernity: Tibetan Medical Theorizing of Women's Health in Lhasa, Tibet." In *Healing Powers and Modernity: Traditional Medicine, Shamanism, and Science in Asian Societies*. Ed. L. Connor and G. Samuel. Westport, CT: Bergin and Garvey, 222–46.

———. 2001b. "The Sacred in the Scientific: Ambiguous Practices of Science in Tibetan Medicine." *Cultural Anthropology* 164:542–75.

———. 2002a. "Establishing Proof: Translating 'Science' and the State in Tibetan Medicine." In *New Horizons in Medical Anthropology: Essays in Honour of Charles Leslie*. Ed. M. Nichter and M. Lock. London: Routledge, 200–220.

———. 2002b. "Randomized Controlled Crime: Postcolonial Sciences in Alternative Medicine Research." *Social Studies of Science* 32(5–6): 959–90.

———. 2005a. "Moral Orgasm and Productive Sex: Tantrism Faces Fertility Control in Lhasa, Tibet (China)." In *Sex in Development: Science, Sexuality, and Morality in Global Perspective*. Ed. V. Adams and S. L. Pigg. Durham, NC: Duke University Press, 207–39.

———. 2005b. "Saving Tibet? An Inquiry into Modernity, Lies, Truths, and Beliefs." *Medical Anthropology* 24(1): 71–110.

———. 2011. "Evidence of the Tibetan Body: Making the Subtle Winds Visible in an Evidence Economy." Presentation given at the American Anthropological Association Annual Meetings, Montreal, Canada, November 16–20, 2011.

Adams, V., R. Dhondup, P. V. Le. 2010. "A Dharmic Way of Science: Revisioning Biomedicines as Tibetan Practice." In *Medicine between Science and Religion: Explorations on Tibetan Grounds*. Ed. V. Adams, M. Schrempf, and S. Craig. London: Berghahn Books, 107–26.

Adams, V., and F. Li. 2008. "Integration or Erasure: Modernization at the Mentsikhang." In *Tibetan Medicine in the Contemporary World: Global Politics of Medical Knowledge and Practice*. Ed. L. Pordié. London: Routledge, 105–31.

Adams, V., S. Miller, J. Chertow, S. Craig, A. Samen, and M. Varner. 2005b. "Having a 'Safe' Delivery: Conflicting Views from Tibet." *Health Care for Women International* 26(9): 821–51.

Adams, V., S. Miller, S. Craig, A. Samen, Nyima, Lhakpen, Sonam, Droyoung, and M. Varner. 2005a. "The Challenge of Cross-Cultural Clinical Trials Research: Case Report from the Tibet Autonomous Region, People's Republic of China." *Medical Anthropology Quarterly* 19(3): 267–89.

Adams, V., S. Miller, S. Craig, Sonam, Nyima, Droyoung, P. V. Le, and M. Varner. 2007. "Informed Consent in Cross-Cultural Perspective: Clinical Research in the Tibetan Autonomous Region, PRC." *Culture, Medicine, and Psychiatry* (31): 445–72.

Adams, V., M. Schrempf, and S. Craig. 2010. "A gso ba rig pa Sensibility." In *Medicine between Science and Religion: Explorations on Tibetan Grounds*. London: Berghahn Books, 1–30.

Agamben, G. 2005. *State of Exception*. Chicago: University of Chicago Press.

Agrawal, A. 2005. *Environmentality: Technologies of Government and the Making of Subjects*. Durham, NC: Duke University Press.

Ahern, E. M. 1979. "The Problem of Efficacy: Strong and Weak Illocutionary Acts." *Man* 14(1): 1–17.

Alter, J. S. 2005. *Asian Medicine and Globalization*. Philadelphia: University of Pennsylvania Press.

Anand, D. 2008. *Imagining Geopolitical Exotica: Tibet in Western Imagination*. Minneapolis: University of Minnesota Press.

Anderson, R. 1992. "The Efficacy of Ethnomedicine: Research Methods in Trouble." In *Anthropological Approaches to the Study of Ethnomedicine*. Ed. M. Nichter. Philadelphia: Gordon and Breach Science Publishers, 3–17.

Appadurai, A. 1986. "Introduction: Commodities and the Politics of Value." In *The Social Life of Things: Commodities in Cultural Perspective*. Ed. A. Appadurai. Cambridge, UK: Cambridge University Press, 3–63.

Arya, P.Y. 1989. *Dictionary of Tibetan Materia Medica*. Delhi: Motilal Banarsidass Publishers.

Aschoff, J., and T. Y. Tashigang. 2001. *Tibetan Precious Pills: A Tantric Healing System*. Ulm, Germany: Fabri Verlag.

AsiaInfo Services. 2008. "China's Tibetan Medicines Go Global." http://business .highbeam.com/436093/article-1G1-178659302/china-tibetan-medicines-go -global. Accessed March 19, 2012.

Baer, H. M. Singer, and I. Susser. 2002. *Medical Anthropology and the World System*. Westport, CT: Praeger.

Banerjee, M. 2009. *Power, Knowledge, Medicine: Ayurvedic Pharmaceuticals at Home and in the World*. New Delhi: Orient BlackSwan.

Barnes, L. 2005. "American Acupuncture and Efficacy: Meaning and Its Points of Insertion." *Medical Anthropology Quarterly* 19(3): 239–66.

Bassini, P. 2007. "Heart Distress on the Sino-Tibetan Frontier: History, Gender, Ecology and Ritual Practice in Tibetan Popular Perceptions and Experiences of Heart Distress (snying nad) in Amdo." D.Phil. dissertation, Oxford University.

Basso, K. 1996. *Wisdom Sits in Places: Landscape and Language among the Western Apache*. Albuquerque: University of New Mexico Press.

Bates, D. 1995. "Scholarly Ways of Knowing: An Introduction." In *Knowledge and the Scholarly Medical Traditions*. Ed. D. Bates. Cambridge, UK: Cambridge University Press, 1–22.

———. 2002. "Why Not Call Modern Medicine 'Alternative'?" *Annals of the American Academy of Political and Social Science* 583:12–28.

Bateson, G. (1972) 2000. *Steps to an Ecology of Mind*. Chicago: University of Chicago Press.

Bauer, K. 2004. *High Frontiers: Dolpo and the Changing World of Himalayan Pastoralists*. New York: Columbia University Press.

Beckwith, C. 1979. "The Introduction of Greek Medicine into Tibet in the Seventh and Eighth Centuries." *Journal of the American Oriental Society* 99(2): 297–313.

Berlin, B. 1992. *Ethnobiological Classification: Principles of Categorization of Plants and Animals in Traditional Societies*. Princeton, NJ: Princeton University Press.

Berlin, B., D. E. Breedlove, and P. H. Raven 1973. "General Principles of Classification and Nomenclature in Folk Biology." *American Anthropologist* 75:214–42.

Berry, N. 2010. *Unsafe Motherhood: Mayan Maternal Mortality and Subjectivity in Post-war Guatemala*. London: Berghahn Books.

Besch, F. 2007. "Making a Medical Living: On the Monetisation of Tibetan Medicine in Spiti." In *Soundings in Tibetan Medicine: Anthropological and Historical Perspectives*. Ed. M. Schrempf. Leiden: Brill, 155–70.

Besch, F., and I. Guerin. In press. "On the Implications of Amchi Medicine Development Activities." In *Healing at the Periphery: Ethnographies of Tibetan Medicine in India*. Ed. L. Pordié. Durham, NC: Duke University Press.

Biehl, J. 2005. *Vita: Life in a Zone of Social Abandonment*. Berkeley: University of California Press.

Blaikie, C. 2011. "Critically Endangered? Himalayan Medicinal Plant Conservation and Diversity in Medical Cultures." In *Asian Medicine: Tradition and Modernity* 5(2): 243–72.

———. In press. "Where There Are No *Amchi*." In *Healing at the Periphery: Ethnographies of Tibetan Medicine in India*. Ed. L. Pordié. Durham, NC: Duke University Press.

Blaikie, C., S. Craig, B. Gerke, and T. Hofer, 2012. "Producing Efficacious Medicines: Reflections on a Remarkable Event." IASTAM Newsletter.

Bloom, G., and G. Xingyuan. 1999. "Health Sector Reform: Lessons from China." *Social Science and Medicine* 45(3): 351–60.

Bode, M. 2006. "Taking Traditional Knowledge to the Market: The Commoditization of Indian Medicine." *Anthropology and Medicine* 13(3): 225–36.

———. 2008. *Taking Traditional Knowledge to the Market: The Modern Image of the Ayurvedic and Unani Industry, 1980–2000*. New Delhi: Orient BlackSwan.

Bodeker, G., C. K. Ong, C. Grundy, G. Burford, and K. Schein, eds. 2005. *WHO Global Atlas of Traditional, Complementary and Alternative Medicine*. Kobe: World Health Organisation Centre for Health Development.

Boesi, A. 2005. "Plant Knowledge among Tibetan Populations." In *Wildlife and Plants in Traditional and Modern Tibet*, ed. A. Boesi and F. Cardi. *Memorie della Società Italiana di Scienze Naturali e del Museo Civico di Storia Naturale di Milano* special issue 33(1): 33–48.

———. 2006. "Plant Categories and Types in Tibetan Materia Medica." *Tibet Journal* 30(4) and 31(1): 67–92.

Boesi, A., and F. Cardi. Ed. 2006. *Tibet Journal* special issue 30(4).

Bookchin, M. 1996. *The Philosophy of Social Ecology: Essays on Dialectical Naturalism*. Montreal: Black Rose Books.

Bourdieu, P., and L. Wacquant. 1992. *An Invitation to Reflexive Sociology*. Chicago: University of Chicago Press.

Bowker, G. C., and S. L. Star. 1999. *Sorting Things Out: Classification and Its Consequences*. Cambridge, MA: MIT Press.

Bradley, S. E. K., N. Prata, N. Young-Lin, and D. M. Bishai. 2007. "Cost-effectiveness of Misoprostol to Control Postpartum Hemorrhage in Low-resource Settings." *International Journal of Gynecology and Obstetrics* 97:52–56.

Bronfenbrenner, U. 1979. *The Ecology of Human Development*. Cambridge, MA: Harvard University Press.

Cameron, M. 2008. "Modern Desires, Knowledge Control and Physician Resistance: Regulating Ayurvedic Medicine in Nepal." *Asian Medicine* 4(1): 86–112.

———. 2009. Healing Landscapes: Sacred and Rational Nature in Nepal's Ayurvedic Medicine. In *Symbolic Ecologies: Culture, Nature and Society in the Himalaya*. Ed. Arjun Guneratne. New York: Routledge.

Cant, S., and U. Sharma. 2005. *A New Medical Pluralism? Alternative Medicine, Patients, Doctors, and the State*. Oxford: Taylor and Francis.

Cardi, F. 2005. "Evolution of Tibetan Medical Knowledge in the Socio-economic Context: The Exploitation of Medicinal Plants among Traditional Doctors." In *Wildlife and Plants in Traditional and Modern Tibet*, ed. A. Boesi and F. Cardi. *Memorie della Societa Italiana di Scienze Naturali e del Museo Civico di Storia Naturale* special issue 34(1–2): 19–32.

———. 2006. "Principles and Methods of Assembling Tibetan Medicaments." *Tibet Journal* 30(4) and 31(1): 91–108.

Carpenter-Song, E. 2009. "Caught in the Psychiatric Net: Meanings and Experiences of ADHD, Pediatric Bipolar Disorder, and Mental Health Treatment among Families in the United States." *Culture, Medicine and Psychiatry* 33(1): 61–85.

Carrin, G., A. Ron, Y. Hui, W. Hong, and Z. Tuohong. 1999. "The Reform of the Rural Cooperative Medical System in the People's Republic of China: Interim Experience in 14 Pilot Counties." *Social Science and Medicine* 48:961–72.

Chen, N. 2005. "Mapping Science and Nation in China." In *Asian Medicine and Globalization*. Ed. J. Alter. Philadelphia: University of Pennsylvania Press, 107–19.

Childs, G. 2008. *Tibetan Transitions: Historical and Contemporary Perspectives on Fertility, Family Planning, and Demographic Change*. Leiden: Brill.

China Daily. 2004. "Tibetan Medicine Packed with Unusual Properties." Accessed August 18. 2004 (no current url available).

———. 2005. "New Rural Medical Cooperatives under Scrutiny." February 11, 2005. www.chinadaily.com.cn/english/doc/2005-11/02/content_489869 .htm. Accessed August 14, 2011.

———. 2006. "Firm Preserves Ancient Cures." December 10, 2006. www .chinadaily.com.cn/bizchina/2006-10/12/content_706519.htm. Accessed October 23, 2011.

China Tibet Information Center. 2006. "Tibetan Medical Institutions Lighten Burden for Rural People." www.tibet.cn/en/news/tin/t20061212_188005 .htm. Accessed March 19, 2012.

———. 2007a. "First Batch of Tibetan Medicine Exported." http://eng.tibet.cn/ news/tibet/200801/t20080115_328768.htm. Accessed August 6, 2010.

———. 2007b. "Tibetan Medicine Industry Rapidly Develops." http://info.tibet .cn/en/news/tin/t20070227_212703.htm. Accessed March 19, 2012.

———. 2007c. "Tibetan Medicine to Declare World Intangible Culture Heritage." http://info.tibet.cn/en/news/tin/t20070907_278777.htm. Accessed March 19, 2012.

Chöpel, K. 1993. *bDud rtsi sman gyi 'khrungs dpe legs bshad nor bu'i phreng mdzes*. Lhasa: Bod ljongs mi dmangs dpe skrun khang.

Citrin, D. 2010. "The Anatomy of Ephemeral Health Care: 'Health Camps' and Short-term Medical Voluntourism in Remote Nepal." *Studies in Nepali History and Society* 15(1): 27–72.

Clifford, J., and G. Marcus. 1986. *Writing Culture: The Poetics and Politics of Ethnography*. Berkeley: University of California Press.

Clift, A., C. Morgan, D. Anderson, and M. Toole. 2004. "Alarming Levels of Hepatitis B Virus Detected among Rural Tibetans." *Tropical Doctor* 34(3): 156–57.

Coelius, R. L., A. Stenson, J. L. Morris, M. Cuomu, C. Tudor, and S. Miller. 2012. "The Tibetan Uterotonic Zhi Byed 11: Mechanisms of Action, Efficacy, and Historical Use for Postpartum Hemorrhage." *Evidence Based Complementary and Alternative Medicine*. Online. Doi: 10.1155/2012/794164.

Cohen, L. 1998. *No Aging in India: Alzheimer's, the Bad Family, and Other Modern Things*. Berkeley: University of California Press.

Craig, S. 2002. "Place, Work, and Identity between Mustang, Nepal and New York City." *Studies in Nepali History and Society* 7(2): 355–403.

———. 2004. A Tale of Two Temples: Culture, Capital, and Community in Mustang, Nepal. *European Bulletin of Himalayan Research* 27:11–36.

————. 2007. "A Crisis of Confidence: A Comparison between Tibetan Medical Education in Nepal and Tibet." In *Soundings in Tibetan Medicine: Anthropological and Historical Perspectives.* Ed. M. Schrempf. Leiden: Brill, 127–54.

————. 2008a. *Horses Like Lightning: A Story of Passage through the Himalayas.* Boston: Wisdom Publications.

————. 2008b. "Place and Professionalisation: Navigating *Amchi* Identity in Nepal." In *Exploring Tibetan Medicine in the Contemporary Context.* Ed. L. Pordié. London: Routledge, 62–90.

————. 2009. "Pregnancy and Childbirth in Tibet: Knowledge, Perspectives, and Practices." In *Childbirth across Cultures.* Ed. H. Selin. New York: Springer, 145–60.

————. 2010a. "Between Empowerments and Power Calculations: Notes on Efficacy, Value, and Method." In *Medicine between Science and Religion: Explorations on Tibetan Grounds.* Ed. V. Adams, M. Schrempf, and S. Craig. London: Berghahn Books, 215–42.

————. 2010b. "No Hidden Kingdom." Op-ed. *Kathmandu Post,* October 15.

————. 2011a. " 'Good' Manufacturing by Whose Standards? Global Governance and the Production of Tibetan Pharmaceuticals." *Anthropological Quarterly* 84(2): 331–78.

————. 2011b. "Migration, Social Change, Health, and the Realm of the Possible: Women's Stories from Nepal to New York." *Anthropology and Humanism* 36(2): 196–214.

————. 2011c. "Not Found in Tibetan Society: Culture, Childbirth and a Politics of Life on the Roof of the World." *Himalaya* 30(1–2): 101–14.

Craig, S., and V. Adams 2008. "Global Pharma in the Land of Snows: Tibetan Medicines, SARS, and Identity Politics across Nations." *Asian Medicine: Tradition and Modernity* 4:1–28.

Craig, S., and G. Bista. 2005. "Himalayan Healers in Transition: Professionalization, Identity, and Conservation among Practitioners of *gso ba rig pa* in Nepal." In *Himalayan Medicinal and Aromatic Plants: Balancing Use and Conservation.* Ed. Y. Thomas, M. Kharki, K. Gurung, and D. Parajuli. Kathmandu: WWF Nepal Program, 411–34.

Craig, S., L. Chase, and T. N. Lama. 2010. "Taking the MINI to Mustang, Nepal: Methodological and Epistemological Translations of Illness Narrative Interviews." *Anthropology and Medicine* 17(1): 1–26.

Craig, S., and D. Glover. 2011. "Cultivation, Conservation and Commoditization of Himalayan and Tibetan Medicinal Plants." *Asian Medicine: Tradition and Modernity* 5(2): 219–42.

Csordas, T. J., and A. Kleinman. 1996. "The Therapeutic Process." In *Medical Anthropology: Contemporary Theory and Method.* Ed. C. F. Sargent and T. Johnson. Westport, CT: Praeger, 3–21.

Cuomu, M. 2010. "Qualitative and Quantitative Research Methodology in Tibetan Medicine." In *Medicine between Science and Religion: Explorations on Tibetan Grounds.* Ed. V. Adams, M. Schrempf, and S. Craig. London: Berghahn Books, 245–64.

———. 2011. Social and Cultural Factors in Developing a Tibetan Public Health System. Ph.D. dissertation, Humboldt University, Central Asian Seminary, Berlin.

Czaja, O. 2010. "The Four Tantras and the Global Market: Changing Epistemologies of Drä versus Cancer." In *Medicine between Science and Religion: Explorations on Tibetan Grounds.* Ed. V. Adams, M. Schrempf, and S. Craig. London: Berghahn Books, 265–96.

Dakpa, T. 1997. *Tibetan Medicinal Plants.* New Delhi: Paljor.

Dash, V. B. 1994. *Pharmacopoeia of Tibetan Medicine.* New Delhi: Sri Satguru.

Davis-Floyd, R., and C. Sargent 1997. *Childbirth and Authoritative Knowledge: Cross-Cultural Perspectives.* Berkeley: University of California Press.

Dawa, D. 2011. "Materia Medica of Tibetan Medicine: Identification, Quality Check, and Protection Measures." *Asian Medicine: Tradition and Modernity* 5(2): 407–32.

Des Chene, M. 2002. "In the Name of Bikas." *Studies in Nepali History and Society* 7(2): 259–70.

Dhungel, R. 2002. *The Kingdom of Lo (Mustang).* Kathmandu: Lo Gyalpo Jigme Foundation.

Dickerson, T., D. Fernandez, Topgyal, A. Samen, Geleg, Nyima, G. Pelto, S. Craig, and T. Dye. 2007. "From Butter Tea to Pepsi: A Rapid Appraisal of Food Preferences, Procurement Sources, and Dietary Diversity in a Contemporary Tibetan Township." *Ecology of Food and Nutrition* 47(1): 229–53.

Dickie, M. 2004. "Tibet Looks to Its Traditional Medicine as Economic Cure." *Financial Times,* July 3.

Diemberger, H. 2005. "Female Oracles in Modern Tibet." In *Women in Tibet: Past and Present.* Ed. J. Gyatso and H. Havnevik. New York: Columbia University Press, 113–68.

Dilmar, T. P., and Y. T. Tashi. 1970. *Principles of Lamaist Pharmacognosy: Being the Texts of the Dri med shel gong, Dri med shel phreng, and the Lang len gces bsdus of Dil-dmar Dge-bshes Bstan-'dzin-phun-tshogs. Reproduced by Photographic Process from the Lhasa Chakpori Blocks by Tashi Yangphel Tashigang.* Leh, India: S. W. Tashigangpa.

Dodin, T., and H. Rather. 2006. *Imagining Tibet: Perceptions, Projections, and Fantasies.* Boston: Wisdom Publications.

Dorje, G, 1995. '*Khrungs dpe dri med shel gyi me long.* Lhasa, Tibet: People's Publishing House.

———. 2011. "An Investigation into the Advisability of Translating Names of Tibetan Medicine into Other Languages." *Asian Medicine: Tradition and Modernity* 5(2): 394–406.

Dorje, R. and K. Stewart. 2009. "Seating, Money, and Food at an Amdo Village Funeral." *Asian Highlands Perspectives* 1:237–94.

Douglas, M. 1966. *Purity and Danger.* London: Taylor and Francis.

Durkheim, É., and M. Mauss. (1903) 1963. *Primitive Classification.* Chicago: University of Chicago Press.

ENS Newswire. 2005. "Tibetans, Chinese Battle over Access to Medicinal Fungus." www.ens-newswire.com/ens/jun2005/2005-06-02-01.asp. Accessed March 14, 2012.

Ernst, W. 2002. "Plural Medicine, Tradition and Modernity. Historical and Contemporary Perspectives: Views from Below and from Above." In *Plural Medicine, Tradition and Modernity, 1800–2000*. Ed. W. Ernst. London: Routledge, 1–18.

Etkin, N. 1988. "Cultural Constructions of Efficacy." In *The Context of Medicines in Developing Countries*. Ed. S. van der Geest and S. Whyte. Dordrecht: Kluwer Academic Publishers, 299–326.

———. 1992. "'Side Effects': Cultural Constructions and Reinterpretations of Western Pharmaceuticals." *Medical Anthropology Quarterly* 6(2): 99–113.

Evans-Pritchard, E. E. 1976. *Witchcraft, Oracles and Magic among the Azande*. Oxford: Clarendon Press.

Fan, R., and I. Holliday. 2006. "Policies for Traditional Medicine in Peripheral China." *Journal of Alternative and Complementary Medicine* 12(5): 238–487.

———. 2007. "Which Medicine? Whose Standard? Critical Reflections on Medical Integration in China." *Journal of Medical Ethics* 33:454–61.

Farmer, P. 1997. "On Social Suffering and Structural Violence." In *Social Suffering*. Ed. A. Kleinman, V. Das, and M. Lock. Berkeley: University of California Press, 261–84.

———. 2001. *Infections and Inequalities: The Modern Plagues*. Berkeley: University of California Press.

———. 2004. *Pathologies of Power: Health, Human Rights, and the New War on the Poor*. Berkeley: University of California Press.

Farquhar, J. 1994. *Knowing Practice: The Clinical Encounter of Chinese Medicine*. Boulder, CO: Westview Press.

———. 1995. "Re-writing Traditional Medicine in Post-Maoist China." In *Knowledge and the Scholarly Medical Traditions*. Ed. D. Bates. Cambridge, UK: Cambridge University Press, 251–76.

Ferguson, J. 1999. *Expectations of Modernity: Myths and Meanings of Urban Life on the Zambian Copperbelt*. Berkeley: University of California Press.

Fischer, A. M. 2005. *State Growth and Social Exclusion in Tibet: Challenges of Recent Growth*. Copenhagen: Nordic Institute of Asian Studies Press.

———. 2008a. "'Population Invasion' versus Urban Exclusion in the Tibetan Areas of Western China." *Population and Development Review* 34(4): 631–62.

———. 2008b. "Subsistence and Rural Livelihood Strategies in Tibet under Rapid Economic and Social Transition." In K. Bauer, G. Childs, A. M. Fischer, and D. Winkler eds., *Journal of the International Association of Tibetan Studies*, 4. www.thlib.org/collections/texts/jiats/#jiats=/04/fischer/.

Fisher, J. 1978. Introduction in *Himalayan Anthropology: The Indo-Tibetan Interface*. Ed. J. Fisher. Paris: Mouton, 1–3.

Fjeld, H. and T. Hofer. Forthcoming. "Women and Gender in Tibetan Medicine: An Introduction." In *Asian Medicine: Tradition and Modernity* special issue 6(2): 1–34.

Foucault, M. 1973. *The Birth of the Clinic: An Archaeology of Medical Perception.* New York: Pantheon Books.

———. 1980. *Power/Knowledge: Selected Interviews and Other Writings, 1972–1977.* New York: Pantheon.

———. 1988. "Technologies of the Self." In *Technologies of the Self.* Ed. L. Martin, H. Gutman, and P. Hutton. Amherst: University of Massachusetts Press, 16–49.

———. 1991. "Governmentality." Trans. Rosi Braidotti. In *The Foucault Effect: Studies in Governmentality.* Ed. G. Burchell, C. Gordon, and P. Miller. Chicago: University of Chicago Press, 87–104.

———. 2007. *Security, Territory, Population: Lectures at the College de France.* Hampshire, UK: Palgrave Macmillan.

Fox, R. C., and J. Swazy. 2008. *Observing Bioethics.* New York: Oxford University Press.

Garrett, F. 2009. "The Alchemy of Accomplishing Medicine: Situating the *Yuthog Heart Essence* Ritual Tradition." *Journal of Indian Philosophy* 37(3): 207–30.

Garrett, F., and V. Adams. 2008. "The Three Channels in Tibetan Medical and Religious Texts, Including a Translation of Tsultrim Gyaltsen's 'Treatise on the Three Channels in Tibetan Medicine.'" *Traditional South Asian Medicine* 8:86–115.

Gerke, B. 2010. "Correlating Biomedical and Tibetan Medical Concepts in *Amchi* Medical Practice: An Ethnographic Example from the Darjeeling Hills." In *Medicine between Science and Religion: Explorations on Tibetan Grounds.* Ed. V. Adams, M. Schrempf, and S. Craig. London: Berghahn Books, 127–53.

———. 2012. *Long Lives and Untimely Deaths: Life-span Concepts and Longevity Practices among Tibetans in the Darjeeling Hills, India.* Leiden: Brill Academic Publishers.

Ghimire, S., G. Bista, W. Lama, T. Darkye, N. Lama, M. Phunchok, T. Choedon, and T. N. Lama. 2010. "Integrating *Amchis'* Traditional Knowledge and Practices for Medicinal Substitutes and Conservation of Threatened Species in the Himalaya." Final Technical Report. Critical Ecosystems Partnership Fund, Kathmandu: WWF Nepal Program.

Ghimire, S. K. 2008. "Sustainable Harvesting and Management of Medicinal Plants in the Nepal Himalaya: Current Issues, Knowledge Gaps and Research Priorities." In *Medicinal Plants in Nepal: An Anthology of Contemporary Research.* Ed. P. K. Jha, S. B. Karmacharya, M. K. Chhetri, C. B. Thapa, and B. B. Shrestha. Nepal: Ecological Society, 25–42.

———. 2010. *Integrating Amchis' Traditional Knowledge and Practices for Medicinal Substitutes and Conservation of Threatened Species in the Himalaya.* Final Technical Report. WWF-CEPF, Kathmandu.

Ghimire, S. K., Y. C. Lama, and G. R. Tripathi. 2001. *Conservation of Plant Resources, Community Development and Training in Applied Ethnobotany at Shey-Phoksumdo National Park and Its Bufferzone, Dolpa.* Kathmandu: WWF Nepal Program.

Ghimire, S. K., D. McKey, and Y. Aumeeruddy-Thomas. 2005a. "Conservation of Himalayan Medicinal Plants: Harvesting Patterns and Ecology of Two Threatened Species, Nardostachys Grandiflora DC and Neopicrorhiza Scrophulariiflora (Pennell) Hong." *Biological Conservation* 124(4): 463–75.

———. 2005b. "Heterogeneity in Ethnoecological Knowledge and Management of Medicinal Plants in the Himalayas of Nepal: Implications for Conservation." *Ecology and Society* 9(3): 6. www.ecologyandsociety.org/vol9/iss3/art6/.

Glover, D. 2006. "Tibetan Medicine in Gyalthang." *Tibet Journal* 30(4) and 31(1): 31–54.

———. 2010. "Classes in the Classics: Historical Changes in Plant Classification in Two Tibetan Medical Texts." In *Socio-historical Studies of Medical Pluralism in Tibetan Contexts.* Ed. S. Craig, F. Garrett, M. Schrempf, and M. Cuomu. Halle: International Institute for Tibetan and Buddhist Studies, 255–78.

Goldberg, A. B., M. B. Greenberg, and P. D. Darney. 2001. "Misoprostol and Pregnancy." *New England Journal of Medicine* 344(1): 38–47.

Goldstein, M. 1989. *A History of Modern Tibet, 1913–1951: The Demise of the Lamaist State.* Berkeley: University of California Press.

———. 1997. *The Snow Lion and the Dragon: China, Tibet, and the Dalai Lama.* Berkeley: University of California Press.

Goldstein, M. C., B. Jiao (Benjor), C. M. Beall, and P. Tsering. 2002. "Fertility and Family Planning in Rural Tibet." *China Journal* 47:19–39.

Grard, P., and L. Pordié. 2005. "Rethinking Taxonomy in the Age of Technology: Perspectives and Limitations of a New Informatics Tool for Conservation in the Himalayas." In *Himalayan Medicinal and Aromatic Plants: Balancing Use and Conservation.* Ed. Y. Thomas, M. Karki, K. Gurung, and D. Parajuli. Kathmandu: WWF Nepal Program, 514–18.

Greenwood, D., and M. Levin. 2006. *Introduction to Action Research.* 2nd ed. Thousand Oaks, CA: Sage.

Groleau, D., A. Young, and L. Kirmayer. 2006. "The McGill Illness Narrative Interview (MINI): An Interview Schedule to Elicit Meanings and Modes of Reasoning Related to Illness Experience." *Transcultural Psychiatry* 43(4): 671–91.

Gutschow, K. 2010. "From Home to Hospital: The Extension of Obstetrics in Ladakh." In *Medicine between Science and Religion: Explorations on Tibetan Grounds.* Ed. V. Adams, M. Schrempf, and S. Craig. London: Berghahn Books, 185–241.

Gyaltsen, K., C. Gewa, H. Greenlee, J. Ravetz, M. Aikman, and A. Pebley. 2007. "Socioeconomic Status and Maternal Child Health in Rural Tibetan Villages." California Center for Population Research Online Working Paper Series. http://repositories.cdlib.org/ccpr/olwp/CCPR-Special-07.

Gyatso, J. 2003. "Mapping the Body with Buddhism: Shifting Fortunes of the Tantric Channel System in Tibetan Medical Anatomy." Presentation at the

10th Annual International Association of Tibetan Studies Conference, September 6–12.

———. 2004. "The Authority of Empiricism and the Empiricism of Authority: Medicine and Buddhism in Tibet on the Eve of Modernity." *Comparative Studies of South Asia, Africa, and the Middle East* 24(2): 84–96.

———. 2010. "The Ethics of the Way of Humans: Before, within, and beyond Tibetan Buddhism." Plenary presentation at the 12th Conference of the International Association of Tibetan Studies, Vancouver, August 24–26.

———. n.d. *The Way of Humans in a Buddhist World: An Intellectual History of Medicine in Early Modern Tibet.*

Gyatso, Y. 2006. "*Nyes pa:* A Brief Review on Its English Translation." *Tibet Journal* 30(4) and 31(1): 109–18.

Gynunity. 2006. *Annotated Bibliography on Misoprostol Alone for Early Abortion.* Gynunity Health Projects, New York.

Hacking, I. 1990. *Scientific Revolutions.* Oxford: Oxford University Press.

Halliburton, M. 2009. *Mudpacks and Prozac: Experiencing Ayurvedic, Biomedical, and Religious Healing.* Walnut Creek, CA: Left Coast Press.

Harper, I. 2010. "Extreme Condition, Extreme Measures? Compliance, Drug Resistance and the Control of Tuberculosis." *Anthropology & Medicine* 17(2): 201–14.

Harper, I., and B. Kohrt. 2008. "Navigating Diagnoses: Understanding Mind-Body Relations, Stigma and Mental Health in Nepal." *Culture, Medicine and Psychiatry* 32: 462–91.

Harper, I., and B. Maddox. 2008. "The Impossibility of Wellbeing: Development Language and the Pathologisation of Nepal." In *Culture and Well-being: Anthropological Approaches to Freedom and Political Ethics.* Ed. A. C. Jimenez. London: Pluto Press, 35–52.

Harper, J. 2002. *Endangered Species: Health, Illness, and Death in Madagascar.* Durham, NC: Carolina Academic Press.

Harrell, S. 2001. *Ways of Being Ethnic in Southwest China.* Seattle: University of Washington Press.

Hawley, A. H. 1950. *Human Ecology: A Theory of Community Structure.* New York: Ronald Press.

Healcy, D. 2006. "The New Medical Oikumene." In *Global Pharmaceuticals: Ethics, Markets, Practices.* Ed. A. Petryna, A. Lakoff and A. Kleinman. Durham, NC: Duke University Press, 61–84.

Heggenhoughen, K. 1997. "Perceptions of Efficacy and the Uses of Traditional Medicine, with Examples from Tanzania." *Curare* 20(1): 5–13.

Hillman, B. 2003. "Paradise under Construction: Minorities, Myths, and Modernity in Northwest Yunnan." *Asian Ethnicity* 4(2): 175–88.

Ho, L. S. 1995. "Market Reforms and China's Health Care System." *Social Science and Medicine* 41(8): 1065–72.

Höfer, A. 1979. "The Caste Hierarchy and the State in Nepal: A Study of the Muluki Ain of 1854." In *Khumbu Himal.* Innsbruck: Universitatsverlag Wagner, 31–238.

Hofer, T. 2006. "Conference Report: Harmonisation of Traditional and Modern Medicine." IASTAM Newsletter, December, 6–16.

————. 2008. "Rinchen Rilbu for the Rich? Socio-economic Dimensions of Tibetan Medicine in the Tibet Autonomous Region, China." *Asian Medicine: Tradition and Modernity* 4(1–2): 29–52.

————. 2011a. "'Essential Drugs'? On the Uses of Antibiotics in Rural Tibet." Presentation for Beyond the Magic Bullet: Reframing History of Antibiotics conference, University of Oslo, March.

————. 2011b. *The Inheritance of Change: Transmission and Practice of Tibetan Medicine in Ngamring*. Vienna: Wiener Studien zur Tibetologie und Buddhismuskunde.

————. 2011c. "Tibetan Medicine on the Margins: 20th Century Transformations of the Traditions of Sowa Rigpa in Central Tibet." D.Phil. dissertation, University College London, Dept. of Anthropology.

————. Forthcoming. "Changing Representations of the Female Tibetan Medical Doctor Khandro Yangkar (1907–1973)." In *Buddhist Himalayas*. Ed. A. McKay and A. Balicki-Denjongpa. Gangktok, India: Sikkim.

Høg, E., and E. Hsu. 2002. Introduction to *Anthropology and Medicine*. Special issue 9(3): 205–21.

Hogan, M. C, K. J. Foreman, M. Naghavi, S. Y. Ahn, M. Wang, S. M. Makeda, A. D. Lopez, R. Loranzo, C. J. L. Murray. 2010. "Maternal Mortality for 181 Countries, 1980–2008: A Systematic Analysis of Progress toward Millennium Development Goal 5." *The Lancet*. Online April 12. Doi:10.1016/S0140-6736(10)60518-1

Hsu, E. 1999. *The Transmission of Chinese Medicine*. Cambridge, UK: Cambridge University Press.

————. 2001. *Innovations in Chinese Medicine*. New York: Cambridge University Press.

————. 2008a: "The History of Traditional Chinese Medicine in the People's Republic of China and Its Globalization." In *The Globalization of Chinese Medicine and Meditation Practices*. ed. E. Hsu. *East Asian Science and Technology Studies* special issue 2:465–84.

————. 2008b. "A Hybrid Body Technique: Does the Pulse Diagnostic *cun guan chi* Method Have Chinese and Tibetan Origins?" *Gesnerus* 65:5–29.

————. 2009. "Chinese Propriety Medicines: An Alternative Modernity? The Case of the Anti-malarial Substance Artemisinin in East Africa." *Medical Anthropology* 28(2): 111–40.

Hsu, E., and S. Harris eds. 2010. *Plants, Health, and Healing: On the Interface of Ethnobotany and Medical Anthropology*. London: Berghahn Books.

Huang, F. 2006. "Traditional Inheritance and Modern Development of Tibetan Medicine." China Tibet Information Center.

Huber, T. 1991. "Traditional Environmental Protectionism in Tibet Reconsidered." *Tibet Journal* 16(3): 63–77.

————. 1997. "Green Tibetans: A Brief Social History." In *Tibetan Culture in the Diaspora*. Ed. F. J. Korom. Vienna: Verlag der österreichischen Akademie der Wissenschaften, 103–19.

Igoe, J. 2004. *Conservation and Globalization: A Study of National Parks and Indigenous Communities from East Africa to South Dakota (Case Studies on Contemporary Issues)*. Independence, KY: Wadsworth.

———. 2010. "The Spectacle of Nature in the Global Economy of Appearances: Anthropological Engagements with the Spectacular Mediations of Transnational Conservation." *Critique of Anthropology* 30(4): 375–97.

Igoe, J., and D. Brockington. 2007. "Neoliberal Conservation: A Brief Introduction." *Conservation and Society* 5(4): 432–49.

Immel, B. 2000. "A Brief History of the GMPs: The Power of Storytelling." *BioPharm*, August, 1–6.

Ingold, T. 2000. *The Perception of the Environment: Essays on Livelihood, Dwelling and Skill*. London: Routledge.

Institute of Medicine. 2005. *Complementary and Alternative Medicine in the United States*. Washington, DC: National Academic Press.

Jacobson, E. 2002. "Panic Attack in a Context of Comorbid Anxiety and Depression in a Tibetan Refugee." *Culture, Medicine and Psychiatry* 26:259–79.

Janes, C. 1995. "The Transformations of Tibetan Medicine." *Medical Anthropology Quarterly* 9(1): 6–39.

———. 1999a. "The Health Transition and the Crisis of Traditional Medicine: The Case of Tibet." *Social Science and Medicine* 48:1803–20.

———. 1999b. "Imagined Lives, Suffering and the Work of Culture: The Embodied Discourses of Conflict in Modern Tibet." *Medical Anthropology Quarterly* 13:391–412.

———. 2001. "Tibetan Medicine at the Crossroads: Radical Modernity and the Social Organization of Traditional Medicine in the Tibet Autonomous Region, China." In *Healing Powers and Modernity: Traditional Medicine, Shamanism, and Science in Asian Societies*. Ed. L. H. Connor and G. Samuel. Westport, CT: Bergin and Garvey, 197–221.

———. 2002. "Buddhism, Science, and Market: The Globalization of Tibetan Medicine." *Anthropology and Medicine* 9(3): 267–89.

Janes, C., and O. Chuluundorj. 2004. "Free Markets and Dead Mothers: The Social Ecology of Maternal Mortality in Post-Socialist Mongolia." *Medical Anthropology Quarterly* 18(2): 230–57.

Johannessen, H., and I. Lazar. 2006. *Multiple Medical Realities: Patients and Healers in Biomedical, Alternative, and Traditional Medicine*. London: Berghahn Books.

Justice, J. 1986. *Policies, Plans, and People*. Berkeley: University of California Press.

Kaptchuk, T. 1998. "Powerful Placebos: The Dark Side of the Randomized Controlled Trial." *Lancet* 351:1722–25.

———. 2001. "The Double-Blind, Randomized, Placebo-Controlled Trial: Gold Standard or Golden Calf?" *Journal of Clinical Epidemiology* 54(6): 541–49.

———. 2002. "The Placebo Effect in Alternative Medicine: Can the Performance of a Healing Ritual Have Clinical Significance?" *Annals of Internal Medicine* 136(11): 817–25.

Karnay, S. 1998. *The Arrow and the Spindle: Studies in History, Myths, Rituals and Beliefes in Tibet*. Kathmandu: Mandala Book Point.

Kleinman, A. 1980. *Patients and Healers in the Context of Culture*. Berkeley: University of California Press.

———. 1988. *The Illness Narratives: Suffering, Healing, and the Human Condition.* New York: Basic Books.

———. 2006. *What Really Matters: Living a Moral Life amidst Uncertainty and Danger.* Oxford: Oxford University Press.

Kletter, C., and M. Kriechbaum. 2001. *Tibetan Medicinal Plants.* London: Medpharm Scientific.

Kloos, S. 2010. "Tibetan Medicine in Exile: The Ethics, Politics and Science of Cultural Survival." Ph.D. dissertation, University of California–Berkeley, Dept. of Anthropology.

———. In press. "Good Medicines, Bad Hearts: The Social Role of the Amchi in a Buddhist Dard Community." In *Healing at the Periphery: Ethnographies of Tibetan Medicine in India.* Ed. L. Pordié. Durham, NC: Duke University Press.

Knauft, B. 2001. "Critically Modern: An Introduction." In *Critically Modern: Alternatives, Alterities, Anthropologies.* Ed. B. Knauft. Bloomington: University of Indiana Press.

Knauss, J. 1998. *Orphans of the Cold War.* Washington, DC: Public Affairs.

Kohrt, B., and I. Harper. 2008. "Navigating Diagnoses: Understanding Mindbody Relations, Stigma and Mental Health in Nepal" *Culture, Medicine, and Psychiatry* 32:462–91.

Koirala, R. R. 2007. *Country Monographs on Traditional Systems of Medicine.* Kathmandu: Ministry of Health and Population.

Kuhn, T. (1962) 1996. *The Structure of Scientific Revolutions.* Chicago: Chicago University Press.

Lama, Y., and Y. Thomas. 2005. "High Altitude Himalayan Medicinal Plants Conservation: Linkages with Health Care Development and Trade in Shey Phoksundo National Park, Dolpo, Nepal." In *Himalayan Medicinal and Aromatic Plants: Balancing Use and Conservation.* Ed. Y. Thomas, M. Karki, K. Gurung, and D. Parajuli. Kathmandu: His Majesty's Government of Nepal Ministry of Forests and Soil Conservation, 362–78.

———. 2008. "Tibetan Medicine and Biodiversity Management in Dolpo, Nepal. Negotiating Local and Global Worldviews, Knowledge and Practices." In *Tibetan Medicine in the Contemporary World: Global Politics of Medical Knowledge and Practice.* Ed. L. Pordié. Abingdon, UK: Routledge, 360–82.

Lama, Y. C., S. K. Ghimire, and Y. A. Thomas. 2001. *Medicinal Plants of Dolpo. Amchis' Knowledge and Conservation.* Kathmandu: People and Plants Initiative, WWF Nepal Program.

Lampland, M., and S. L. Star. 2009. *Standards and Their Stories: How Quantifying, Classifying, and Formalizing Practices Shape Everyday Life.* Ithaca, NY: Cornell University Press.

Langford, J. 1999. "Medical Mimesis: Healing Signs of a Cosmopolitan 'Quack.'" *American Ethnologist* 26(1): 24–46.

———. 2002. *Fluent Bodies: Ayurvedic Remedies for Postcolonial Imbalance.* Durham, NC: Duke University Press.

Langwick, S. 2010. "From Non-Aligned Medicines to Market-Based Herbals: China's Relationship to the Shifting Politics of Traditional Medicine in Tanzania." *Medical Anthropology* 29(1): 1–29.

Larsen, K., and A. Sinding-Larsen. 2001. *The Lhasa Atlas: Traditional Tibetan Architecture and Townscape.* Boston: Shambhala.

Latour, B. (1979) 1986. *Laboratory Life: The Construction of Scientific Facts.* Princeton, NJ: Princeton University Press.

———. 1993. *We Have Never Been Modern.* Cambridge, MA: Harvard University Press.

Law, J. 2006. *Big Pharma: Exposing the Global Health Care Agenda.* New York: Carroll & Graff.

Law, W., and J. Salick. 2005. "Human Induced Dwarfing of Himalayan Snow Lotus." *PNAS* 102:10218–220.

———. 2007. "Comparing Conservation Priorities for Useful Plants among Botanists and Tibetan Doctors." *Biodiversity Conservation* 16:1747–59.

Lévi-Strauss, C. 1964. *The Raw and the Cooked.* Vol. 1. New York: Harper and Row.

———. 1967. "The Sorcerer and His Magic." In. *Magic, Witchcraft, and Curing.* Ed. J. Middelton. New York: AMNH Press, 167–85.

Li, T. 2007. *The Will to Improve: Governmentality, Development, and the Practice of Politics.* Durham, NC: Duke University Press.

Litzinger, R. 1998. "Memory Work: Reconstituting the Ethnic in Post-Mao China." *Cultural Anthropology* 13(2): 224–55.

———. 2006. "Contested Sovereignties and the Critical Ecosystem Partnership Fund." *Political and Legal Anthropology Review* 29(1): 66–87.

Lo Bue, E. 2011. *Wonders of Lo: The Artistic Heritage of Mustang.* Gaithersburg, MD: Marg Publications.

Lock, M. 1990. "Rationalization of Japanese Herbal Medication: The Hegemony of Orchestrated Pluralism." *Human Organization* 49:41–47.

Lock, M., and V. K. Nguyen 2010. *An Anthropology of Biomedicine.* Oxford: Wiley-Blackwell.

Lock, M., and N. Scheper-Hughes. 1987. "The Mindful Body: A Prolegomenon to Future Work in Medical Anthropology." *Medical Anthropology Quarterly* 1(1): 6–41.

Lopez, D. 1998. *Prisoners of Shangri La.* Chicago: University of Chicago Press.

Low, S. 1981. "Culturally Interpreted Symptoms or Culture-Bound Syndromes: A Cross-cultural Review of Nerves." *Social Science and Medicine* 21(2): 187–96.

Lowe, C. 2006. *Wild Profusion: Biodiversity Conservation in an Indonesian Archipelago.* Princeton, NJ: Princeton University Press.

Lurhman, T. 2001. *Of Two Minds.* New York: Knopf.

Marshall, P. 2007. *Ethical Challenges in Study Design and Informed Consent for Health Research in Resource-Poor Settings.* Geneva: WHO, TDR/SDR/SEB/ST/07.1, special topics No. 5.

May, S. 2010. "Rethinking Anonymity in Anthropology: A Question of Ethics." *Anthropology News* 51(4): 10–13.

Mayer, K., and H. F. Pizer 2007. *The Social Ecology of Infectious Disease.* Amsterdam: Elsevier ebook.

McElroy, A., and P. Townsend. 2003. *Medical Anthropology in Ecological Perspective.* Boulder, CO: Westview Press.

McGranahan, C. 2010. *Arrested Histories: Tibet, the CIA, and Memories of a Forgotten War.* Durham, NC: Duke University Press.

McKay, A. 2007. *Their Footprints Remain.* Amsterdam: IIAS Publications

———. 2010. "Biomedicine in Tibet at the Edge of Modernity." In *Medicine between Science and Religion: Explorations on Tibetan Grounds.* Ed. V. Adams, M. Schrempf, and S. Craig. London: Berghahn Books, 33–56.

McKay, A., and D. Wangchuk. 2005. "Traditional Medicine in Bhutan." *Asian Medicine* 1(1): 204–18.

Meyer, F. 1995. "Theory and Practice of Tibetan Medicine." In *Oriental Medicine: An Illustrated Guide to the Asian Arts of Healing.* Ed. J. van Alphen and F. Meyer. London: Serendia, 109–42.

Millard, C. 2002. "Learning Processes in a Tibetan Medical School." Ph.D. dissertation, University of Edinburgh, Dept. of Social Anthropology.

———. 2006. "Man and Glud: Standard Tibetan Medicine and Ritual Medicine in a Bon Medical School and Clinic in Nepal." *Tibet Journal* 30(4) and 31(1): 1–20.

———. 2007. "Tibetan Medicine and the Classification and Treatment of Mental Illness." In *Soundings in Tibetan Medicine: Anthropological and Historical Perspectives.* Ed. M. Schrempf. Leiden: Brill, 247–84.

———. 2008. "The Integration of Tibetan Medicine in the UK: The Clinics of the Tara Rokpa Institute." In *Tibetan Medicine in the Contemporary World: Global Politics of Medical Knowledge and Practice.* Abingdon, UK: Routledge, 189–214.

Miller, S., P. V. Le, S. Craig, V. Adams, C. Tudor, Sonam, Nyima, Droyoung, M. Cuomu, Lhakpen, and M. Varner. 2007a. "How to Make Consent Informed: Possible Lessons from Tibet." *Hastings Review / IRB Ethics and Human Research,* November-December issue, 7–14.

Miller, S., C. Tudor, Nyima, V. R. Thorsten, Sonam, Droyoung, S. Craig, P. Le, L. L. Wright, and M. W. Varner. 2007b. "Maternal and Neonatal Outcomes of Hospital Vaginal Deliveries in Tibet." *International Journal of Obstetrics and Gynecology* 98(3): 217–21.

Miller, S., C. Tudor, V. Thorsten, Nyima, Kalyang, Sonam, Lhakpen, Droyoung, K. Quzong, T. Dekyi, T. Hartwell, L. L. Wright, and M. Varner. 2009. "Randomized Double Masked Trial of *Zhi Bhed 11,* a Tibetan Traditional Medicine, versus Misoprostol to Prevent Postpartum Hemorrhage in Lhasa." *Journal of Midwifery and Women's Health* 54(2): 133–41.

Mintz, S. 1986. *Sweetness and Power.* New York: Penguin.

Mitchell, T. 2002. *Rule of Experts: Egypt, Techno-politics, Modernity.* Berkeley: University of California Press.

Moerman, D. 2002. *Meaning, Medicine, and "the Placebo Effect."* Cambridge, UK: Cambridge University Press.

Myers, F. 2001. "Introduction: The Empire of Things." In *The Empire of Things. Regimes of Value and Material Culture.* Ed. F. Myers. Oxford: School of American Research Press, 3–61.

———. 2002. *Painting Culture: The Making of an Aboriginal High Art.* Durham, NC: Duke University Press.

Nandy, A., and S. Visvanathan. 1990. "Modern Medicine and Its Non-Modern Critics: A Study in Discourse." In *Dominating Knowledge*. Ed. F. Apffel Marglin and S. Marglin. Oxford: Clarendon Press, 145–84.

Narayan, K. 1999. "Anthropology and Fiction: Where Is the Border?" *Anthropology and Humanism* 24(2): 134–47.

———. 2007. "Tools to Shape Texts: What Creative Nonfiction Can Offer Ethnography." *Anthropology and Humanism* 32(2): 130–44.

Nichter, M. 2008. *Global Health: Why Cultural Perceptions, Social Representations, and Biopolitics Matter*. Tucson: University of Arizona Press.

Norbu, K. 2004. *Clear Mirror of Medicinal Plants [sngo sman gsal ba'I me long]*. Lhasa: Tibet People's Publishing house [bod ljongs mi dmangs dpe skrun khang].

Olsen, C., and N. Bhattarai. 2005. "A Typology of Economic Agents in the Himalayan Plant Trade." *Mountain Research and Development* 25(1): 37–43.

Olsen, C. S., and H. O. Larsen. 2003. "Alpine Medicinal Plant Trade and Himalayan Mountain Livelihood Strategies." *Geographical Journal* 169:243–54.

Osterman, J., and J. T. V. M. de Jong. 2007. "Culture and Trauma." In *Handbook of PTSD: Science and Practice*. New York: Guilford Press, 425–46.

Parsons, T. (1951) 1964. *The Social System*. New York: The Free Press/Macmillan.

People's Daily. 2004. "Tibetan Medicine Industry Developing Steadily." August 15. http://english.peopledaily.com.cn/200408/15/eng20040815_153105.html. Accessed March 19, 2012.

Petryna, A. 2002. *Life Exposed: Biological Citizens after Chernobyl*. Princeton, NJ: Princeton University Press.

———. 2009. *When Experiments Travel: Clinical Trials and the Global Search for Human Subjects*. Princeton, NJ: Princeton University Press.

Petryna, A., and A. Kleinman. 1995. "Acronyms and Effacement: Traditional Medical Practitioners (TMP) in International Health Development." *Social Science and Medicine* 41(1): 47–68.

———. 1997. "'Found in Most Traditional Societies': Traditional Medical Practitioners between Culture and Development." In *International Development and the Social Sciences: Essays on the History and Politics of Knowledge*. Ed. F. Cooper and R. Packard. Westport, CT: Praeger, 259–90.

———. 2001. "Languages of Sex and AIDS in Nepal: Notes on the Social Production of Commensurability." *Cultural Anthropology* 16(4): 481–541.

———. 2006. "The Pharmaceutical Nexus." In *Global Pharmaceuticals: Ethics, Markets, Practices*. Durham, NC: Duke University Press.

Pigg, S. L. 1992. "Inventing Social Categories through Place: Social Representations and Development in Nepal." *Comparative Studies in Society and History* 34(3): 491–513.

———. 1995. "Acronyms and Effacement: Traditional Medical Practitioners (TMP) in International Health Development. *Social Science and Medicine* 41(1): 47–68.

———. 1996. "The Credible and the Credulous: The Question of 'Villagers' Beliefs' in Nepal." *Cultural Anthropology* 11(2): 160–201.

———. 1997. "Found in Most Traditional Societies": Traditional Medical Practitioners Between Culture and Development." In F. Cooper and R. Packard, eds. *International Development and the Social Sciences: Essays on the History and Politics of Knowledge.* Berkeley: University of California Press.

———. 2001. "Languages of Sex and AIDS in Nepal: Notes on the Social Production of Commensurability." *Cultural Anthropology* 16(4): 481–541.

Pinto, S. 2008. *Where There Is No Midwife: Birth and Loss in Northern India.* London: Berghahn Books.

Pordié, L. 2002. "La pharmacopée comme expression de société: Une étude himalayenne." In *Des sources du savoir aux médicaments du futur.* Ed. J. Fleurentin, G. Mazars, and J. M. Pelt. Paris: Editions IRD–SFE, 183–94.

———. 2005. "Claims for Intellectual Property Rights and the Illusion of Conservation: A Brief Anthropological Unpacking of a 'Development' Failure." In *Himalayan Medicinal and Aromatic Plants: Balancing Use and Conservation.* Ed. Y. Thomas, M. Kharki, K. Gurung, and D. Parajuli. Kathmandu: WWF Nepal Program, 394–410.

———. 2007. "Buddhism in the Everyday Medical Practice of the Ladakhi *Amchi.*" *Indian Anthropologist* 37(1): 93–116.

———. 2008a. "Hijacking Intellectual Property Rights: Identities and Social Power in the Indian Himalayas." In *Tibetan Medicine in the Contemporary World: Global Politics of Medical Knowledge and Practice.* Ed. L. Pordié. Abingdon, UK: Routledge, 132–59.

———. 2008b. "Reformulating Ingredients: Outlines of a Contemporary Ritual for the Consecration of Medicines in Ladakh." In *Modern Ladakh: Anthropological Perspectives on Continuity and Change.* Ed. M. van Beek and F. Pirie. Leiden: Brill, 152–74.

———. 2008c. *Tibetan Medicine in the Contemporary World: Global Politics of Medical Knowledge and Practice.* Abingdon, UK: Routledge.

Pordié, L., and P. H. Petitet. In press. "Birth in Shun Shade: Notes on the Role of the *Amchi* Regarding Childbirth." In *Healing at the Periphery: Tibetan Medicine and Himalayan Societies in India.* Ed. L. Pordié. Durham, NC: Duke University Press.

Prost, A. 2006. "The Problem with 'Rich Refugees': Sponsorship, Capital, and the Informal Economy of Tibetan Refugees. *Modern Asian Studies* 40:233–53.

———. 2008. *Precious Pills: Medicine and Social Change among Tibetan Refugees in India.* London: Berghahn Books.

Quah, S. 2003. "Traditional Healing Systems and the Ethos of Science." *Social Science and Medicine* 57:1997–2012.

Ramble, C. 1997. "Tibetan Pride of Place: Or, Why Nepal's Bhotia Are Not an Ethnic Group." In *Nationalism and Ethnicity in a Hindu Kingdom.* Ed. D. Gellner, J. Pfaff-Czarnecka, and J. Whelpton. Amsterdam: Harwood Academic Publishers, 379–412.

———. 2008. *The Navel of the Demonness.* Oxford: Oxford University Press.

Rechung, R. 1973. *Tibetan Medicine.* London: Wellcome Institute of the History of Medicine.

Reeler, A. 1990. "Injections: A Fatal Attraction?" *Social Science and Medicine* 31(10): 1119–25.

Ritenbaugh, C., M. Verhoef, S. Fleishman, H. Boon, and A. Leis. 2003. "Whole Systems Research: A Discipline for Studying Complementary and Alternative Medicine." *Alternative Therapies Health Medicine* 9(4): 32–36.

Rose, N., and C. Novas. 2005. "Biological Citizenship." In *Global Assemblages*. Ed. A. Ong and S. Collier. Oxford: Wiley-Blackwell, 439–63.

Sachs, W. 1992. *The Development Dictionary: A Guide to Knowledge as Power*. London: Zed Books.

Salick, J., A. Byg, and A. Amend. 2006. "Tibetan Medicine Plurality." *Economic Botany* 60(3): 227–53.

Sallon, S., T. Namdul, S. Dolma, P. Dorjee, D. Dolma, T. Sadutshang, P. Ever-Hadani, T. Bdolah-Abram, S. Apter. S. Almog and S. Roberts. 2006. "Mercury in Traditional Tibetan Medicine: Panacea or Problem?" *Human and Experimental Toxicology* 25(7): 405–12.

Samuel, G. 1993. *Civilized Shamans: Buddhism in Tibetan Societies*. Kathmandu: Mandala Book Point.

———. 1999. "Religion, Health, and Suffering among Contemporary Tibetans." In *Religion, Health, and Suffering*. Ed. J. Hinnell and R. Porter. London: Kegan Paul International.

———. 2001. "Tibetan Medicine in Contemporary India: Theory and Practice." In *Healing Powers and Modernity: Traditional Medicine, Shamanism, and Science in Asian Societies*. Ed. L. H. Connor and G. Samuel. Westport, CT: Bergin and Garvey, 247–68.

———. 2006. "Tibetan Medicine and Biomedicine: Epistemological Conflicts, Practical Solutions." *Asian Medicine: Tradition and Modernity* 2(1): 72–85.

———. 2007. "Spirit Causation and Illness in Tibetan Medicine." In *Soundings in Tibetan Medicine: Anthropological and Historical Perspectives*. Ed. M. Schrempf. Leiden: Brill, 213–24.

———. 2010. "A Short History of Into-Tibetan Alchemy." In *Studies of Medical Pluralism in Tibetan History and Society*. Proceedings of the 11th Seminar of the International Association of Tibetan Studies, Bonn 2006. Ed. S. Craig, M. Cuomu, F. Garrett, and M. Schrempf. Halle: International Institute for Tibetan and Buddhist Studies, 221–34.

Saxer, M. 2010a. "Manufacturing Tibetan Medicine: The Creation of an Industry and the Moral Economy of Tibetanness." Manuscript in preparation for publication as a book, based on 2010 Ph.D. dissertation, University of Oxford.

———. 2010b. "Tibetan Medicine and Russian Modernities." In *Medicine between Science and Religion: Explorations on Tibetan Grounds*. Ed. V. Adams, M. Schrempf, and S. Craig. London: Berghahn Books, 57–80.

———. 2011. "Herbs and Traders in Transit: Border Regimes and the Contemporary Trans-Himalayan Trade in Medicinal Plants." *Asian Medicine: Tradition and Modernity* 5(2): 317–39.

Scheid, V. 2002. *Chinese Medicine in Contemporary China: Plurality and Synthesis*. Durham, NC: Duke University Press.

———. 2007. *Currents of Tradition in Chinese Medicine, 1626–2006*. Seattle, WA: Eastland Press.

Scheper-Hughes, N. 2000. "The Global Traffic in Human Organs." *Current Anthropology* 41(2): 191–211.

———. 2007. "Nervios." In *Beyond the Body Proper*. Ed. M. Lock and J. Farquhar. Durham, NC: Duke University Press, 459–68.

Scheper-Hughes, N., and M. Lock. 1987. "The Mindful Body: A Prolegomenon to Future Work in Medical Anthropology." *Medical Anthropology Quarterly* 1(1): 6–41.

Schrempf, M. 2007. "Bon Lineage Doctors and the Local Transmission of Knowing Medical Practice in Nagchu." In *Soundings in Tibetan Medicine: Anthropological and Historical Perspectives*. Ed. M. Schrempf. Leiden: Brill, 91–126.

———. 2010. "Between Mantra and Syringe: Healing and Health Seeking Behavior in Contemporary Amdo." In *Medicine between Science and Religion: Explorations on Tibetan Grounds*. Ed. V. Adams, M. Schrempf, and S. Craig. London: Berghahn Books, 157–84.

———. Forthcoming. "Experiences of Fertility, Family Planning and Reproductive Health among Amdo Tibetan Women." *Asian Medicine: Tradition and Modernity* special issue 6(2).

Schwabl, H. 2011. "It Is Modern to Be Traditional: Tradition and Tibetan Medicine in the European Context." *Asian Medicine: Tradition and Modernity* 5(2): 373–84.

Scott, J. 1998. *Seeing Like a State: How Certain Schemes to Improve the Human Condition Have Failed*. New Haven, CT: Yale University Press.

———. 2010. *The Art of Not Being Governed: An Anarchist History of Upland Southeast Asia*. New Haven, CT: Yale University Press.

Sharma, S. P. 2010. "Politics and Corruption Mar Health Care in Nepal." *Lancet* 375:2063–64.

Shneiderman, S. 2008. "Living Practical Dharma: A Tribute to Chomo Khandru and the Bonpo Women of Lubra Village, Mustang, Nepal." In *Nuns, Yoginis, Saints and Singers: Women's Renunciation in South Asia*. Ed. Meena Khandelwal and Sondra L. Hausner. Delhi: Zubaan.

———. 2010. "Are the Central Himalayas in Zomia? Some Scholarly and Political Considerations across Time and Space." *Journal of Global History* 5:289–312.

———. Forthcoming. "Himalayan Border Citizens: Living the Nepal—Tibetan Autonomous Region (China) Border Zone." *Political Geography*.

Shrestha, S. M., N. Takeda, F. Tsuda, H. Okamoto, S. Shrestha, and V. M. Shrestha. 2002. "High Prevalence of Hepatitis B Virus Infection amongst Tibetans in Nepal." *Tropical Gastroenterology* 23(2): 63–65.

Shrestha, T. B., and R. M. Joshi. 1996. *Rare, Endemic and Endangered Plants of Nepal*. WWF Nepal Program, Kathmandu.

Sihlé, N. 1995. "Pour le bien des êtres et de la doctrine: L'action altruiste dans la culture tibétaine à travers l'exemple du religieux et médecin Ts'ampa Ngawang (Jomsom, Nord du Népal)." Master's thesis, University of Paris X–Nanterre, Dept. of Ethnology and Comparative Sociology.

Snellgrove, D. 1967. *The Nine Ways of Bon: Excerpts from the gZi-brjid*. London: Oxford University Press.

———. 1981. *Himalayan Pilgrimage*. Boston: Shambhala.

Sontag, S. *Illness as Metaphor and AIDS and its Metaphors*. New York: Picador.

Stockoks, D., J. Allen, and R. L. Bellingham. 1996. "The Social Ecology of Health Promotion: Implications for Research and Practice." *American Journal of Health Promotion* 10:247–51.

Stokols, D. 1996. "Translating Social Ecological Theory into Guidelines for Community Health Promotion." *American Journal of Health Promotion* 10:282–98.

Stone, L. 1986. "Primary Health Care for Whom? Village Perspectives from Nepal." *Social Science and Medicine* 22(3): 293–302.

Strathern, M. 2000. *Audit Cultures: Anthropological Studies in Accountability, Ethics, and the Academy*. London: Routledge.

Subedi, B. 2006. *Linking Plant-Based Enterprises and Local Communities to Biodiversity Conservation in Nepal Himalayas*. New Delhi: Adroit.

Sung W. and Yi-Ming L. 1998. "Illegal Wildlife Trade in the Himalayas." In *Ecoregional Cooperation for Biodiversity Conservation in the Himalayas: Report on the International Meeting on Himalaya Ecoregional Cooperation*. United Nations Development Program, New York, 187–213.

Sweeney, B. 2009. "Traditional Medical Regulation in the UK and EU." Paper presented at the 7th Congress of IASTAM, Thimphu, Bhutan, September 7–11.

Taussig, 1983, *The Devil and Commodity Fetishism in South America*. Durham, NC: University of North Carolina Press.

Taylor, K. 2005. *Chinese Medicine in Early Communist China, 1945–1963: A Medicine of Revolution*. London: Routledge.

Terry, B. 2009. *Blue Heaven: Encounters with the Blue Poppy*. Seattle, WA: Touchwood.

Thomas, Y., and Y. Lama. 2008. "Tibetan Medicine and Biodiversity Management in Dolpo, Nepal: Negotiating Local and Global Worldviews, Knowledge and Practices." In *Tibetan Medicine in the Contemporary World: Global Politics of Medical Knowledge and Practice*. Ed. L. Pordié. Abingdon, UK: Routledge, 160–85.

Tibet Information Network. 2004. *Tibetan Medicine in Contemporary Tibet: Health and Health Care in Tibet, II*. London: Tibet Information Network Press.

Tsering, T. 2005. "Outstanding Women in Tibetan Medicine." In *Women in Tibet*. Ed. J. Gyatso and H. Havnevik. London: Hurst, 169–94.

Tsing, A. 1993. *In the Realm of the Diamond Queen*. Princeton, NJ: Princeton University Press.

Tso, D. 2011. "Perspectives and Experiences on the Training of Tibetan Medicine Practitioners." In *Socio-historical Studies of Medical Pluralism in Tibetan Contexts*. Ed. S. Craig, F. Garrett, M. Schrempf, and M. Cuomu. Halle: International Institute for Tibetan and Buddhist Studies, 179–88.

Tucci, G. 1980. *The Religions of Tibet*. Berkeley: University of California Press.

Tudor, C., S. Miller, Nyima, Droyoung, Sonam, Lhakpen, L. Wright, and M. Varner. 2006. "Preliminary Progress Report: Randomized Double-Blind Trial of Zhijé 11, a Tibetan Traditional Medicine, versus Misoprostol to Prevent Postpartum Hemorrhage in Lhasa." *International Journal of Gynecology and Obstetrics* 94 (supplement 2): 145–46.

UNICEF. 2001. *Progress since the World Summit for Children: A Statistical Review*. New York: United Nations Children's Fund.

Unschuld, P. 1985. *Medicine in China: A History of Ideas*. Berkeley: University of California Press.

van der Geest, S., and S. Whyte. 1989. "The Charm of Medicines: Metaphors and Metonyms." *Medical Anthropology Quarterly* 3(4): 345–67.

van der Geest, S., S. Reynolds Whyte, and A. Hardon. 1996. "The Anthropology of Pharmaceuticals: A Biographical Approach." *Annual Review of Anthropology* 25:153–78.

van der Geest, S., and S. Whyte, eds. 1988. *The Context of Medicines in Developing Countries*. Dordrecht: Kluwer Academic Publishers.

Vargas, I. 2011. "Legitimizing Demon Disease in Tibetan Medicine: The Conjoining of Religion, Medicine, and Ecology." In *Socio-historical Studies of Medical Pluralism in Tibetan Contexts*. Ed. S. Craig, F. Garrett, M. Schrempf, and M. Cuomu. Halle: International Institute for Tibetan and Buddhist Studies, 379–404.

Verhoef, M., G. Lewith, C. Ritenbaugh, K. Thomas, H. Boon, and V. Fønnebø. 2005. "Whole Systems Research: Moving Forward." *Focus on Alternative and Complementary Therapies* 9(2): 87–90.

Villar, M. D., A. M. Gülmezoglu, G. J. Hofmeyr, and F. Forna. 2002. "Systematic Review of Randomized Controlled Trials of Misoprostol to Prevent Postpartum Hemorrhage." *Obstetrics & Gynecology* 100(6): 1301–12.

Waldram, J. 2000. "The Efficacy of Traditional Medicine: Current Theoretical and Methodological Issues." *Medical Anthropology Quarterly* 14(4): 603–25.

———. 2009. "Comparative Perspectives on Efficacy between Canadian First Nations and Indigenous Communities in Belize." Presentation at the American Anthropological Association Annual Meetings, Washington DC, November.

West, P. 2006. *Conservation Is Our Government Now: The Politics of Ecology in Papua New Guinea*. Durham, NC: Duke University Press.

White, S. 2001. "Medicines and Modernities in Socialist China: Medical Pluralism, the State, and Naxi Identities in the Lijiang Basin." In *Healing Powers and Modernity: Traditional Medicine, Shamanism, and Science in Asian Societies*. Ed. L. Connor and G. Samuel. Westport, CT: Bergin and Garvey, 171–96.

Whyte, S. R., S. van der Geest, and A. Hardon. 2002. *Social Lives of Medicines*. Cambridge Studies in Medical Anthropology. Cambridge, UK: Cambridge University Press.

Williams, D. M. 1996. "The Barbed Walls of China: A Contemporary Grassland Drama." *Journal of Asian Studies* 55(3): 665–91.

Williams, T. T. 2008. *Finding Beauty in a Broken World*. New York: Pantheon Books.

Winkler, D. 2005. "Yartsa Gunbu—*Cordyceps sinensis*: Economy, Ecology, and Ethno-Mycology of a Fungus Endemic to the Tibetan Plateau." In *Wildlife and Plants in Traditional and Modern Tibet*. Ed. A. Boesi and F. Cardi. *Memorie della Societa Italiana di Scienze Naturali e del Museo Civico di Storia Naturale* special issue 34(1–2): 69–86.

———. 2011. "Caterpillar Fungus Production and Sustainability on the Tibetan Plateau and in the Himalayas." *Asian Medicine: Tradition and Modernity* 5(2): 291–316.

Witt, C. 2009. "Efficacy, Effectiveness, Pragmatic Trials: Guidance on Terminology and the Advantages of Pragmatic Trials." *Forsch Komplementmed* 16:292–94.

Witt, C., S. Craig, B. Graz, M. Heinrich, H. Schwabl and M. Cuomu. In press. "White Paper: Clinical Research on Tibetan Medicine. Where Do We Go? Where Do We Stand?" In *Clinical Reearch on Tibetan Medicine: Challenges and Points of Consensus*. Ed. C. Witt. Berlin: CVC/Essen, with support from Hans-Görtz-Stiftungsinstitut.

World Health Organization. 2005a. *National Policy on Traditional Medicine and Regulation of Herbal Medicines: Report of a WHO Global Survey*. Geneva: World Health Organization.

———. 2005b. *The World Health Report 2005: Make Every Mother and Child Count*. Geneva: World Health Organization.

———. 2008. "Address Given at the WHO Congress on Traditional Medicine by Dr. Margaret Chan and Beijing Declaration." Adopted by the WHO Congress on Traditional Medicine, Beijing, November 8.

Wujastyk, D., and F. M. Smith. 2008. *Modern and Global Ayurveda: Pluralism and Paradigms*. Albany: State University of New York Press.

Wyatt, H. V. 1984. "The Popularity of Injections in the Third World: Origins and Consequences for Poliomyelitis." *Social Science and Medicine* 19:911–15.

Wylie, T. 1959. "A Standard System of Tibetan Transcription." *Harvard Journal of Asiatic Studies* 22:261–67.

Xie, X. 2007. "The Main Differences between Chinese GMP and the International GMP-ICH Q7." *Journal of GMP Compliance*, July 1.

Xinhua News Agency. 2004. "Age-old Tibetan Medicines in Predicament to Get Accepted outside World." http://english.peopledaily.com.cn/200509/07/eng20050907_207132.html. Accessed March 19, 2012.

Xu Y. Q., Zhou Y. D., Bii S. L. 2005. "Preliminary Study on Genotype of Hepatitis B Virus Detected from Tibetans in China" (in Chinese). *Zhonghua Shi Yan He Lin Chuang Bing Du Xue Za Zhi* 19(2): 118–20.

Yangga. 2010. "Tibetan Medicine and Galenic Medicine." Ph.D. dissertation, Harvard University, Dept. of Religion.

Yeh, E. 2000. "Forest Claims, Conflicts, and Commodification: The Political Ecology of Tibetan Mushroom-Harvesting Villages in Yunnan Province, China." *China Quarterly* 161:212–26.

———. 2007. "Tropes of Indolence and the Cultural Politics of Development in Lhasa, Tibet." *Annals of the Association of American Geographers* 97(3): 593–612.

———. 2009. "From Wasteland to Wetland: Nature and Nation in China's Tibet." *Environmental History* 14(1): 103–37.

Yi, Y. 2003. "Modern Medicines to Make Use of Tibetan Traditions." *China Daily*, September 23. www.chinadaily.com.cn/en/doc/2003-09/23/content _266435.htm. Accessed November 4, 2011.

Zhan, M. 2009. *Other-Worldly: Making Chinese Medicine through Transnational Frames*. Durham, NC: Duke University Press.

Zhang, X. 2005. *Global and Regional Perspectives on Development of Traditional Medicine*. Document No. 5, World Health Organization.

Zhang, Z., G. C. Roman, Z. Hong, C. Wu, Q. Qu, J. Huang, B. Zhou, Z. Geng, J. Wu, H. Wen, H. Zhao, and G. Zahner. 2005. "Parkinson's Disease in China: Prevalence in Beijing, Xian, and Shanghai." *Lancet* 365(9459): 595–97.

Zschocke, S., T. Rabe, J. L. S. Taylor, A. K. Jäger, and J. van Staden. 2000. "Plant Part Substitution: A Way to Conserve Endangered Medicinal Plants?" *Journal of Ethnopharmacology* 71:281–92.

Index

abortion, induced: with misoprostol, 222, 283n6; with *zhijé 11*, 221–22, 223
Aconitum spp. *(bongkar)*, 44
acupressure, 15
acupuncture, 15, 39, 66, 115; golden needle *(ser khab)*, 140; in Qinghai clinic, 117, 120
Adapt to the Holy Land Capsule, 176, 178, 187
agar 8, 226
agar 15, 223
agar 20, 223, 226
Agrawal, A., 214
akar kara (Anacyclus pyrethrum), 42, 64
Akhong Rinpoche, 201–2; story of boiling leather soles for sustenance, 202, 282n12
alcohol use, 126, 134
Allium przewalskianum (zimbu), 42
Alternative Health Act proposal, 80
alternative medicine, 23, 93; as traditional medicine, 80; whole systems research on, 61
amchi, 2, 3, 11, 15–16, 18, 33; certification of, 82; clinical records of, 31, 37–39; collaboration with World Wildlife Fund, 193–200; cultivation of medical plants, 40–41; daily life in Mustang District, 21–22, 27–47; diversity of, 104; donations supporting, 193,

195–200; education and training of, 35–36, 82, 84, 85, 87–88, 102–8, 257; efficacy of, 84; grades of, 82, 113; in Himalayan Amchi Association, 101–10; interaction with conservation policies and projects, 25, 193–200; languages used by, 84, 96, 103–4, 110, 111; legitimacy of, 23; marginalization of, 15, 88; medicinal substitutions used by, 208; medicine preparation by, 131*fig*; Nepal Alternative Health Council documents describing, 81–82; payment for services of, 10, 34, 36–37, 135; pulse reading by, 113*fig*; state recognition of, 14, 15, 79, 81, 84–88, 107; therapeutic encounters in Kathmandu clinic of Darkye, 112–17; traditional and modern approaches of, 10, 32, 45; in twenty-first century, 93–101; use of term, 12; women as, 90–91; and women's health, 39–40; *zhijé 11* used by, 219, 220. *See also* Himalayan Amchi Association
Anacyclus pyrethrum (akar kara), 42, 64
animal products, 206–7
Annapurna Conservation Area, 27, 194–95, 277n2(ch1)
anweichi, 243–44. *See also* placebos in research
Appadurai, A., 250, 251
arura (Terminalia chehula), 230, 255

TEXT
10/13 Sabon

DISPLAY
Sabon

COMPOSITOR
Westchester Book Group

PRINTER AND BINDER
Maple-Vail Book Manufacturing Group